A Sociology of Mental Health and Illness

Fifth Edition

A Sociology of Mental Health and Illness

Fifth Edition

Anne Rogers and David Pilgrim

Mc Graw Hill Education Open University Press

Open University Press
McGraw-Hill Education
McGraw-Hill House
Shoppenhangers Road
Maidenhead
Berkshire
England
SL6 2QL

email: enquiries@openup.co.uk
world wide web: www.openup.co.uk

and Two Penn Plaza, New York, NY 10121-2289, USA

First published 1993
Second edition published 1999
Third edition published 2005
Fourth edition published 2010
First published in this fifth edition 2014

A catalogue record of this book is available from the British Library

ISBN-13: 978-0-335-26276-2
ISBN-10: 0-335-26276-7
eISBN: 978-0-335-26277-9

Library of Congress Cataloging-in-Publication Data
CIP data applied for

Typeset by Aptara, Inc.
Printed and bound in Great Britain by Bell & Bain Ltd, Glasgow

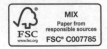

Praise for this book

"Rogers and Pilgrim go from strength to strength! This fifth edition of their classic text is not only a sociology but also a psychology, a philosophy, a history and a polity. It combines rigorous scholarship with radical argument to produce incisive perspectives on the major contemporary questions concerning mental health and illness. The authors admirably balance judicious presentation of the range of available understandings with clear articulation of their own positions on key issues. This book is essential reading for everyone involved in mental health work."

Christopher Dowrick, Professor of Primary Medical Care, University of Liverpool, UK

"Pilgrim and Rogers have for the last twenty years given us the key text in the sociology of mental health and illness. Each edition has captured the multi-layered and ever changing landscape of theory and practice around psychiatry and mental health, providing an essential tool for teachers and researchers, and much loved by students for the dexterity in combining scope and accessibility. This latest volume, with its focus on community mental health, user movements criminal justice and the need for inter-agency working, alongside the more classical sociological critiques around social theories and social inequalities, demonstrates more than ever that sociological perspectives are crucial in the understanding and explanation of mental and emotional healthcare and practice, hence its audience extends across the related disciplines to everyone who is involved in this highly controversial and socially relevant arena."

Gillian Bendelow, School of Law Politics and Sociology, University of Sussex, UK

"From the classic bedrock studies to contemporary sociological perspectives on the current controversy over which scientific organizations will define diagnosis, Rogers and Pilgrim provide a comprehensive, readable and elegant overview of how social factors shape the onset and response to mental health and mental illness. Their sociological vision embraces historical, professional and socio-cultural context and processes as they shape the lives of those in the community and those who provide care; the organizations mandated to deliver services and those that have ended up becoming unsuitable substitutes; and the successful and unsuccessful efforts to improve the lives through science, challenge and law."

Bernice Pescosolido, Distinguished Professor of Sociology, Indiana University, USA

For Steven and Jack (again!)

Contents

Preface to the fifth edition

In this latest edition of our book, which began life in 1993, we have made a number of changes to update the text and respond, where possible, to feedback from readers. Updating has meant including new material and citations. A chapter has been added on mental health and prisons, which means that legal aspects are now covered in two chapters, not the single one of previous editions. We have disposed of some older references but many remain. New is not always and necessarily 'good' nor is old necessarily 'bad', and so we have made decisions during the editing process about what remains relevant to any new reader. As a consequence, we are aware that our reference list at the end of the book has become fairly lengthy; indeed, there are enough words for two whole chapters. However, this also now constitutes a weighty bibliography for the student of our topic.

In previous editions we have commented on the scope and disciplinary context of the title. It remains 'A' not 'The' sociology of mental health and illness. Theoretical and empirical diversity in social science means that we consider that this is a logical necessity, with aspirations of certainty and definitive accounts always being dashed. At the same time, the inherent contentiousness we are dealing with makes it an interesting intellectual exercise for students of sociology. It also raises important ethical and political challenges for trainees in 'mental health work'.

A quick scan of the lengthy reference list reveals that the singular role of sociology, as a discipline, in illuminating this exercise remains far from clear. Much of the time in our text we do our best to offer a sociological framing, and discussion, of material drawn from diverse disciplinary sources. For example, there is much we deal with from journals such as the *Sociology of Health and Illness, Social Science & Medicine, Social Theory and Health, Health Sociology Review* and *Sociology*. However, not only are some of those articles at times outputs from non-sociologists, the work of sociologists also appear in other journals, which we cite from medicine, psychology, nursing, geography and health services research. Our own work in interdisciplinary contexts over the years confirms this inevitable academic complexity, and this experience ensures that our choice of title remains appropriately humble. It also has meant that while we adopt a realist perspective in our own work, we are mindful of other perspectives from social science and so do our best to represent them in the text.

Anne Rogers and David Pilgrim

1 Perspectives on mental health and illness

Chapter overview

This chapter will explore some of the different perspectives and arguments about conceptualizing mental health and illness. We make some necessary conceptual clarifications about the question of terminology. Our assumption at the outset is that terminology remains a controversial issue for the sociology of mental health and illness because there are markedly differing ways of speaking about mental normality and abnormality in contemporary society.

The chapter will first cover the following perspectives outwith sociology:

- psychiatry;
- psychoanalysis;
- psychology.

Both the lay perspective and that of labelling theory will also be dealt with at the end of the book in the chapter on stigma and recovery. In this chapter we cover the following four perspectives within sociology:

- social causation;
- hermeneutics;
- social constructivism;
- social realism.

Clinical perspectives on mental health and illness

Psychiatry

We start with psychiatry because it has been the dominant discourse. Accordingly, it has shaped the views of others or has provoked alternative or opposing perspectives. While psychiatric patients (Rogers *et al.* 1993) and those in multi-disciplinary mental health teams (Colombo *et al.* 2003) evince a complex range of views about the nature of mental disorder, each of these models competes for recognition and authority alongside the traditional and dominant medical approach deployed by psychiatry.

Psychiatry is a specialty within medicine. Its practitioners, as in other specialties, are trained to see their role as identifying sick individuals (diagnosis), predicting the future course of their illness (prognosis), speculating about its cause (aetiology) and prescribing a response to the condition, to cure it or ameliorate its symptoms (treatment). Consequently, it would be surprising if psychiatrists did not think in terms of illness when they encounter variations in conduct which are troublesome to people (be they the identified patient or those upset by them). Those psychiatrists who have rejected this illness framework, in whole or in part, tend to have been exposed to, and have accepted, an alternative view derived from another discourse (psychology, philosophy or sociology).

As with other branches of medicine, psychiatrists vary in their assumptions about diagnosis, prognosis, aetiology and treatment. This does not imply, though, that views are evenly spread throughout the profession, and as we will see later in the book, modern Western psychiatry is an eclectic enterprise. It does, however, have dominant features. In particular, diagnosis is considered to be a worthwhile ritual for the bulk of the profession and biological causes are favoured along with biological treatments.

This biological emphasis has a particular social history, which is summarized in Chapter 8. However, this should not deflect our attention from the capacity of an illness framework to accommodate multiple aetiological factors. For instance, a psychiatrist treating a patient with antidepressant drugs may recognize fully that living in a high-rise flat and being unemployed have been the main causes of the depressive illness, and may assume that the stress this induces has triggered biochemical changes in the brain, which can be corrected by using medication.

The illness framework is the dominant framework in mental health services because psychiatry is the dominant profession within those services. However, its dominance should not be confused with its conceptual superiority. The illness framework has its strengths in terms of its logical and empirical status, but it also has weaknesses. Its strengths lie in the neurological evidence: bacteria and viruses have been demonstrably associated with madness (syphilis and encephalitis). Such a neurological theory might be supported further by the experience and behaviour of people with temporal lobe epilepsy, who may present with anxiety and sometimes florid psychotic states. The induction of abnormal mental states by brain lesions, drugs, toxins, low blood sugar and fever might all point to the sense of regarding mental illness as a predominantly biological condition.

The question raised is: what has medicine to do with that wide range of mental problems that elude a biological explanation? Indeed, the great bulk of what psychiatrists call 'mental illness' has no proven bodily cause, despite substantial research efforts to solve the riddle of a purported or assumed biological aetiology. These 'illnesses' include anxiety neuroses, reactive depression and functional psychoses (the schizophrenias and the affective conditions of mania and severe or endogenous depression). While there is some evidence that we may inherit a vague predisposition to nervousness or madness, there are no clear-cut laws evident to biological researchers as yet. Both broad dispositions run in families, but not in such a way as to satisfy us that they are biologically caused. Upbringing in such families might equally point to learned behaviour and the genetic evidence from twin studies remains contested (Marshall 1990).

It may be argued that biological treatments that bring about symptom relief themselves point to biological aetiology (such as the lifting of depression by electroconvulsive therapy (ECT) or the diminution of auditory hallucination by major tranquillizers). However, this may not follow: thieving can be prevented quite effectively by chopping off the hands of perpetrators, but hands do not cause theft. Likewise, a person shocked following a car crash may feel better by taking a minor tranquillizer, but their state is clearly environmentally induced. The thief's hands and the car crash victim's brain are merely biological mediators in a wider set of personal, economic and social relationships. Thus, effective biological treatments cannot be invoked as necessary proof of biological causation.

A fundamental problem with the illness framework in psychiatry is that it deals, in the main, with symptoms, not signs. That is, the judgements made about whether or not a person is mentally ill or healthy focus mainly (and often singularly) on the person's communications. This is certainly the case in the diagnosis of neurosis and the functional psychoses. Even in organic conditions, such as dementia, brain damage is not always detectable post-mortem. In the diagnosis of physical illness the diagnosis can often be confirmed using physical signs of changes in the body (e.g. the visible inflammation of tissue as well as the patient reporting pain).

However, it is possible to overdraw the distinctions between physical and mental illness. For example, an internal critic of psychiatry, Thomas Szasz (1961), has argued that mental illness is a myth. He says that only bodies can be ill in a literal sense and that minds can only be sick metaphorically (like economies). And yet, as we noted earlier, physical disturbances can sometimes produce profound psychological disturbances. Given that emotional distress has a well-established causative role in a variety of psychosomatic illnesses, like gastric ulcers and cardiovascular disease, the mutual inter-play of mind and body seems to be indicated on reasonable grounds.

It is true (following Szasz 1961) that the validity of mental diagnosis is undermined more by its over-reliance on symptoms and by the absence of detectable bodily signs, but this can apply at times even in physical medicine. For instance, a person may feel very ill with a headache but it may be impossible to appeal to signs to check whether or not this is because of a toxic reaction, for instance a 'hangover', or a brain tumour. Also, people with chronic physical problems have much in common, in terms of their social role, with psychiatric patients – both are disabled and usually not valued by their non-disabled fellows.

The absence of a firm biological aetiology is true of a number of physical illnesses, such as multiple sclerosis. Moreover, mental illnesses often lack treatment specificity (i.e. the diagnosis does not always imply a particular treatment and the same treatments are used across different diagnostic categories) but this is also true of some physical conditions, such as rheumatoid arthritis (which attract analgesics, anti-inflammatories and even anti-cancer drugs). Thus, the conceptual and empirical uncertainties that Szasz draws our attention to, legitimately, about mental illnesses, can apply also to what he considers to be 'true illnesses'.

A final point to note about the biological emphasis in psychiatry is that it has been repeatedly challenged by a minority of psychiatrists, including but not only Szasz. For example, some retain diagnosis but reject narrow biological explanations. They prefer to offer a bio-psycho-social model which takes into account social circumstances and biographical nuances (Engel 1980; Pilgrim 2002a; Pilgrim et al. 2008). Others have argued that madness is intelligible provided that the patient's social context is fully understood (Laing and Esterson 1964). More recently some psychiatrists have embraced social constructivism and argued that their profession has no privileged understanding of mental disorder. This emerging 'post-psychiatry' 'emphasizes social and cultural contexts, places ethics before technology and works to minimize medical control of coercive interventions' (Bracken and Thomas 2001: 725).

Thus although a biomedical approach in clinical psychiatry is common (focusing on the twin fetish of diagnosis and medication), not all psychiatrists conform to its logic (Pilgrim and Rogers 2009). Many are committed to alternative perspectives, such as social causationism and social constructivism (see later) or the next approach to be discussed.

Psychoanalysis

Psychoanalysis was the invention of Sigmund Freud. It has modern adherents who are loyal to his original theories but there are other trained analysts who adopt the views of Melanie Klein; others take a mixed position, borrowing from each theory. Thus, psychoanalysis is an eclectic or fragmented discipline. Its emphasis on personal history places it in the domain of biographical psychology. Indeed, Freud's work is sometimes called depth or psychodynamic psychology, along with the legacies of his dissenting early group such as Jung, Adler and Reich. Depth psychology proposes that the mind is divided between conscious and unconscious parts and that the dynamic relationship between these gives rise to psychopathology.

Like other forms of psychology, psychoanalysis works on a continuum principle – abnormality and normality are connected, not disconnected and separate. To the psychoanalyst we are all ill to some degree. However, the medical roots of psychoanalysis and the continued dominance of medical analysts within its culture have, arguably, left it within a psychiatric, not psychological, discourse. It still uses the terminology of pathology ('psychopathology' and its 'symptoms'); assessments are 'diagnostic' and its clients 'patients'; people do not merely have ways of avoiding human contact, they have 'schizoid defences'; and they do not simply get into the habit of angrily blaming others all of the time, instead they are 'fixated in the paranoid position'. The language of psychoanalysis is saturated with psychiatric terms. Thus, the discipline of psychoanalysis stands somewhere between psychiatry and psychology.

Psychoanalysis, arguably, has two strengths. First, it offers a comprehensive conceptual framework about mental abnormality. Once a devotee accepts its strictures, it offers the comfort of explaining, or potentially explaining, every aspect of human conduct. Second, there is asymmetry between its causal theory and its corrective programme. That which has been rendered unconscious by past relationships can be rendered conscious by a current relationship with a therapist.

Its first weakness is the obverse of biological psychiatry. The latter tends to reduce psychological phenomena to biology, whereas psychoanalysis tends to psychologize everything (i.e. the biological and the social as well as the personal). A person with temporal lobe epilepsy or a brain tumour would be helped little by a psychoanalyst. The brain-damaged patient would certainly give the analyst plenty to interpret, but the analyst would be wrong to attribute a psychological, rather than a neurological, cause. Likewise, socially determined deviance (like prostitution emerging in poor or drug-using cultures) may be explained away psychoanalytically purely in terms of individual history (Pilgrim 1992; 1998). A second weakness of psychoanalysis as a frame of reference is that it can do no more than be wise after the event. It has never reached the status of a predictive science.

Psychoanalysis has been part of a picture of internal division within psychiatry (see Box 1.1 on page 15), with medical psychoanalysts offering different perspective on the development of mental disorder than orthodox biological psychiatry. Because of its speculative interpretive emphasis, which goes beyond consciousness (about the unconscious), its role in academic psychology has been contested and marginal, but undoubtedly it is a form of psychology. But from the outset, Freud and his followers largely made a living as therapists and so they were also incorporated into psychiatry despite offering a version of normal psychology or 'the psychopathology of everyday life'. For psychoanalysts we are in a sense all ill.

Psychology

Because psychology, as a broad and eclectic discipline, focuses, in the main, on 'normal' conduct and experience, it has offered concepts of normality as well as abnormality. Buss (1966) suggests that psychologists have put forward four conceptions of normality/abnormality:

1   the statistical notion;
2   the ideal notion;
3   the presence of specific behaviours;
4   distorted cognitions.

The statistical notion

The statistical notion simply says that frequently occurring behaviours in a population are normal – so infrequent behaviours are not normal. This is akin to the notion of norms in sociology. Take as an example the tempo at which people speak. Up to a certain speed, speech would be called normal. If someone speaks above a certain speed they might be considered to be 'high' in ordinary parlance or 'hypomanic' or suffering from 'pressure of thought' in psychiatric language. If someone speaks below a certain speed they might be described as depressed. Most people would speak at a pace between these upper and lower points of frequency.

A question raised, of course, is who decides on the cut-offs at each end of the frequency distribution of speech speed and how are those decisions made? In other words, the notion of frequency in itself tells us nothing about when a behaviour is to be adjudged normal or abnormal. Value judgements are required on the part of lay people or professionals when punctuating the difference between normality and abnormality. Also, a statistical notion may not hold across cultures, even within the same country: for example, slow speech might be the norm in one culture, say in rural areas, but not in another, such as the inner city. The statistical notion of normality tells us nothing in itself about why some deviations are noted when they are unidirectional rather than bidirectional. The example of speech speed referred to bidirectional judgements. Take, in contrast, the notion of intelligence. Brightness is valued at one end of the distribution but not at the other. Being bright will not lead, in itself, to a person entering the patient role, but being dim may well do so.

In spite of these conceptual weaknesses, the statistical approach within abnormal psychology remains strong. Clinical psychologists are trained to accept that characteristics in any population follow a normal distribution and so the statistical notion has a strong legitimacy for them. This acceptance of the normal distribution of a characteristic in a population means that in psychological models there is usually assumed to be an unbroken relationship between the normal and abnormal. However, this notion of continuity of, say, everybody being more or less neurotic, may also assume a discontinuity from other variables. For instance, in Eysenck's (1955) personality theory neurosis and psychosis are considered to be personality characteristics that are both normally distributed but separate from one another.

The ideal notion

There are two versions of this notion: one from psychoanalysis and the other from humanistic psychology. In the former case, normality is defined by a predominance of conscious over unconscious characteristics in the person (Kubie 1954). In the latter case, the ideal person is one who fulfils their human potential (or 'self-actualizes'). Jahoda (1958) drew together six criteria for positive mental health to elaborate and aggregate these two psychological traditions:

1   balance of psychic forces;
2   self-actualization;
3   resistance to stress;
4   autonomy;
5   competence;
6   perception of reality.

The problem is that each of these notions is problematic as a definition of normality (and, by implication, abnormality). The first and second are only meaningful to those in a culture who subscribe to their theoretical premises (such as psychoanalytical or humanistic psychotherapists).

The resistance-to-stress notion is superficially appealing, but what of people who fail to be affected by stress at all? We can all think of situations in which anxiety is quite normal and we would wonder in such circumstances why a person fails to react in an anxious manner. Indeed, the absence of anxiety under high-stress conditions has been one defining characteristic of 'primary psychopathy' by psychiatrists. Likewise, those who are excessively autonomous (i.e. avoid human contact) might be deemed to be 'schizoid' or be suffering from 'simple schizophrenia'.

As for competence, this cannot be judged as an invariant quality. Norms of competence vary over time and place, likewise with perceptions of reality. In some cultures, seeing visions or hearing voices is highly valued, and yet it would be out of sync with the reality perceived by most in that culture. In other cultures the hallucinators may be deemed to be suffering from alcoholic psychosis or schizophrenia.

The presence of specific behaviours

The emergence of psychology as a scientific academic discipline was closely linked to its attention to specifiable aspects of conduct. It emerged and separated from speculative philosophy on the basis of these objectivist credentials. Behaviourism, the theory that tried to limit the purview of psychology to behaviour and eliminate subjective experience as data, no longer dominates psychology but it has left a lasting impression. Within clinical psychology, behaviour therapy and its modified versions are still common practices. Consequently, many psychologists are concerned to operationalize in behavioural terms what they mean by abnormality.

The term 'maladaptive behaviour' is part of this psychological discourse, as is 'unwanted' or 'unacceptable' behaviour. The strength of this position is that it makes explicit its criteria for what constitutes abnormality. The weakness is that it leaves values and norms implicit. The terminology of specific behaviours still raises questions about what constitutes 'maladaptive'. Who decides what is 'unwanted' or 'unacceptable'? One party may want a behaviour to occur or find it acceptable but another may not. In these circumstances, those who have more power will tend to be the definers of reality. Thus, what constitutes unwanted behaviour is not self-evident but socially negotiated. Consequently, it reflects both the power relationships and the value system operating in a culture at a point in time.

Distorted cognitions

The final approach suggested by Buss emerged at a time when behaviourism was becoming the dominant force within the academic discipline. However, during the 1970s this behavioural emphasis declined and was eventually displaced by cognitivism. As a result, psychologists began to treat inner events as if they were behaviours (forming the apparently incongruous hybrid of a 'cognitive-behavioural' approach to mental health problems) or they increasingly incorporated constructivist, systemic and even psychoanalytical views (e.g. Bannister and Fransella 1970; Guidano 1987; Ryle 1990). It is not clear even now whether the ascendancy of 'cognitive therapy' within clinical psychology during the 1980s was driven by cognitivism or was merely legitimized by it. So much of the seminal writing on cognitive therapy came not from academic psychology but from clinicians, some of whom were psychiatrists, not psychologists, offering a pragmatic and a-theoretical approach to symptom reduction (e.g. Beck 1970; Ellis 1970; Pilgrim and Carey 2010).

Since the outline by Buss was offered, we can also note that in the field of mental health humanistic psychology has become more evident as a political force, within clinical psychology, counselling psychology and psychotherapy. Humanistic psychology emphasizes the inherent capacity of human beings to seek and find meaning, including during periods which are distressing for people. Humanistic psychology emerged from North American philosophy (William James and James Dewey) and was developed in the field of mental health by Abraham Maslow, Carl Rogers and Rollo May. It has affinities with European existentialism, which joined humanistic approaches to mental health problems in anglophone countries with the work of existential psychiatry (especially from Victor Frankl and Ludwig Binswanger) after the Second World War.

A particularly important variant of humanistic psychology has been that of 'positive psychology', which emphasizes strengths and solutions rather than deficits and problems (the dominant tradition in clinical work) (Ryan and Deci 2001). Psychology is thus a highly variegated discipline and this diverse character is at its most obvious in relation to the wide range of psychological approaches to mental health problems.

Discussion of the clinical perspectives

The expert clinical perspectives on mental health and illness all have some persuasiveness. Equally, we have noted some credibility problems that each encounters. The illness framework emphasizes discontinuity (people are ill/disordered or they are not) whereas the other perspectives tend to emphasize continuity. It is a matter of opinion whether a continuous or discontinuous model of normality and abnormality fits our knowledge of people's conduct and whether one or the other is morally preferable. Traditional psychiatrists might argue that, unlike psychoanalysts, they do not see abnormality everywhere. Psychoanalysts might argue that the pervasive condition of mental pain connects us all in a common humanity.

Generally psychological approaches (including psychoanalysis) agree on the need to be aware of the *continuity* between normal and abnormal states. This implies the need for context specific formulations, rather than the de-contextualized diagnoses favoured by biological psychiatry, of this sort: 'Why is this person presenting with this particular problem or complaint at this point in their life?' However, because psychology itself is a contested discipline (a point made more obvious if we include psychoanalysis and then contrast it with behaviourism) then *which* form of formulation to believe becomes a moot point.

Our concern here is not to resolve these questions but to record them in order to demonstrate that the topic of mental health and illness is highly contested. There are no benchmarks that experts from different camps can agree on and discuss. Thus 'mental disorder' or 'mental illness' or 'maladaptive behaviour' or simply being 'loony' do not necessarily have a single referent. It is not only a matter of terminology, although it is in part. It is not simply like the difference between speaking of motor cars and automobiles. In our discussion, each perspective may be warranting certain types of reality but not others. What we have is a fragmented set of perspectives, divided internally and from one another, which occasionally overlap and enter the same world of discourse.

The clinical perspectives have difficulty in sustaining notions of mental health and illness, which are stable, certain or invariant. In each case, the caveat of social relativism has to be registered. Judgements about health and illness (physical as well as mental) are value-laden and reflect specific norms in time and place. The formulations of psychoanalysts and psychologists can be adapted to include social context. For this reason it is the claims about the global objective and trans-historical 'nature' of psychiatric diagnosis, in the Diagnostic and Statistical Manual of Mental Disorders (DSM) and International Classification of Disease (ICD) systems, which remain most controversial in the field of mental health. A diagnostic approach predominates but is also the one that has witnessed most public controversy.

Also we need to be mindful of the ways that ordinary words start to take on different meanings in our field of inquiry. For example, in clinical research the word 'validity' refers to whether a fact being claimed is true in some sense. Does a diagnosis or formulation refer to or measure what it is supposed to refer to or measure? Does it predict accurately a state of affairs, such as the treated or untreated outcome for a patient (in medicine this is called 'prognosis')? By contrast, in clinical work and research, 'reliability' refers to consistency over time or agreement between raters or diagnosticians. This use of terminology can be contrasted with everyday language and legal understandings. For example, we talk of a person being a 'reliable witness' and whether a fact being claimed is reliable. Thus in everyday and legal understandings 'reliability' and 'validity' tend to overlap but not so in clinical work and research. We return to this point about ordinary language in Chapter 10.

Perspectives within sociology

Having discussed perspectives about mental health and illness from outside sociology, we now turn to contributions within the latter academic discipline. Before that we can note that a cross-cutting matter above which overlaps with the perspectives described below relates to versions of holism, which have been particularly evident in US social science (Bateson 1980) and US culture more generally. Disciplinary perspectives and variants within each discipline generate claims at times of holistic understandings. For example, the bio-psycho-social model was mentioned as a variant of the medical model. (Some writers add a spiritual dimension to these three levels of integrative enquiry.) General systems theory is another example used across the natural and social sciences and has been obvious recurrently in sociology (Parsons 1951;

Offe 1993; Habermas 1975). In clinical work this can at times be seen in complementary approaches to mental health care, with the challenge from alternative therapies, or the incorporation of Eastern 'ways' or antiquarian philosophy into therapy. An example of the latter is the blending of Buddhism and Stoicism into versions of psychotherapy, including so-called 'Third Wave' CBT.

Holistic preferences are also evident in service user demands (more on this in Chapter 12). One lobbying response came from the Hearing Voices Network (HVN), which in its press release (20 May 2013: para 2) said:

> psychiatric diagnoses are both scientifically unsound and can have damaging consequences. HVN suggest that asking 'what's happened to you?' is more useful than 'what's wrong with you?' Concerned that essential funds are being wasted on expensive and futile genetic research, HVN call for the redirection of funds to address the societal problems known to lead to mental health problems and provide the holistic support necessary for recovery.

The emphasis on the inclusion of both personal meanings and social causes in this statement reflect a balancing act within sociological perspectives as we will now see.

An outline of four sociological perspectives

Four major sociological perspectives will be outlined: social causation, hermeneutics, social constructivism and social realism. (Societal reaction or labelling theory will be considered separately in Chapter 11.) Taken together, these perspectives bear the imprints of major contributions from Durkheim, Weber, Freud, Foucault and Marx. These influences are not linear but cross-cut and are mediated by the work of contributors such as Sartre and Mead. Different theoretical perspectives have been popular and influential at different times. However, it is important to acknowledge that there is no set of boundaries to neatly periodize disciplinary trends. Rather, there are sedimented layers of knowledge, which overlap unevenly in time and across disciplinary boundaries and professional preoccupations. The social causation thesis arguably peaked in the 1950s, when a number of large-scale community surveys of the social causes of mental health problems and of the large psychiatric institutions were undertaken. It has seen a resurgence recently in the longitudinal epidemiological work of some clinical psychologists looking at the role of childhood adversity as a predictor of adult mental health problems (Read and Bentall 2012).

However, one of its most quoted exemplars appeared in the late 1970s and early 1980s (Brown and Harris 1978), and studies in the social causation tradition were set to proliferate in the late 1990s with an explicit government policy agenda designed to tackle the social, economic and environmental causes of mental health problems (Department of Health 1998). Similarly, there is no absolute distinction between sociological knowledge and other forms of knowledge. In relation to lay knowledge/perspective, some sociological perspectives (such as symbolic interactionism) in large part draw on the meaning and understandings of lay people. More recently, and in line with a rediscovered enthusiasm for psychoanalytical approaches applied to sociology, the sociological perspective of 'social constructionism' within sociology has been treated 'as if it were a client presenting itself for psychoanalysis' (Craib 1997). According to Craib, social constructionism (discussed in more detail later):

> can be seen as a manic psychosis – a defense against entering the depressive position . . . Sociologists find it difficult to recognize the limitations of their discipline – the depressive position – one reason being that we do not actually exercise power over anybody; social constructionism enables us to convince ourselves that the opposite is true, that we know everything about how people become what they are, that we do not have to take account of

other disciplines or sciences, but we can explain everything . . . a non-psychotic theory is one which knows its own limitations.

(Craib 1997: 1)

With this caution in mind, each of the four sociological perspectives will now be considered.

Social causation

This response from sociologists essentially accepts constructs, such as 'schizophrenia' or 'depression', as legitimate diagnoses. They are given the status of facts in themselves. Once these diagnoses are accepted, questions are then asked about the role of socially derived stress in their aetiology.

The emphasis within a social causation approach is upon tracing the relationship between social disadvantage and mental illness. Given that many sociologists have considered the main indicator of disadvantage to be low social class and/or poverty, it is not surprising that studies investigating this relationship have been a strong current within social studies of psychiatric populations (see Chapter 2). Social class has not been the only variable investigated within this social causation perspective. Disadvantages of other sorts, related to race, gender and age have also been of interest. The implications of these studies are discussed in subsequent chapters.

The advantage of this psychiatric epidemiological perspective is that it provides the sort of scientific confidence associated with objectivism and empiricism (methodological assurances of representativeness and pointers towards causal relationships). However, four main disadvantages of the approach can be identified:

- First, pre-empirical conceptual problems associated with psychiatric knowledge are either not acknowledged or are evaded (see for example Brown and Harris 1978).
- Second, psychiatric epidemiology investigates correlations between mental illness and antecedent variables. However, correlations are not necessarily indicative of causal relationships. This caution also applies within biological psychiatry to genetic studies of mental disorders.
- Third, the investigation of large subpopulations cannot illuminate the lived experience of mental health problems or the variety of meanings attributed to them by patients and significant others. Aggregate data and averages tell us little or nothing about the *particular experiences of individuals* with mental health problems.
- Fourth, medical epidemiology attempts to map the distributions of causes of diseases, not merely the cases of disease. Because most psychiatric illnesses are described as 'functional' (i.e. they have no known biological marker, and causes are either not known or contested), then psychiatric epidemiology cannot fulfil the general expectation of mapping causes.

Despite these cautions, social causationist arguments do reveal tendencies. For example, as we will see in later chapters, not only does social group membership predict, to some extent, mental health status, with poverty being a prime example, causal processes operate within social group distinctions. This is particularly the case with familial differences: benign family cultures buffer the child against immediate and subsequent mental health problems, whereas abusive and neglectful families increase the probability of those problems.

Hermeneutics

Hermeneutics is the science of making interpretations. Some social scientists and therapists specialize in this approach, but arguably it is a routine aspect of social interaction in all human societies. Indeed, some versions of social science, such as social phenomenology, ethnomethodology, symbolic interactionism and existentially or psychoanalytically informed models of social inquiry, focus on our capacity to interpret ourselves and others. This focus is so salient in these approaches that meaning- and sense-making are the main forms of data generation. However, for this to be a sociological (rather than clinical or psychological) exercise, then social context must also be a central consideration in hermeneutics. The influence of symbolic interactionism in the field of mental health is clear in labelling theory, which we consider in Chapter 11. That is inherently about the exchange of meanings in their particular social contexts. For this reason the roots of that approach in the work of Weber and Cooley reflect one variant of a social form of hermeneutics.

During the twentieth century, a number of writers attempted to account for the relationship between socio-economic structures and the inner lives of individuals. One example was the work of Sartre (1963) when he developed his 'progressive-regressive method'. This method was an attempt to understand biography in relation to its social context and understand social context via the accounts of people's lives. This existential development of humanistic Marxism competed with another and more elaborate set of discussions about the relationship between unconscious mental life and societal determinants and constraints.

Within Freud's early circle, a number of analysts took an interest in using their psychological insights in order to illuminate societal processes. This set a trend for later analysts, some of whom tended to reduce social phenomena to the aggregate impact of psychopathology (e.g. Bion 1959). The dangers of psychological reductionism were inevitable in a tradition (psychoanalysis) that had a starting focus of methodological individualism. Moreover, the individuals studied by psychoanalysis were from a peculiar social group (white, middle-class, European neurotics).

Out of this tradition emerged a group of Freudo-Marxists who came to be known as 'critical theorists', most of whom were associated with the Frankfurt Institute of Social Research, which was founded in 1923 and led after 1930 by Horkheimer (Slater 1977). This group accordingly came to be known as the 'Frankfurt School'. The difference between the work of the Frankfurt School and most of clinical psychoanalysis was the focus on the inter-relationship between psyche and society. In an early address to the Institute, Horkheimer (1931: 14) set out its mission as follows:

> What connections can be established, in a specific social group, in a specific period in time, in specific countries, between the group, the changes in the psychic structures of its individual members and the thoughts and institutions that are a product of that society, and that have, as a whole, a formative effect upon the group under consideration?

These inter-relationships between the material environment of individuals and their cultural life and inner lives were subsequently explored by a number of writers in the Institute, including Marcuse, Adorno and Fromm. In addition, there were contributions from Benjamin (who was a marginal and ambivalent Institute member) and Reich, a Marxist psychoanalyst and outsider. These explorations had an explicit emancipatory intent and were characterized by anti-Stalinist as well as anti-fascist themes. Within the Frankfurt School, Freudianism was accepted as the only legitimate form of psychology which was, potentially at least, philosophically compatible with Marxism. (Both Freud and Marx were atheists and materialists, although Freud's materialism was barely historical.) The compatibility was explored and affirmed, though, by one member in particular who was a psychoanalyst – Eric Fromm. The integration of Freudianism was selective and critical, filtering out or querying elements such as the death instinct (a revision of classical psychoanalytical theory by Freud himself (Freud 1920)) and questioning the mechanistic aspect of instinctual drive-theory.

The role of this group of critical theorists in social science has been important and seemingly paradoxical. For a theory that drew heavily, if selectively, upon clinical psychoanalysis, the raft of work associated with the Frankfurt School (which was largely relocated in the USA with the rise of Nazism) focused not on mental illness but instead upon what Fromm called the 'pathology of normalcy'. It was only seemingly paradoxical because psychoanalysis was (and still is) concerned with the notion that we are all ill – psychopathology for Freud and his followers was ubiquitous, varying between individuals only in degree and type. Accordingly, the concerns of this group of Freudo-Marxists were about life-negating cultural norms associated with authoritarianism and the capitalist economy and the ambiguous role of the super-ego as a source of conformity and mutuality. These norms were said to be mediated by the intra-psychic mechanism (especially the repression) highlighted in Freud's theory of a dynamic unconscious.

Critical theory is exemplified in studies of the authoritarian personality (Adorno *et al.* 1950), the mass psychology of fascism (Reich 1933; Fromm 1942) and the psychological blocks attending the transitions from capitalist to socialist democracy (Fromm 1955). When Habermas (1989) came to review the project of the early Frankfurt School, he suggested a six-part programme of topic focus: forms of integration in post-liberal societies, family socialization and ego development, mass media and culture, the social psychology behind the cessation of protest, the theory of art, and the critique of positivism and science.

The problems of critical theory have been twofold. First, as was indicated earlier, the theoretical centre of gravity of this project (the Frankfurt School) fragmented. Second, the meaningfulness of any hybrid of dialectical materialism and psychoanalysis requires social scientists to accept the legitimacy of both of its component parts and their conceptual and practical integration. This requires a triple act of faith or theoretical commitment that leaves many unconvinced, dubious or even hostile to the expectation.

The German version of Freudo-Marxism (the Frankfurt School) emerged in the first half of the twentieth century and its traces in social science, with the exception of Habermas and Offe, tend recently to be faint and influenced by other theoretical positions. For example, the long list of post-war American and British writers cited above have been part of a theoretical tradition which is still psychoanalytically orientated but reflects changes such as the impact of Klein and later object-relations theorists. Another Freudo-Marxian hybrid can be found in French intellectual life, especially following the work of Althusser and Lacan (Elliot 1992). This current moved in a different direction from the Frankfurt School and contributed to the emergence in the 1970s of post-structuralism; a variant of the next perspective we summarize.

Social constructivism

One of the most influential theoretical positions in the sociology of health and illness since the 1980s has been social constructivism – as mentioned earlier, it sometimes appears as 'social constructionism'. A central assumption within this broad approach is that reality is not self-evident, stable and waiting to be discovered, but instead it is a product of human activity. In this broad sense all versions of social constructivism can be identified as a reaction against positivism and naïve realism. Brown (1995) suggests three main currents within social constructivism:

1   The first approach is not concerned with demonstrating the reality or otherwise of a social phenomenon but with the social forces which define it. The approach is traceable to sociological work on social problems (Spector and Kitsuse 1977). To investigate a social problem, such as drug misuse or mental illness, is to select a particular aspect of reality and implicitly, concede the factual status of reality in general (Woolgar and Pawluch 1985). In particular, the lived experience of social actors, those inside deviant communities or those working with and labelling them, are the focus of sociological investigation. The social problems emphasis, which gave rise to this version of social constructivism, has been associated, like societal reaction theory, with methodologies linked to symbolic interactionism and ethnomethodology.

2   The second approach is tied more closely to the post-structuralism of Foucault and is concerned with deconstruction – the critical examination of language and symbols in order to illuminate the creation of knowledge, its relationship to power and the unstable varieties of reality which attend human activity ('discursive practices'). Foucault's early work on madness, however, was not about such discursive concerns (Foucault 1965). The latter have been the focus of interest of later post-structuralists (see below).

3   The third approach is associated neither with the micro-sociology of social problem definition nor with deconstruction but with understanding the production of scientific knowledge and the pursuit of individual and collective professional interests (Latour 1987). This science-in-action version of sociology is concerned with the illumination of interest work. This version of social constructivism examines the ways in which scientists and other interested parties develop, debate and use facts. It is thus interested in the networks of people involved in these activities. Unlike the post-structuralist version of social constructivism noted earlier, it places less emphasis upon ideas and more upon action and negotiation (e.g. Bartley et al. 1997). This approach is thus compatible with both symbolic interactionism and social realism (see next section).

These three versions of constructivism are not neatly divided within many studies within medical sociology. Bury (1986) notes that the notion of social constructivism subsumes many elements, some of which are contradictory. However, certain core themes can be detected across the three main types described by Brown. The first is that if reality is not rejected as an epiphenomenon of human activity (as in very strict constructivism) it is nonetheless problematized to some degree – hence the break with positivism. The second relates to the importance of reality being viewed, in whole or part, as a product of human activity. What constructivists vary in is whether this activity is narrowly about the cognitive aspects of human life (thought and talk), or it is conceived in a broader sense in relation to the actions of individuals and collectivities. The third is that power relationships are inextricably bound up with reality definition. Whether it is the power to define or the power to influence or the power to advance some interests at the expense of others, this political dimension to constructivism is consistent.

When we come to examine sociological work on mental health and illness these three core elements are evident. Constructivists problematize the factual status of mental illness (e.g. Szasz 1961). They analyse the ways in which mental health work has been linked to the production of psychiatric knowledge and the production of mental health problems (e.g. Parker et al. 1995). Also, they establish the links which exist in modern society with the coercive control of social deviance by psychiatry on the one hand and the production of selfhood by mental health expertise on the other (e.g. Miller and Rose 1988).

The final point to be made about social constructivism is that it does not necessarily have to be set in opposition to social realism (the view that there is an independent existing reality) or social causationism (the view that social forces cause measurable phenomena to really exist). It is certainly true that strong social constructivism challenges both of these positions (see e.g. Gergen 1985). However, a number of writers who accept some constructivist arguments point out that, strictly, it is not reality which is socially constructed but our theories of reality (Greenwood 1994; Brown 1995; Pilgrim 2000). So much of the apparent opposition between constructivist and realist or causationist arguments in social science results from a failure to make this distinction. This brings us to our next perspective.

Social realism

The final perspective to be discussed in this chapter is that of social realism – a perspective held by the authors (Pilgrim and Rogers 1994; Pilgrim 2013) as well as others working in the field of mental health and the social psychology of emotions and human agency (Greenwood 1994; Archer 1995; Williams 1999; Bendelow 2009). Bhaskar (1978; 1989) outlines the philosophical basis of realism and we will draw out, briefly, the implications of his work for a sociology of mental health and illness. His version is called 'critical realism'. Thus here we are using the term 'social realism' to denote the sociological *application* of the philosophy of critical realism.

As the name implies, critical realism accepts that reality really does exist (contra strict constructivism, which dwells overwhelmingly on the representations or constructions of reality). However, the 'critical' prefix suggests that it diverges from social causationism. The latter follows the Durkheimian view that external social reality impinges on human action and shapes human consciousness. The Weberian view emphasizes the opposite process – that human action intersubjectively constructs reality. Critical theory, following Freud, emphasizes the role of unconscious processes, especially repression, and is rooted in methodological individualism (clinical psychoanalysis). By contrast to all of these, critical realism attends to conscious action or agency and is critical of methodological individualism.

Social realists consider that human action is neither mechanistically determined by social reality nor does intentionality (voluntary human action) simply construct social reality. Instead, society exists prior to the lives of people but they become agents who reproduce or transform that society. Material reality (the biological substrate of actors and the material conditions of their social context) *constrains* action but does not simply determine it. Social science and natural science warrant different methodologies and social phenomena cannot be reduced to natural phenomena, even though the latter may exert an influence on the former and are a precondition of their existence.

Bhaskar (1989: 79) highlights the difference between natural and social science in the light of this basic starting point. Here we quote three major differences between natural and social structures and then draw out the implications for the topic of this book:

1   Social structures, unlike natural structures, do not exist independently of the activity they govern.
2   Social structures, unlike natural structures, do not exist independently of the agents' conceptions of what they are doing in their activity.
3   Social structures, unlike natural structures, may be only relatively enduring so that the tendencies they ground may not be universal in the sense of a space-time invariant.

Thus realism in social science can be of two forms. The first is naïve realism or positivism. The second is critical realism. Both are committed to the view that reality exists independently of its observers or commentators. This then is an *ontological* emphasis. The difference between them is that positivism accepts its current views about empirical investigations without question and privileges objective over subjective data. What is currently known empirically by dominant forms of inquiry ('actualism') is deemed scientifically to define reality, thereby demoting the meanings and legitimacy of other forms of knowledge. Naïve realism also aspires to separate facts from values in order to generate 'disinterested' objective truth claims.

By contrast critical realism is interested in the relationship between subjective and objective data and assumes that both are generated by, and evaluated within, particular social contexts, which must be part of any comprehensive social inquiry. For this reason values and interests are part of any critical realist informed inquiry. Thus critical realism can be distinguished by its *epistemological* emphasis, once the centrality of ontology to its concerns is understood.

It can be viewed (though some critical realists are not always happy with this depiction) as a *weak* form of constructivism because it takes concepts and their social generation seriously. However, it does not dwell singularly on meanings (the emphasis of hermeneutics) because causes may operate beyond the experience of social actors. It also goes beyond constructs or social representations (the emphasis of radical social constructivism). Also, for critical realists constructs are personal or shared *concepts* (for example shared in a particular culture and time). This then is about *construing* the world not about *constructing* the world. The latter is an active verb meaning 'building', when for critical realists the world is built already, independent of human minds and action. These are implicated though in agency, which is a real presence that can and does reproduce or transform reality. By contrast, radical constructivists privilege 'perspectivism' (hence their priority of epistemology) and not an independent reality (the critical realist's priority of ontology).

For social realists, causes ('generative mechanisms') may be biological, psychological or social, a position compatible with a bio-psycho-social model noted earlier. However, as Pilgrim (2013) notes, most developments of that model have naïvely accepted medical constructs and tended to privilege the biological. We will see in Chapter 11 that symbolic interactionism in labelling theory also accepts multi-level causation and so an alignment with social realism is possible. However, the emphasis on meanings of that model tends to push causes into the background. By contrast social realism places causes ('generative mechanism') at the centre of its analysis, with the meanings that human agents then bring to bear on those mechanisms also being taken into consideration in any full social analysis of a topic.

A final point about social realism is that it can accommodate several factors existing concurrently in society as an open system. In the case of mental health problems and their management, then the complex reality of the economic, socialization and welfare systems are all relevant for understanding it (Pilgrim 2012). The economic system both generates stressors, and profits from the amelioration of the impact of those stressors. The socialization system determines the adoption of social norms during childhood and then offers corrective interventions of secondary socialization if those norms are transgressed in adulthood (mental health work). The welfare system employs mental health workers and contains systems of regulation to ameliorate distress and control the disruptions to socio-economic order and efficiency.

Discussion of the clinical and sociological perspectives

We can see then across sociological perspectives that the balance between causes and meanings is always apparent. The other balance evident from perspective to perspective is the type of scepticism or criticism, offered or implied, of the clinical perspectives discussed in the first part of the chapter. With the exception of (naïve) social causationism, sociological perspectives problematize the diagnostic perspective on mental disorder. The force of these arguments can be seen in the continuing debates both within sociology and increasingly from across other disciplines, particularly those who encounter mental distress and interpersonal dysfunction in their everyday work. Various forms of ambivalence are evident on all sides. Social realists can still 'do business' with psychiatry, particularly if a bio-psycho-social model is deployed and investigated in a spirit of genuine interdisciplinary collaboration. The interdisciplinary project of 'social psychiatry' describes this convergence of disciplinary interests. We also mentioned the tendency for some critical psychiatrists and other professional groups to embrace social constructivism. Some sociologists have gone some way to legitimize the core business of psychiatry by accepting that the psychoses are 'true' illnesses, while designating 'common mental disorders' as being forms of social deviance (not illnesses). Horwitz argues that 'a valid definition of mental disorder should be narrow and should not encompass many of the presumed mental disorders of diagnostic psychiatry, especially appropriate reactions to stressful social condition and many culturally patterned forms of deviant behaviour' (2002: 15). A problem with this partial validation of psychiatric diagnosis is that it relies too readily on immediate social intelligibility. That is, stress reactions and cultural context warrant attributions of non-pathology, whereas psychosis does not. We return to this point in Chapter 4.

Some medical practitioners have rejected the concept of mental illness but not in the way that was evident in the Szaszian critique noted earlier. Baker and Menken (2001) suggest that the term 'mental illness' must be abandoned because it is an erroneous label for true brain disorder. They are dismissive of the countless critiques and ambiguities previously identified by dissenting psychiatrists and sociological critics. Instead they argue for a clear philosophical assertion that all mental illnesses are brain disorders as 'an essential step to promote the improvement of human health' from within clinical medicine:

> We suggest that it is unscientific, misleading and harmful to millions of people worldwide to declare that some brain disorders are not physical ailments. Neurology and psychiatry must end the twentieth century schism that has divided their fields.
>
> (Baker and Menken 2001: 937)

This assertion, about biodeterminism seems to discard all of the sociological theorizing about mental disorder in favour of medical jurisdiction and paternalism, purportedly in service of the common good. However, this medical confidence evades an obvious point: the bulk of what are called 'mental disorders' still have no definitive proven biological cause. The only aspects of the social this medical view leaves intact are the environmental factors, which might putatively contribute to the aetiology of illness. However, this stance is one reflection of a deeper problem for both medicine and sociology; the problem of mind/body dualism.

Baker and Menken create a unity between mind and body by asserting the single centrality of the skin-encapsulated body out of which each and every form of human ill emerges. Radical social constructivism generates another unitary position by arguing instead that 'everything is socially constructed'. In this view, reality, truth claims and causes are all dismissed just as readily as Baker and Menken dismiss the conceptual objections facing the concept of mental illness. This goes further than labelling theory which left the ontological status of primary deviance intact. It ascribed to it a basic reality and permitted a variety of causes. Radical social constructivism does not make this concession, and primary not just secondary deviance is examined critically.

The constructivist position is not consistent though. For example, Szasz deconstructed the representations of mental illness in order to render it a 'myth'. At the same time he accepted uncritically the reality of physical illness. Carpenter (2000) notes the proliferation of diagnostic categories after the appearance of the third edition of the American Psychiatric Association's Diagnostic and Statistical Manual (DSM-III). Box 1 summarizes the DSM-5 controversy in the historical context of diagnostic psychiatry.

Box 1.1 The DSM controversy

In 1918, after the First World War, the American Medico-Psychological Association, which became the American Psychiatric Association (APA) in 1921, produced the 'Statistical Manual for the Use of Institutions of the Insane'. This was the starting point in 1952 for DSM-I (Grob 1991), and it reflected the dominance at the time of psychoanalytical and social psychiatric ideas in both the academy and the clinic in the USA. Three main factions within the APA were emerging in the postwar period: biological psychiatrists, medical psychoanalysts and social psychiatrists.

By the 1970s biological psychiatrists had consolidated their relationship with the pharmaceutical industry in the wake of the putative 'pharmacological revolution' of the 1950s (Healy 1997). They consolidated the bio-reductionist medical tradition of assuming that brain diseases explained all mental illness (Kraepelin 1883). This group of 'neo-Kraepelinians' formed an 'invisible college' of like-minded researchers at Washington University, St Louis and in New York that captured control of the DSM committee within the APA (Blashfield 1982; Bayer and Spitzer 1985; Wilson 1993).

This neo-Kraepelinian project shifted the DSM emphasis from its assumptions about bio-graphical context to one based upon discrete disease entities, with their proposed scientific equiv-alence to categories in physical medicine. The neo-Kraepelinian rationale was that abnormalities in neurotransmitters caused mental illnesses, which were then amenable to specific medicinal responses or 'magic bullets'. The dominance of the drug-company-backed neo-Kraepelinians from DSM-III onwards (DSM-IV appeared in 1994) meant that they could expand their jurisdiction and scientific claims. The number of categories virtually tripled from around a hundred in DSM-I to nearly 300 in DSM-IV.

In 2013 DSM-5 was issued and met much criticism; an organized campaign had already emerged in 2011 in opposition to it. The Society of Humanistic Psychologists (Division 32 of the American Psychological Association) began to lobby against the inherent de-humanization of psychiatric diagnosis. In an open letter to the APA it argued that 'it is time for psychiatry and psychology collaboratively to explore the possibility of developing an alternative approach to the conceptualization of emotional distress' (Society of Humanistic Psychologists 2011). The letter drew upon the hostile response issued by the British Psychological Society:

> The putative diagnoses presented in DSM-V are clearly based largely on social norms, with 'symptoms' that all rely on subjective judgments, with little confirmatory physical 'signs' or evidence of biological causation. The criteria are not value-free, but rather reflect current normative social expectations. . . . [Taxonomic] systems such as this are based on identifying problems as located within individuals. This misses the relational context of problems and the undeniable social causation of many such problems.
>
> (British Psychological Society 2011)

At this point an Anglophone consensus (across the USA, Australia and the UK) was negoti-ated that connected the range of objections listed above, and website set up containing a petition opposed to DSM: 'Is the DSM-5 safe?' (http://dsm5response.com). Contributors to this campaign included psychiatrists, psychologists and service users. In translation the campaign was extended to Spanish- and French-speaking countries.

The launch of DSM-5 has flushed out a range of positions about psychiatric diagnosis and its social context. The National Institute of Mental Health in the USA criticized it for not being biologi-cal *enough* and suggested that a different research framework should be used. From the other side of this biological reductionism, dissident psychiatrists, hostile psychologists and radical service users (see Box 1.1) complained about four main problems.

First, unrelenting diagnostic proliferation in DSM has been criticized. For example, Wykes and Callard (2010) warned that after 2013 'the pool of "normality" would shrink to a mere puddle'. With the lowering of thresholds, what was previously normal would become abnormal. Previous editions of DSM explicitly discounted grief as a mental disorder; in DSM-5 it was included. In the run up to the DSM revision, book-length critiques appeared pointing out that normal sadness was being turned into illness after DSM-III (Horwitz and Wakefield 2007) and that habitual shyness was being framed as a form of personality disorder (Lane 2008).

Second, particular concerns were expressed about the pathologization of childhood, when ipso facto primary socialization is not complete and so normative judgements about psychological health are particularly problematic (Timimi 2002). The Western Australian MP Martin Whitely had led national campaigns against the introduction into DSM-5 of 'psychosis risk disorder', and he has been critical of the over-diagnosis of 'attention deficit hyperactivity disorder' with the concomitant prevalence of stimulant medication for the condition.

Third, and arising from the above, many objectors to DSM-5 were alert to the ever-presence of marketed 'magic bullets' and their risks. For example, if a teenager is deemed to be at risk of psychosis and is then medicated before they develop symptoms, then they will be exposed to the iatrogenic risks of anti-psychotic drugs (Bentall and Morrison 2002).

Fourth, some objections reflected an opposition to the point of diagnosis in principle. Some medical psychoanalysts have offered such criticisms (e.g. Szasz 1961; Laing 1967) but it has also been evident within the Meyerian tradition that has been influential in the development of social psychiatry (Double 1990; Pilgrim 2013). Latterly the influence of French post-structuralism in some criticisms from psychiatrists about expert knowledge is also now a consideration (Bracken and Thomas 2001).

Various sociological commentators have pointed to how interests, agencies and technology have promoted the medicalization and institutionalization of certain diagnostic categories, such as 'post-traumatic stress disorder', 'depression' and 'eating disorders'. Lyons (1996) points to activities of the drug companies in promoting Prozac as an acceptable drug to make life better for all – almost a recreational drug. Such a trend is reinforced in primary care, where depression has come to be accepted as more of a legitimate condition amenable to a technical fix. Identifying technologies (e.g. antidepressant medication and counselling) as a means of management located within primary care is likely to have contributed to increasing medicalization and acceptability of depression as a valid presenting problem in GP consultations (May et al. 2004).

In response to this proliferation of diagnostic categories and the medicalization of everyday suffering Horwitz (2002) argues that only symptoms that reflect psychological dysfunctions, considered to be universally inappropriate, should warrant being labelled as true mental diseases. The advantage of this approach is that it is an attempt to overcome the void left by the relativistic nihilism characteristic of some post-modernist approaches to the conceptualization of mental health problems.

On the face of things, this line of reasoning follows those sociologists of mental health and illness who have aligned themselves with a critical realist position (i.e. presenting a weak social constructivist argument without abandoning the notion of mental illness and undermining the notion that mental distress exists). However, this argument may precariously be introducing another essentialist view of psychiatric disorder. Implying some self-evident and natural distinction between true mental illness and varieties of socially generated mental distress is akin to some older psychiatric classifications that distinguished mental illness from distressing environmental reactions (Fish 1968).

From a critical realist perspective it is clearly the case that pressure groups and drug companies also do much to promote and maintain all diagnostic categories (Pilgrim 2007a); profit makes none of the distinctions considered or asserted by Horwitz. Moreover the criterion of 'universal inappropriateness' is difficult to sustain for any diagnostic category. For example, 'hearing voices' has been associated with the diagnostic category of 'schizophrenia' but it would fail to fit the categorization of 'universally inappropriate'. Not only is voice-hearing evident in the general population (including in those without a diagnosis of psychosis), in some cultures it provides evidence of spiritual superiority. Hallucinations have no universal meaning – they might occur universally but what they mean varies from place to place.

Another difficulty for sociology trying to define the unique and troublesome features of mental illness is the tendency to leave physical illness non-problematized (the Szaszian error). The focus on mental disorder means that sociologists have at times claimed for mental health what applies more generically. For example, Horwitz's key argument about the proliferation of psychological categories (Horwitz 2002) clearly includes examples which are considered to be essentially physical (even though they may also be identified with certain psychological tendencies). In accepting mind/body dualism, sociologists, like those in other disciplines, may disregard or dismiss physical health problems as unproblematic and fail to consider the common social processes shaping the definition and causes of all illness behaviour and experience.

The ontological status of musculoskeletal disease, as an essentially physical entity, provides an interesting point of comparison of the way in which the mind/body dualism has overridden the experience and conceptualizations of people's pain and distress provided in a study in which:

> respondents' conceptualizations of the physical body emphasized fragility and paralysis. This view of the body resonates with an understanding of incapacity, or of not being able to act as desired, which emerges from a sense of ineptness, weakness and pain. . . . Descriptions of an amorphous sense of pain which accompanied this sense of precariousness seemed to suggest a lack of demarcation between pain located in specific parts of the body and concerns in broader social and personal worlds and in this respect pain and suffering transcended the commonly understood notion of the physical body and extended to include other personal disappointments.
>
> (Rogers and Allison 2004: 81)

Ironically, in failing to construct alternative models of illness in general, both sociologists and medical practitioners may remain trapped in forms of mind/body dualism or offer implausible assertions to impose a unity, such as medical naturalism or radical social constructivism.

Finally, it may seem, at first reading, that sociology is somehow a separate and recent commentator on mental health and illness. This is only partially true. Since the mid-twentieth century newly trained sociologists have contributed to knowledge about psychiatry and the mental patient, but this may give the false impression that sociology is merely responding to the dominant discourse on health and illness coming from health professionals.

However, 'social science' existed at the beginnings of medicine. Before the latter settled down to become preoccupied with individual bodies and their parts, social medicine had emerged in the eighteenth century as a programme of political intervention to prevent ill health (Rosen 1979). Indeed, Foucault (1980) argues that medical surveys of society in the early nineteenth century were the true roots of modern sociology, not its reputed fathers such as Comte, Marx, Durkheim and Weber. (For a wider discussion of this topic see Kleinman (1986) and Turner (1990).)

In the particular case of mental health, so much research of the epidemiological variety was intertwined with medical research. The discipline of social psychiatry demonstrates this overlap (Goldberg and Morrison 1963; Warner 1985). Also, some of the groundbreaking epidemiological work of the 1950s and 1960s involved the collaboration of sociologists (e.g. Hollingshead and Brown) with psychiatrists (e.g. Redlich and Wing).

However, it is also true that the more recent response of sociologists has been seen as oppositional by those inside clinical psychiatry. During the late 1960s, sociologists became part of 'antipsychiatry' or 'critics of psychiatry', according to leaders of the offended profession, such as Roth (1973). Thus, sociologists are in an ambivalent relationship to psychiatry. On the one hand, they have contributed to an expanded theory of aetiology, in tracing the social causes of mental illness; on the other, they have set up competing ways of conceptualizing mental abnormality.

The bulk of the work we have reviewed in this chapter reflects a dominant sociological interest in mental abnormality and in psychiatry. By comparison, since the beginning of the twentieth century, there has been much less sociological (and for that matter general social scientific) interest in ordinary emotional life, non-deviant conduct and professional knowledge outside of the governance of psychiatric experts. However, this is changing, as we discuss in depth in the final chapter of this book. One major shift about this became evident in the work of poststructuralists (e.g. Rose 1986; 1990). Although this had mental health experts as a central focus (the 'psy complex'), it did demonstrate, under the prompt of Foucault, the diffused and widespread influence of 'the confessional' and other personalizing discourses in everyday life.

Outside of post-structuralist frameworks we find a more pluralistic sociological interest in ordinary emotions (Elias 1978; Hochschild 1983; Freund 1988; James 1989; Giddens 1992; Beck and Beck-Gersheim 1995; Bendalow and Williams 1998). This range itself may reflect an aspect of post-modernity. Diverse commentaries on personal life are becoming increasingly legitimate and demanded with resonances of psychoanalytical ideas about ordinary emotional life and those which bridge psychoanalysis and social constructionism (Craib 1998; Lupton 1998).

Within this shift in social science, there has developed an interest in the ways in which society has followed the trend of the fast-food chain McDonald's in a whole range of cultural process (including sexual activity, health care 'delivery' and dying). This 'McDonaldization thesis' (Ritzer 1995; 1997) reflects a shift in society towards consumerism, which suggests that the emotions, like food, have become subject to both commercial prepackaging and increasing everyday interest to ordinary people.

Moreover, some commentators have argued that the USA is exporting its own version of psychiatric classification to the whole world, and with it forms of medicinal treatment specificity, exploiting new pharmaceutical markets in the developing world. This case is made by Watters in his *Crazy Like Us: The Globalization of the American Psyche* (Watters 2010). Moreover, this criticized tendency has been positively endorsed by some psychiatric reformers pushing for 'global mental health' (Collins *et al.* 2011). But that zeal has been criticized by some of their colleagues for its cultural imperialism as being insensitive to local and service user knowledge (Das and Rao, 2012), as well as having a flimsy evidence base (Summerfield 2008).

Discussion

The emphasis in this chapter has been on sociological ideas about the definition and shifting knowledge claims about what constitutes mental health and illness. Sociological analyses can also influence other disciplines at times in their revisions about the nature of mental health and illness. The weak validity of 'depression' as a biological notion has been challenged not only by sociological studies (e.g. Brown and Harris 1978) but by re-formulations based on observations in routine clinical practice. The need to transcend current classifications has become a mainstream controversy for clinicians, with the observation that categories such as 'depression' and 'anxiety' in population groups do not have distinct features (Das-Munshi *et al.* 2008). These observations in clinical practice confirm conceptual critiques offered by critical realists (e.g. Pilgrim and Bentall 1999). It is clear now that there is little evidence to support 'depression' as a discrete biological entity. Clinical research about the 'management of depression' suggests that there is a major overlap in practice with a wide range of 'unexplained symptoms', and there is a recurring conflation of social difficulties and the individual experience of distress experienced by patients (Chew-Graham *et al.* 2008).

The practical challenges for clinicians are not the analytical and empirical challenges for sociologists. The former have to personally engage and 'manage' people with mental health problems. Nonetheless, in working out how best to do this, sociological concepts inform these formulations and the formulations that are suggested in turn feed into sociological ideas. This is evident in the analyses put forward by Dowrick (2004) and Gask *et al.* (2000) when examining the personal and social circumstances of miserable patients. In response to this extensive conceptual doubt, the lack identified by medical researchers is not better medical diagnostic categories but rather a lack of an adequate theory of self. Dowrick (2009) suggests that what is required in practice is the generation of a new set of metaphors to guide practice 'which are dynamic and temporal offering possibilities of hope, action and purpose'. What is clearly evident is that in response to the philosophical debates about the conceptual underpinnings of what constitutes mental health and illness a number of theoretical frameworks underpin approaches to psychiatry and mental health work more generally. We return to these in Chapter 7, on professions.

This chapter has rehearsed and summarized a set of perspectives about mental health and illness both inside and outside of sociology. The existence of such a wide range of viewpoints highlights that the field of mental health and illness is highly contested. As a result, any discussion of the topic cannot take anything for granted – one's own assumptions, and those of others, need to be checked at the outset and at each stage of a dialogue or analysis thereafter.

Questions

1 What are the strengths and weaknesses of psychological perspectives on mental illness?
2 Compare and contrast two approaches to mental health and illness within sociology.
3 Discuss the relevance of the Frankfurt School to contemporary discussions about mental health.
4 Compare and contrast social constructivism with social realism when conducting sociological studies of mental health and illness.
5 Discuss recent developments in the sociology of the emotions.
6 How have sociology and psychiatry dealt with the mind/body dualism?

For discussion

Consider your own views about mental health and illness. How do they relate to the range of perspectives offered in this chapter?

2   Social stratification and mental health

Chapter overview

Whether we use the term 'social class' or 'socio-economic status', there is no dispute that differentials of wealth, power and status are considered to be of recurring importance for sociologists. The study of mental health accords with this trend. Arguably the relationship between social class and mental health is the most consistent one to be demonstrated in sociological research. This chapter will explore various aspects of that consistent relationship. It will cover:

- the general relationship between social class and health status;
- the relationship between social class and diagnosed mental illness;
- social capital and mental health;
- the relationship between poverty and mental health status;
- social class and mental health professionalism;
- lay views about mental health and social class.

The general relationship between social class and health status

Establishing the relationship between social and economic conditions and poor mental health has been a dominant trend in social psychiatry and sociology. As we discussed in the last chapter, a close association between sociology and medicine is traceable to nineteenth-century social medicine (Kleinman 1986). Historically it went on to form the bases of joint projects between the two disciplines. One of the earliest studies in psychiatric epidemiology, which sought to establish a link between schizophrenia and social class (Faris and Dunham 1939), was associated with the development of 'human ecology', a theoretical trend within the Chicago School of Sociology (Park 1936). Since then some sociologists have continued to collaborate with psychiatrists in ways in which a link between social conditions and milieu has been made.

This focus also appears in the developing area of the 'sociology of emotions' and the links being made between the unconscious dimensions of human experience and identity in post-modern societies (discussed at the end of Chapter 1). Mental health is part of a wider topic (health) and so first we will examine this wider relationship between social class and ill health.

In Chapter 1 we noted the social causation position in medical sociology. The empirical case for this position is at its strongest in relation to the correlations that have been established between social class and ill health. Link and Phelan (1995: 81) summarized work in medical sociology that has supported the social causation of disease by noting that:

> Lower SES [socio-economic status] is associated with lower life expectancy, higher overall mortality rates and higher rates of infant and perinatal mortality. Moreover, low SES is associated with each of the 14 major cause-of-death categories in the International Classification of Diseases as well as many other health outcomes including major mental disorders.

However, the authors go on to note that the social causation case is not limited to considerations of class and other social variables are implicated, such as life stage.

The life-course perspective on social class and mental health

The relevance of a life-course perspective in understanding the determinants of inequalities in mental and physical health is succinctly put by Bartley and her colleagues (1998: 573):

> The more data we have which show how early circumstances contribute to health in later life, the clearer it becomes that 'social class' at any given point is but a very partial indicator of a whole sequence, a 'probabilistic cascade' of events which need to be seen in combination if the effects of social environment on health are to be understood. Different individuals have arrived at any particular level of income, occupational advantage or prestige which have different life histories behind them. Variables such as height, education and ownership of additional consumer goods act as indicators of these past histories.

Health indicators comparing community samples over time consistently show a class gradient on a number of indicators throughout the life-span. For example, individuals who are considered to be more physically attractive at age of 15 have higher social mobility by the age of 36 than those considered less attractive (Benzeval *et al.* 2013). This life-span approach is able to suggest factors that are influential at different points or over periods of time in relation to mental health. From the analysis of a Scottish longitudinal survey we find that increased levels of psychological distress occurring over 10 years among young women is linked to elevated levels of stress as a result of increased, educational expectations and the impact of concerns about personal identity (West and Sweeting 2004).

Understanding personal factors influential at one point in the life course, how they are shaped by class position and the interactive impact on emotional well-being reflects a range of aspects of the dynamic relationship between inequality and mental health. There is evidence that attachment style in childhood can affect the prospects of social mobility and mental health in later years. Family-specific attachment styles are part of parenting experienced in early childhood, which can act as a source of resilience or vulnerability in the face of adversity, and which can affect educational achievement and emerging self-confidence. Longitudinal research has suggested that the presence of secure and absence of an anxious or avoidant (trying not to get attached) attachment style acts as a form of protection (resilience), and enables middle-aged men to overcome the disadvantage of a lower level of educational attainment and career progression.

Traditionally, inequalities in both physical and mental health have been explained with reference to four main factors, which have their origins in the Black Report (DHSS 1980).

- *Artefact explanations* suggest that inequalities are an artefact of the way in which official statistics have been collated (Illsley 1986). By implication the artefact explanation attacks the assumption that health inequalities exist at all and that there is a causal relationship between social conditions and health. However, methods available for validating the existence of class inequalities, using longitudinal census data on health inequalities and linking these to death certification and cancer registration, have confirmed that health inequalities are not likely to be due to statistical bias (Bartley *et al.* 1998).
- *Selection explanations* suggest that long-term illness or 'health capital' in early life constrains social mobility and continued inequalities in illness in adulthood (Power *et al.* 1996). In other words health status determines socio-economic position (Illsley 1986) (as in the 'social drift' hypothesis discussed in more detail later).
- *Cultural/behavioural explanations* suggest that lifestyle and health-related behaviours (such as cigarette smoking, poor diet and lack of exercise among manual groups) lead to health inequalities.

- *Materialist explanations* emphasize the differential exposure to health threats inherent in society over which people have little control. This explanation suggests that a person's socio-economic position, and material deprivation in particular, leads to poorer health among people in lower social classes.

These explanations about health inequalities and ill health, and the extent to which one is favoured over another, are influenced by theoretical developments and research in the field (see below). However, to a degree they have also been influenced by the politicized context within which social and medical research has been undertaken. During the 1980s, ideological pressure, intended perhaps to gloss over the persistent and growing inequalities between rich and poor, found expression in a change of official terminology. There was also a seeming imbalance between work that prioritized cultural individual and artefact explanations, and work that focused on material deprivation (Davey Smith *et al.* 1990). During this period, the term 'inequalities' was replaced by the preferred official (Conservative) government term 'variations' in health. With an incoming health (Labour) administration in 1997, there was a reversal to the previous terminology, and a Green Paper with the aim of tackling inequalities and unmet need (Department of Health 1998). This point about terminology also reminds us of the vulnerability of only conducting debates about health within a framework of constructivism – there is a risk that these debates are only about what we call the world rather than about the reality of that world.

Over time there have been elaborations of this fourfold typology and the introduction of new variables and factors. The debates about the causes of inequalities in health and illness have moved beyond simplistic unitary explanations. They have incorporated more complex theories and concepts from mainstream sociology and the sub-discipline of the sociology of health and illness, as well as from other disciplines such as social epidemiology). The use of other indicators and proxies for social class (e.g. the use of housing tenure and car ownership), which have produced similar socio-economic gradients in health, has lessened the strength of the artefact explanation (Davey Smith *et al.* 1990). The importance of time, biography and longitudinal life-course research (Mheen *et al.* 1998; Shaw *et al.* 1998) and of 'place' (e.g. the types of spatial effects which may impact on health status (Macintyre *et al.* 1993; Curtis and Jones 1998)) may act to reinforce a focus on the inequalities in health status and health care operating within a locality.

Analyses which take an inter-sectorial approach draw on cultural and structural factors to gain more of an understanding of how stratification shapes mental health and captures more of the complexity described above. For example, the notion of 'triple jeopardy' points to the combined risks to mental health produced by multiple minority statuses, such as gender, race and class (Rosenfield 2012).

An understanding of mental health in society implicates the interaction of social structure and personal agency: it is a both/and not an either/or form of analysis. It requires notions of social capital, personal identity and the situated actions and decisions made by individuals, when exploring health inequalities in the structural context of a material gradient of wealth and power, associated with class membership. A lack of 'social capital' refers to 'features of social life-networks, norms and trust that enable participants to act together more effectively to pursue shared objectives' (Putnam, cited in Wilkinson 1996: 221) It implies that the quality of social relationships and, most importantly, our perceptions of where we are relative to others in the social structure, are likely to be important psycho-social mediators in the cause of inequalities in health (Wilkinson 1996).

Informed by this multi-factorial approach Nettleton and Burrows (1998) explored the experience of mortgage debt and insecure home ownership. They pointed to the way in which people's notion of home and home ownership are part of their sense of identity and aspirations, which provide a basis for what Laing (1959) called 'ontological security'. A threat to the latter may occur when, for example, mortgage arrears impact negatively on an individual's mental health.

As part of this transition in theorizing about health inequalities more generally, greater importance has been attributed to social-psychological factors as mediators in health inequalities (Williams 1998) and emotions have come to be seen as central to the relationship between social structure and health.

> the fact that socio-economic factors now primarily affect health through psycho-social rather than material pathways, places emotions centre-stage in the social patterning of disease and disorder in advanced Western societies. In this sense, emotions, as existentially embodied modes of being in the world and the *sine qua non* of causal reciprocity and exchange, provide the 'missing link' between 'personal troubles' and broader 'public issues' of social structure.
>
> (Williams 1998: 133)

One final point with regard to the broader research agenda relates to the changing notion of social class and how it should be measured. In Britain there has been a wide recognition that the conventional classification in operation during the late twentieth century now fails to reflect contemporary social divisions or class structure. Not only has occupational structure changed but subjective aspects of class identity were previously ignored. When questions are asked about social, cultural and economic capital together, it is clear that a new classificatory system is implied. This is suggested by the proposition of a seven-class model of social class, which more readily incorporates contemporary social influences on social divisions. It draws heavily on the post-Marxian sociology of Pierre Bourdieu, who describes in addition to economic resources two other important forms of capital: social capital refers to social networks and cultural capital refers to one's education, social skills and confidence and our accumulated cultural artefacts (such as books and art works). The proposed seven-class schema (Savage *et al.* 2013) consists of:

- *Elite:* the most privileged group in the UK, distinct from the other six classes through its wealth. This group has the highest combined levels of economic, social and cultural capital.
- *Established middle class:* the second wealthiest, scoring highly on all three forms of capital. The largest and most gregarious group, scoring second highest for cultural capital.
- *Technical middle class:* a small, distinctive new class group which is prosperous but scores low for social and cultural capital. It is distinguished by its social isolation and relative cultural apathy.
- *New affluent workers:* a young class group which is socially and culturally active, with a middle range of income.
- *Traditional working class:* scores low on all forms of capital, but is not completely deprived. When home owners, its members have reasonably high house values (this is the oldest group).
- *Emergent service workers:* a new, young, urban group which is relatively poor but has high social and cultural capital.
- *Precariat, or precarious proletariat:* the poorest, most deprived class, scoring low for social and cultural capital. This reflects but replaces the older Marxian notion of the 'lumpenproletariat'.

The status of having a mental health problem (usually considered to be a dependent rather independent variable) could also be seen to form a social class of its own. If we take the notion that class is a form of social stratification in which people are grouped into a set of hierarchical social categories then those with mental health problems, particularly those with a diagnosis of schizophrenia, can be accorded a particular shared status of being vulnerable to the vagaries of stigmatization by others in society and limited social opportunities (Pescosolido *et al.* 2013) and having a lower life expectancy from birth and poorer physical health than others (Chang *et al.* 2011). Another version of this proposal is that the social group of people with long-term mental health problems could be seen as a sub-class (of the 'precariat'). The latter may be more plausible because it does not reify dubious diagnostic groups (see Chapter 1) but simply recognizes that psychotic functioning, for example, brings with it particular forms of marginalization and oppression in societies dominated by concerns of rationality and economic efficiency.

The relationship between social class and diagnosed mental illness

Despite attempts to change sociological classification, class remains a predictable correlate of mental ill health, whether we adopt the new version noted above or default to older versions of social stratification. Basically, the poorer a person is the more likely they are to have a mental health problem. A class gradient is evident in mental health status across the bulk of the diagnostic groups but it is not a neat inverse relationship. For example, affective disorders are diagnosed fairly evenly in all social classes, whereas a very strong correlation exists between low social class and the diagnosis of schizophrenia.

Faris and Dunham (1939) studied the intake of patients to hospital from different parts of Chicago. They found higher rates of diagnosed schizophrenia, alcoholism and organic psychosis in those groups from poor areas. The greatest difference was in the diagnosis of schizophrenia (seven times the rate for people from poor inner city districts compared with middle-class suburban areas). The investigators concluded that the combination of poverty plus a lack of social cohesion in a locality precipitated schizophrenic breakdown. They argued that those vulnerable to breakdown are those who, for developmental reasons, became socially isolated during childhood. The stress of poverty and social disorganization then pushes these vulnerable individuals into psychosis. Faris (1944) then elaborated this 'social isolation' theory of schizophrenia.

After the Second World War, Dunham (1957) drew attention to several studies that confirmed the role of social isolation in the aetiology of schizophrenia; there were exceptions, though. Clausen and Kohn (1959) did not find the relationship between isolation and psychosis in the small city of Hagerstown, Maryland. Also, Weinberg (1960), studying the histories of patients with a diagnosis of schizophrenia, did not find a pattern of social isolation. Gerard and Houston (1953) found that divorced and single people who already had a diagnosis of schizophrenia moved to inner city areas. At this stage, the controversy over 'social drift' emerged. Its proponents argued that mentally ill people drift into poverty. Its opponents argued that poverty precipitates illness.

Lapouse et al. (1956) and Hollingshead and Redlich (1958) did not find in their surveys that people diagnosed as schizophrenic drifted into poor areas, but they confirmed the class gradient in the diagnosis of schizophrenia. Overall, the early epidemiological evidence strongly pointed to an over-representation of patients considered to have schizophrenia in lower-class samples (e.g. Tietze et al. 1941; Stein 1957; Goldberg and Morrison 1963). These patients were particularly over-represented at the bottom of the social scale (Dunham 1964). The question is, why does this class gradient exist?

Broadly, there have been two competing hypotheses about why mental illness is diagnosed more in poorer populations. The first is the 'drift' hypothesis and the other is the 'opportunity and stress' hypothesis. The 'drift' hypothesis, which suggests that illness incapacitates social competence, has two aspects. One has already been mentioned – that psychotic patients perhaps drift into poorer urban areas. The other is that patients drift down the social scale. Here the assumption is that patients from all classes above that of the lowest stratum (the unskilled and the unemployed) who become mentally ill cannot maintain their class position (because their impairments make them unable to compete with those who are not patients) and they sink to the bottom of society, in class terms.

The different causal explanations vary according to the type of mental health problem under investigation (Dohrenwend et al. 1992). However, there also appears to be compelling and competing evidence that causation is a more significant influence than selection, in relation to the diagnosis of schizophrenia, which is strongly affected by contextual factors operating in the urban environment (Krabbendam and van Os 2005). Thus when we think of the exogenous impact of the patient's environment, this includes the historical conditions of their family of origin and the current conditions of social stress.

Investigations to date have not resolved the drift versus stress debate. The clear evidence for the complexities of the intervening variables, together with analysis suggesting that *both* are implicated makes this an increasingly irrelevant or irresolvable debate. For example, family of origin is a key intervening variable which could mediate either genetic vulnerability (favouring the social selection thesis) or neglect and abuse (favouring the social causation thesis). And of course both might be operating in interaction in the families which eventually produce patients. Given the mixed evidence for both, there have been some attempts to integrate elements of each of them. For example, the mixed model of Kohn is assessed by Cochrane (1983). The hypothesis relating to stress and opportunities suggests that these differentially affect lower-class people compared with those from the middle and upper classes. The debate is kept alive because favouring one explanation against the other reflects ideological concerns about the nature/nurture implications for politics. For example, a nature focus favours eugenic and socially conservative arguments, whereas a nurture arguments favours those of psycho-social determinism or environmentalism.

Srole *et al.* (1962) and Langer and Michael (1963) in their large-scale community surveys of mental health in the USA found that lower-class people were more likely to have psychotic symptoms and middle-class people were more likely to have neurotic symptoms. They accounted for this difference in part by suggesting that middle-class children are over-inhibited compared with their lower-class equivalents; their sexual and aggressive impulses were considered to be more controlled. This was thought to lead to problems of anxiety and guilt appearing more often in non-lower-class groups. Also, the emphasis on self and identity was found to be a stronger preoccupation during upbringing in non-lower-class families. This may mean that a sense of identity is stronger in these groups. By contrast, identity strength may be lower, on average, in lower-class groups. People starting off in life lower down the social class ladder may be more readily vulnerable to the loss and fragmentation of their sense of self and thus may become psychotic.

These speculations about psychological differences in upbringing and their consequences (which resonate with our earlier discussion about life course and attachment styles) can be added to the strong evidence about the material differences between classes in terms of contingent stress and daily struggle. Poor people have to contend with the particular personal consequences of material deprivation. In their locality they must endure higher stress from crime, traffic and dirt, and their home conditions are more likely to be cramped. Their diet and physical health will tend to be inferior to those further up the class scale. They will be vulnerable to unemployment more often and the jobs they obtain will lack a sense of personal control. All these factors will contribute to lower levels of self-worth and esteem. Such patients are more likely to stay as inpatients for longer periods of time and thus become more severely disabled from re-entering society (Hardt and Feinhandler 1959).

The evidence from social psychiatric follow-ups of patients with diagnoses of schizophrenia shows that the more opportunities individuals have for employment the better their prognoses. Indeed, socio-economic conditions may be a better predictor of recovery than access to treatment; even optimal treatment (Ciompi 1984; Warner 1985; 2003). Also, the point about esteem or relative self-worth has been confirmed in studies looking at quality of life in different classes. While people in all classes have negative experiences, the proportion of these to positive experiences decreases with increasing class position. For instance, Phillips (1968) found no class differences in the reporting of negative experiences. There were, however, significant differences in the presence of positive experiences between high- and low-class respondents. The former were twice as likely as the latter to report feeling excited, proud or interested by an event during the last month than the latter. Phillips then concluded that lower-class people have fewer positive experiences to buffer themselves against life's stresses, which makes them more vulnerable to mental distress.

This is consistent with the findings of the longitudinal study of Myers (1975). It was found that, in all social classes, the greater the number of life events, both positive and negative, the greater the probability of psychiatric symptoms appearing. But non-lower-class people experienced a greater proportion of positive events and this led to them being buffered from symptom formation more often than lower-class people. So, while it can be demonstrated unequivocally that social stress is correlated with social class, the evidence is still not clear about its causal role in schizophrenia. The epidemiological evidence from social psychiatry seems to point strongly at the role of social stress in recovery and relapse, but this is not the same as deducing that social stressors actually cause schizophrenia. As we will see later (Chapter 5), the clear traumatic stress of sexual abuse raises the probability of most forms of psychiatric morbidity except for the diagnosis of schizophrenia. This role of stress in relapse, rather than aetiology, may account for the prevalence of schizophrenia being affected by social stress (but not for the incidence of first episodes) and may explain why lower-class patients recover less frequently.

In the case of depression and anxiety the relationship between current and past adversity seems fairly clear (both past and current adversity increase the chances of symptoms of 'common mental disorders'). However, despite this broad truism there remain methodological debates in this field of inquiry. Socio-economic inequality in depression is heterogeneous and varies according to the way psychiatric disorder is measured, the definition and measurement of socio-economic status, and contextual features, such as region and time (Lorant et al. 2003). There are other differentiations to note as well when we go beyond the general point about social adversity and symptoms. For example, Stansfeld et al. (2003) found that work is the main determinant of inequalities in depressive symptoms in men, and work and material disadvantage are equally important in explaining inequalities in depressive symptoms in women, while health behaviours are more important for explaining inequalities in physical functioning (such as cardiovascular disease).

Wiggins et al. (2004) examined the link between common psychiatric symptoms and work. They found a complex relationship of social class to anxiety and depression linked to changing employment status. They examined three different ways of describing social position: (i) income; (ii) social advantage and lifestyle; and (iii) social class. They found a relationship between mental health and social position, when the latter was combined with employment status. This relation itself varied according to a person's psychological health in recent times. They concluded that the relation between social position and minor psychiatric morbidity depended on whether or not a person was employed, unemployed or economically inactive. The relation was more evident in those with previously poorer psychological health. Among economically active men and women in good health, mental health varied little according to social class, status or income. There was a traditional social gradient in psychiatric symptoms in those in work. However, in the unemployed group, a reverse gradient was found: the impact of unemployment on symptoms was greater for those who were previously in a more advantaged social class position.

Social capital and mental health

In many epidemiological studies there has been a tendency to treat the socio-economic status of individuals as a proxy for the social contexts in which they live (and vice versa). For example, we assume that poor people only live in poor areas and in poor areas there are only poor people. However, this can lead to the 'ecological fallacy' – the mistake of assuming that there are no individual class differences within specified localities. This fallacy may be particularly evident in large cities, such as London, containing many socially 'mixed' areas. We explore the impact of place further in Chapter 6 but here we can note that where we live is one factor that determines the quality and extent of our immediate networks. Relationships are a good predictor of both the emergence and re-emergence of mental health problems (and inversely explain much of the time why people do not develop such problems). Significant others in our lives emerge first in our families and school during childhood and remain in various degrees later in adulthood, when friends, neighbours, work colleagues and others enlarge or displace those developments. We can think of these as social networks and a related favoured concept in sociology is that of social capital.

Social capital is a construct linking social ties with the broader social structure. These ties might be bonds between family members or links with others in a locality or extended community: neighbours, or those with a shared interest in an activity (Portes 1998). At an individual level 'cognitive social capital' describes the values, attitudes and beliefs that produce co-operative behaviour (Colletta and Cullen 2000). Other definitions emphasize structural- or institutional-level processes; for example, 'collective efficacy', 'trust', participation in voluntary organizations and social integration for mutual benefit (Lochner *et al.* 1999). There has been an increasing refinement of what we mean by 'social capital', as it is increasingly used as a measured social determinant of health. There have been distinctions made between 'structural social capital', which refers to social action or what people actually do (e.g. participation in aspects of civil society), and 'cognitive social capital', which refers to what people feel (e.g. the trust one has in other people; reciprocity between people) (Harpham 2008). In relation to mental health specifically, it is the latter that may be more important. For example, a low availability of cognitive social capital, measured by levels of trust, has been associated with depression (Fujiwara and Kawachi 2008).

Notwithstanding these finer grained distinctions, generating or regenerating social capital is assumed broadly to be good for mental health. Focusing on repairing the breakdown of trust networks and relationships in an area is assumed to help reverse the processes of social exclusion. Thus the notion of partnership is commonly advocated – at a structural level between agencies, and between social groups and social agencies. However, the obstacles to this communitarian vision of community healing are power discrepancies and barriers. Individuals within localities may not view community organizations or networks as representative of their interests or needs and therefore may be reluctant to engage in partnerships.

Equally, confidence in the benefits or outcomes of increased social capital is contested. The protective effect vis-à-vis mental health is not necessarily uniform across social groups, leading to counter-intuitive outcomes. For example, Kawachi and Berkman (2001) suggest that gender differences in support derived from social network participation may partly account for the *higher prevalence* of psychological distress among women compared to men. Social connections may paradoxically increase levels of symptoms among women with low resources, especially if such connections entail role strain associated with obligations to provide social support to others.

Probably the most important and recurrent criticism of social capital, as a focus for social reform strategy, is that it diverts attention from the need to reverse structural inequalities. Politicians can use it to claim the credit for social improvements, without any fiscal consequences for spending or political consequences for the ownership of the means of production. Indeed, the linkage of social capital to economic efficiency and its health benefits tempt the politician with the prospect of actual savings for the State. This emphasis on process reform rather than structural reform was a feature of New Labour policies after 1997. An indication that it reflected an adaptation of capitalism is that the political importance of social capital was also endorsed by the World Bank (Colletta and Cullen 2000). Muntaner *et al.* (2001: 214) suggest that social capital:

> presents itself as an alternative to materialist structural inequalities (class, gender and race) and invokes a romanticized view of communities without social conflict . . . social capital is used in public health as an alternative to both state-centred economic re-distribution and party politics, and represents a potential privatization of both economics and policies.

Moreover the causal role of social capital in supporting well-being and preventing mental illness may not be as great as its advocates suggest. Ziersch *et al.* (2005) found that socio-economic factors were of relatively greater importance in determining mental health than social capital variables. Higher-income level and educational achievement were related to better mental health, and mental health was found to be higher within older age groups.

Similarly, Browning and Cagney (2003) found that affluence is a precursor to residential stability and its associated mental health benefits. The class bias is also supported by Stafford *et al.* (2008), who found that the link between neighbourhood social capital and common mental disorders is only evident for those living in deprived circumstances. Bridging social capital (intimate contact among local friends) was found to be associated with *lower* reporting of symptoms, while bonding social capital (where people are attached to their local neighbourhood) was found to be associated with a *higher* reporting of symptoms. This raises the possibility that subjectively this attachment to place might constitute a form of entrapment (the latter being linked to symptom formation). Araya *et al.* (2006) found that the contextual feature of the social and built environment did not have an impact on measures of depression but that trust and social cohesion were correlated with better mental health scores. This suggests that while elements of social capital are likely to be important in protecting against mental health problems in policy terms, initiatives probably need to be targeted on very specific aspects of social capital and to keep centre stage the relationship between socio-economic disadvantage and mental health.

The metaphors and language associated with 'social capital' are also important to consider if they are favoured by sociologists. Cohen and Prusak (2001) claim that the language of 'social capital' denotes the reduction of relationships to their financial value: forms of investment, rather than ordinary human processes. Nonetheless, sociologists continue to use 'capital' in a fluid way, as a linguistic resource. For example, Bourdieu's work on 'habitus' emphasizes the role played by various forms of capital (economic, social, cultural and symbolic) in perpetuating social inequalities (Williams 1995; Bourdieu 1997). Above we noted the influence of Bourdieu in the recent revision of the classification of social class by British sociologists.

The relationship between poverty and mental health status

The discussion above seems to indicate that poverty should remain a strong causal focus in our understanding of mental health status. This focus allows us to explore the interaction between disempowerment and material deprivation. For example, if depressed groups are studied, black people are more severely depressed than their white counterparts with low socio-economic status (Biafora 1995). This could be accounted for by the double impact of oppression in this group (being poor and black).

Evidence of the link between poverty and mental health is evident in relation to other social groupings. A number of empirical examples demonstrate this point. A study in Scotland found that financially deprived young people were twice as likely to commit suicide as their peers in more affluent localities (McLoone 1996). Brown and Moran (1997) found that single mothers had poorer mental health than those with partners. They were also twice as likely to suffer financial hardship even though they were also twice as likely to be in some form of full-time employment. These vulnerable mothers were trapped in conditions of poverty and isolation. Reading and Reynolds (2001) found that anxiety about debt was the best predictor of depressive symptoms in poor families. There is consistent evidence that people facing hunger, debt and living in poor or overcrowded housing have very high levels of mental health problems (Drentea and Reynolds 2012). It is still overwhelmingly the case that, at an individual level, fewer material assets and economic inactivity are strongly associated with depression whatever the country-level income (Rai *et al.* 2013).

An analytical advantage of focusing on poverty, rather than social class *per se*, is that it helps us to clarify a contradiction about mental health service utilization. Generally, in health care there is an 'inverse care law' – that is, access to health care increases with increasing class status. However, the reverse appears to be the case in mental health care systems. While there are problems for disadvantaged groups accessing desirable interventions, such as some psychological therapies (Gask *et al.* 2012), psychiatric services, especially inpatient care, are dominated by patients from low-social-class backgrounds.

Superficially this might suggest that those with the greatest need are being responded to. That is, given that poor people are more likely to be diagnosed as mentally ill, services are responding to their need. However, there is a problem with this logic. While most health care interventions are voluntary and ameliorative in intent in their response to the needs of sick people, in psychiatric services, involuntary detention and treatment are never far away. A proportion of patients are being forcibly detained and treated by the use of therapeutic law, some are notionally voluntary but *de facto* detainees, and others are genuinely voluntary but exist in a service context where the threat of coercion is ever present (Rogers 1993).

In the light of these peculiar features about psychiatry, it might be more accurate to conceptualize mental health work, in part at least, as part of a wider state apparatus which controls the social problems associated with poverty (what has been increasingly called the 'underclass'). Once conceived in this way, it lowers our expectations that service contact should necessarily be about aiming for, or achieving, a gain in the mental health status of service recipients, given that the latent, and sometimes the explicit, function of psychiatry is that of successful coercive social control. The latter entails mental health services serving the interests of parties (such as relatives and strangers in the street) other than the patients they contain and treat.

Thus, poverty is an important focus for understanding the relationship between social class and mental health because it highlights the social control role of psychiatry in response to certain types of social crises and deviance. The social consequences of poverty become a dimension of understanding mental health in society. Poverty is also important in understanding the social antecedents of madness and psychological distress. These antecedents include interactions with other forms of oppression (such as racism, discussed above), the stress of poor living conditions and the impact of labour market disadvantage.

Relative deprivation has a greater impact on morbidity and GP consultation for stress-related conditions such as depression, anxiety and headache/migraine. For all these conditions, higher levels of self-reported morbidity and a greater probability of consulting the doctor are associated with a cluster of social disadvantages – living in rented accommodation, unemployment, younger age and lower educational status.

Labour market disadvantage and mental health

Reviews of the evidence on the impact of labour market disadvantage on mental health have found that unemployment has a predictable negative toll on both the unemployed individuals and their family members (Kasl *et al.* 1998). However, it is not a simple matter of unemployment being bad for a person's mental health and employment being good. Employment can bring with it stressors, as well as buffers, in relation to psychological well-being. Elsewhere (Rogers and Pilgrim 2003) we have explored this complexity, which can be summarized in the following points:

- Optimal mental health is correlated with secure, well-paid work, in which the worker has control over his or her tasks. While unemployed people have poorer mental health, those who are 'inadequately employed' (i.e. poorly paid, insecure and with unsatisfying tasks) have the poorest mental health (Dooley *et al.* 2000).
- This pattern of a hierarchy of mental health in relation to employment status (good work conditions being the best, poor work conditions being the worst and unemployment being in between) has been confirmed by longitudinal studies looking at changes of employment and their mental health impact (Kasl *et al.* 1998).
- Having a mental health problem is correlated with labour market disadvantage. For example, only one in four psychotic patients outside of their acute episodes are in employment

and they are three times more likely to be unemployed than physically disabled people (Sayce 2000).

- The direction of causality between these findings is not always easy to trace, For example, depressed patients may lack the motivation and confidence to work (their primary disability renders them unfit for work). At the same time, there is strong evidence that psychiatric patients who are fit to work face predictable discrimination from employers (Sayce 2000).

The link between labour disadvantage and mental health has gained considerable traction in official mental health policy, with some economists and psychologists arguing that increasing access to psychological therapies is cost-effective. The investment not only ameliorates distress at the individual level if successful but there is an aggregate economic impact; it reduces the costs associated with depression and anxiety caused by increased welfare benefits. Moreover, if the point in the economic cycle is one in which work is available then tax revenues accrue from a return to work of patients and increased productivity created by those previously incapacitated through anxiety or depression (Layard et al. 2006). However, as some have pointed out this sort of policy initiative preceded the global financial crisis of 2008. Moreover, it individualizes and medicalizes distress rather than exploring its intelligibility in its social context (Teghtsoonian 2009; Pilgrim and Carey 2010).

Housing and mental health

The second broad set of antecedent factors relates not to employment status but to accommodation. However, it is important to note that while these are discussed separately here from employment factors for convenience, they are co-present and additive in the lives of many poor people. The following main points can be made about the link between housing and mental health:

- Poor accommodation produces stress reactions in inhabitants (Hunt 1990; Hyndman 1990).
- Some researchers have argued that mental health problems lead to homelessness rather than the poverty on the streets being a stressor which provokes mental ill health (Bassuk et al. 1984). Others argue that the reverse is the case (Hamid 1991).
- Arguments about the direction of causality at times have been driven by professional interests to retain psychiatric beds. Snow et al. (1986) undertook ethnographic fieldwork to assess the mental health status of homeless people and found, using standard diagnostic criteria, that only 15 per cent of a population of 991 were considered to be mentally ill. This empirical picture can be contrasted with the catastrophic discourse about deinstitutionalization in those who lobbied to retain large-scale hospitalization of psychiatric patients which over-emphasized prevalence in homeless populations. For example, one British pressure group in the early 1990s in favour of retaining the mass segregation of patients (Concern) argued that 40–50 per cent of the homeless population was mentally ill and, moreover, that prison populations had grown in response to hospital closure (see Page and Powell 1991). The latter collection also contained articles emphasizing the need to retain the Victorian asylums and the highly dangerous nature of madness (Hollander 1991).
- While homeless people are no more likely to be psychotic than other poor people, they are more likely to suffer from reactive depression (Gory et al. 1990) and they do have high rates of substance misuse (Toro 1998). Indeed, substance misuse seems to be a good predictor of homeless status, whether or not an individual has a mental health problem (note the ambiguity here of 'substance misuse' itself being classified as a mental disorder under DSM and ICD). According to Teeson et al. (2000), in a cross-national review of the topic, 25–50 per cent of women and 50–75 per cent of men who are homeless also abuse substances.

- The small minority of homeless patients who are both psychotic and abuse substances represents a particularly vulnerable group. They are prone to both self-neglect and violence (Soyka 2000).
- Psychiatric epidemiology suggests that homeless populations have different 'symptom profiles' than other poor (housed) groups. Homeless people are more likely to abuse substances and fulfil criteria for anti-social personality disorder (North *et al.* 1997). Moreover, when homeless and housed psychotic patients are studied it is found that the former are more likely to have troubled social histories, including abuse and conduct disorders in childhood, criminal activity and substance misuse (Odell and Commander 2000).
- Homeless young people have higher levels of mental health problems than young people in stable accommodation. This highlights the experience of mental health problems often beginning in childhood with links to family breakdown, parental abuse and violence, and poor levels of educational achievement. Taking a symptom approach to identification and amelioration of mental health problems among homeless people may exacerbate rather than ameliorate mental health problems. Young homeless people do not associate positively with facilities labelled 'mental health services' (O'Reilly *et al.* 2009).

The economic crisis after 2008 pushed to the forefront the role played by the sudden collapse of the lending market on mortgage repayments and its impact on mental health. Indeed, housing market processes ('the sub-prime crisis') have now come to actually constitute the global crisis in popular discourse. This reminds us that the basic need for available shelter for all human beings is a precondition of their well-being.

Social class and mental health professionalism

A set of factors reinforce (rather than singularly create) class differences in mental health status. A number of studies have focused on the impact of the 'cultural gap' which can exist between clients and their treating mental health professionals (Horwitz 1983). The latter concept refers to more than class differences as it can implicate race and ethnicity as well as age, gender and sexuality. However, class is an important consideration when people with mental health problems engage with professional services. Poor patients are more likely to receive a diagnosis of schizophrenia than richer patients, who are more likely to receive a less stigmatizing neurotic label such as one of the affective disorders (depression, mania or manic-depression). Poorer patients are more likely to receive biological treatments than psychological treatments. Poorer patients are less likely to be referred for psychotherapy, are rejected more often on assessment by specialists and drop out of treatment earlier (Pilgrim 1997a). Poorer patients are more likely to be treated coercively than voluntarily.

Some of this picture could be accounted for by the simple issue of raised incidence of severe mental health problems in poor populations – in other words, the more severe mental illness profile of the latter warrants greater levels of coercion and biological treatments in mental health service responses. Sedgwick (1982) warned of the dangers inherent in social constructivist arguments in this regard. He commented that some critics of psychiatry wanted it both ways: on the one hand they argued that adverse material conditions cause severe mental illness (warranting more psychiatric services) and, on the other, they deconstructed, and thereby undermined, the legitimacy of diagnostic data demonstrating this causal relationship. They also complained of the social control role of psychiatric professionals.

However, as we noted in Chapter 1, constructivism and causationism can be reconciled. It is logically quite feasible that the material conditions of poverty raise the probability of mental distress in a population, and that professional interests are at play and, within this, the role and 'world views' of psychiatric professionals. This might include the class and cognitive interests of mental health professionals operating when they respond to low-class patients in contact with services, and formulate this distress in bio-medical terms or in the thinly veiled value judgements of psychological interpretations. For example, clinicians tend to interpret psychometric test responses from lower socio-economic groups as reflecting greater psychopathology than similar responses from middle-class clients. Also, growing conditions of poverty significantly affects how people perform on tests of abstract thinking, intelligence and academic achievement (Franks 1993).

Taken together, these processes point to both causal and constructed influences upon poor clients in service contact. However, the influence of knowledge about the impact of social class on the generation of mental health problems on professional socialization and subsequent management of patients is also evident. A study of GPs' perspectives showed that, rather than a diagnostic category, GPs working in deprived areas conceptualized depression as an everyday problem of practice. For patients living in socio-economically deprived environments, the problems associated with depression were seen to be insoluble, with the presentation of depression viewed as a common and normal response to life events or the environment within which people lived. This compared to GPs serving a less deprived population, who saw depression as a treatable illness and as rewarding work.

Poverty and other class-related phenomena remain neglected areas in the training of mental health professionals, with the latter not being exposed to the narratives of poverty, oppression and daily struggle which would sensitize them to the needs of their client group. Schnitzer (1996) suggests that mental health professionals typically question the responsibility, cognitive competence and moral sensitivity of poorer clients. This may reflect not just the secondary socialization (in their training) of mental health professionals but also their primary socialization (in their class of origin).

A number of commentators have pointed to the absence of notions of class and inequality in disciplinary knowledge which underpin mental health professionals' practice. For example, in mainstream psychiatry and psychology textbooks class, racial and gender inequalities receive little attention. Power inequalities are then marginalized and are seen as having little to do with psychiatric vulnerability or psychiatric management more generally (Horsfall 1997). Ussher (1994) points to the narrow focus of mainstream clinical psychology models, such as behavioural therapy and CBT, which ignore class at the level of both theory and practice.

Lay views about mental health and social class

While there has been a social psychiatric epidemiology which maps the relationship between social variations and mental health, the views of people within different classes about the topic of mental health and social class has, until recently, been a relatively neglected area. As we have outlined above there is an extensive literature which maps and puts forward explanations for differences between groups in the population in terms of mental health status. Traditionally, there has been little interest in how people themselves construed their distress and oppression. However, more recently, there has been a growing interest in the understanding of lay knowledge. One of the arguments for this greater concentration is to augment gaps in professional knowledge about how ordinary people understand their health.

Blaxter (1990) has explored the views that people have about inequalities in health in general. In relation to mental health, lay people tend to adopt a relative, rather than absolute, view of mental health and social causation (Rogers and Pilgrim 1997). People in all social classes tend to view money problems as a central feature of mental well-being – though those from more middle-class backgrounds identify it as being more of a problem for working-class families. Similarly, work stress and stress related to common life events, such as bereavement and birth, were considered by working-class respondents to affect people similarly, albeit in different ways.

Perceptions of lay knowledge about help-seeking are also important. The expectations of patients and prospective patients shape demand for, and use of, formal services. For example, in primary care settings lay people provide accounts of help-seeking about mental health problems which are different from those offered by GPs (Pilgrim *et al.* 1997). Professionals emphasize diagnostic categories (like depression) based upon a symptom approach to presenting problems. By contrast, patients themselves understand their problems within a unique biographical context situated in time and place. These attributions within a life story include factors such as poverty, employment and unemployment, domestic violence and life events (like birth and death in the family).

Blaxter (1997) found that social inequality in health is not a topic that is very prominent in lay presentations, particularly among those who are most likely to be exposed to disadvantaging environments. Blaxter notes the way in which accounts of social identity have the potential to be self-devaluing, through the act of explicitly labelling and acknowledging inequality and poverty. Resistance to talk of class, in her respondents, was displaced by accounts of individual, private experience. Class was discussed though in more impersonal discussions of health as a wider social or political phenomenon.

Blaxter's work lends qualified support to the 'individualization thesis': demonstrable objective inequalities in health are not reproduced subjectively by the actors they apply to, in the personal accounts given in qualitative research or in focus group discussions. Class identity and health are negotiated in lay talk as participants shift argumentatively back and forth between competing positions, and public and private realms, in the attempt to make sense of health and illness (Bolam *et al.* 2004).

Discussion

Some disease categories such as 'schizophrenia' have been subjected to persuasive critical deconstruction. For example, this diagnosis has been criticized for its lack of aetiological specificity, its lack of predictive validity and its lack of inter-rater reliability (Bentall *et al.* 1988). It is a 'disjunctive' diagnosis: that is, two patients called 'schizophrenic' may have no symptoms in common (Bannister 1968). Some historians of the concept (Boyle 1991) have even demonstrated that the symptom profiles recorded in the late nineteenth century – when Kraepelin and Bleuler constructed the disease entity, first called 'dementia praecox' and then 'schizophrenia' – bear little relationship to the first-rank symptoms that psychiatrists currently use in their diagnoses. In other words, the features of patients given the diagnosis of schizophrenia at its conceptual inception were not the same as those with the same label today.

These conceptual problems with 'schizophrenia' are raised in this chapter because the diagnosis has been at the heart of the case for a class gradient in mental health. If the concept of schizophrenia is discredited by the critiques outlined, does this undermine our confidence in social causationist claims from over 60 years of social psychiatric research? Also, we need to be aware, when examining the relationship between social class and mental health, that the concept has itself become increasingly problematized within sociology. With the decline in the centrality of Marxism within social theory and its replacement by a mixture of other currents including feminism and post-structuralism, social class appears less frequently in the literature or is problematized by non-Marxists when discussing social stratification and societal disadvantage. Reflecting this trend, in the first edition of this book in 1993 we provided only a section, not a whole chapter, on the topic. Parker *et al.* (1995: 46) in their social-constructivist critique of psychopathology raised an important point to consider about reducing class to an individualized variable, which can exclude a discussion of social processes. Moreover, sociological descriptions of social class divisions or groupings (poor/rich, employed/unemployed and so on) do not automatically connote inequality.

Turner (1986) pointed out that terms such as 'inequality' or 'oppression' require that empirically described social divisions are then understood within an ideological framework of value judgements. Conservative political values emphasize individual freedom rather than the minimization of social divisions. The notion of 'oppression' is more likely to be individualized within conservative ideology and not seen as a matter of social justice. (For this reason some conservative libertarians might champion the civil liberties of the mad who are constrained by the State.) The notion of 'exploitation' is obvious to the left-wing critic of capitalism but to its conservative supporters it is simply and laudably a matter of employers providing work for others. Earlier we also noted how conservative politicians previously showed a preference for the term 'health variation' rather than 'health inequality'.

These tensions highlight a problem as well for radical social constructivists. A critical realist paradigm would argue that there is an irreducible materiality to poverty, which is not open to semantic manipulation or various constructions, a point made well by Pilger (1989). Pilger highlights the thrust of his argument about poverty by citing the humorist Jules Feiffer thus:

> I used to think that I was poor. Then they told me that I wasn't poor, I was needy. Then they told me it was self-defeating to think of myself as needy. I was deprived. Then they told me deprived was a bad image. I was underprivileged. Then they told me under-privileged was over used. I was disadvantaged. I still don't have a cent but I have a great vocabulary.
>
> (Feiffer, cited in Pilger 1989: 313)

This humorous point is used here seriously to indicate that arguments about the relationship between concepts (or 'constructions') and reality need to be understood in relation to both psychiatry and sociology. Psychiatry may well confuse the map with territory at times (with dubious diagnoses such as 'schizophrenia' or 'depression'). At the same time, lay people as well as professionals can consistently spot when their contemporary rules of social convention are broken and when others are mad or miserable (see Chapter 3). Similarly, Turner may be correct to argue that social divisions do not automatically connote inequality, but empty pockets and empty bellies are material realities.

Currently there is a split between one type of literature on inequalities in mental health status and another on the inequalities that service contact might perpetuate. However, as we have discussed earlier, there is evidence that service contact brings with it risks that can have a sustained negative impact on mental health or indeed be a path for exploring how to reverse inequalities. A better understanding of the relationship between service contact and its impact on quality of life and psychological distress would illuminate further our understanding of one aspect of the multifactorial interaction noted earlier.

Apart from the displacement of Marxism as the central discursive focus of class within sociology, societal changes have brought with them difficulties in thinking simply about the concept and formulating and conducting empirical projects. For example, the traditional use of the Registrar General's classifications system has become less and less meaningful. Women can no longer be conceptualized as sharing their husband's class status – not just because this is now ideologically rejected in the wake of feminism but because marriage has declined in popularity (so it fails to capture the range of forms of interdependent cohabitation). Also women, not men, numerically now dominate the labour market.

Moreover, the old pyramid notion of class structure has been found wanting because of its lack of attention to the relevance of cultural capital and other dimensions other than wealth which are central to contemporary stratification (Savage *et al.* 2013). Thus, the notion of oppression, which was previously associated mainly, or singularly, with low social class within Marxian sociology, has been linked to other social groups independent of their class position – women, black people, people with physical disabilities, people with learning difficulties, gay people, older people and, of particular relevance to this book, people with mental health problems.

Given the conceptual problems within both psychiatric epidemiology, discussed earlier, and the contested concept of class within sociology, we can make only very broad confident statements about social class and mental health. For example, it is safe to say that poverty contains causal influences which both create and exacerbate mental health problems. We cannot say definitively, however, that 'poverty causes schizophrenia'. We can say that being poorly employed or homeless increases the probability of mental health problem development, although we cannot, with certainty, say that this person has a mental health problem because they are poorly employed or homeless. We can say that the oppression and powerlessness, associated with low social class, disadvantage poor people during mental health service contact (they are more likely to have interventions imposed upon them and be treated with biological treatments than those in a higher class position), but we cannot say that these discriminatory service eventualities are only attributable to social class, because other variables, such as race or gender, might be alternative or coexisting determinants of professional action.

Additionally, evidence changes over time and the picture of class inequalities and mental health fluctuates. Greater awareness of social class differences on the part of professionals may act to change the pattern of class bias. For example, in contrast to earlier evidence, a more recent picture provided by Weich *et al.* (2007) suggested that there were few socio-economic differences in the allocation of therapies. This suggests the absence of an inverse care law as far as treatment in primary care is concerned. It maybe the greater awareness of social class differences in primary care (discussed above) means that in this health setting at least social class differences are diminishing over time.

However, notwithstanding the matter of access to therapy, the matter of material disadvantage remains salient. A tacit understanding of the material, psychological and social 'costs' of engagement by patients and health professionals still influence decisions to seek and offer help. These costs are proportionally higher in deprived, marginalized and minority communities, where individual resources are limited and the stigma attached to mental ill-health is higher (Lamb *et al.* 2012).

Questions

1   Does poverty cause schizophrenia?
2   Why are richer people mentally healthier than poorer people?
3   Discuss the relationship between housing and mental health problems.
4   Discuss lay views about mental health and social class.
5   Have changes in sociological interest in social class produced changes in sociological work on mental health and illness?
6   What are the strengths and weaknesses of the concept of 'social capital' in understanding mental health status?

For discussion

Think about people you know who have had mental health problems and discuss ways in which their social class background may have affected their lives.

3   Gender, sexuality and mental health

Chapter overview

Most of the discussion about mental health and gender has tended to focus on women. This chapter reflects this in both the sociological discourse and social psychiatric research reported. However, in addition, the question of men, mental health and psychiatry is addressed. The latter has emerged in recent sociological interest in masculinity. For example, a recent analysis of discourses on suicide has suggested a link with masculinity. In applying the concept of hegemonic masculinity Scourfield (2005) suggests that 'suicidal masculinities' result from men losing access to 'patriarchal privileges' and that important areas for understanding male suicide relate to honour, emotional literacy and control of others.

There are many areas in which gender and mental health intersect. For example, in the area of treatment response, sociologists have shown how gendered categories and responses reveal embodied relations of affect and social conditions that underlie responses to treatment (e.g. 'working on the emotional self'). These differ from the neurochemical narrative favoured by the traditional 'marketized' portrayal of drug response (Fullagar and O'Brien 2013). However, in this chapter we focus on a specific set of mental health topics:

- gender bias and representation of men and women in psychiatric diagnosis;
- the question of whether society causes excessive female mental illness;
- whether female over-representation in statistics about mental health is a measurement artefact;
- whether women are labelled as mentally ill more often than men;
- men, dangerousness and mental health services;
- masculinity and femininity;
- gender and sexuality.

The over-representation of women in psychiatric diagnosis

Although most academic attention about the topic of this chapter has focused on women and mental health, the study of gender is a comparative exercise in which the relationship of men and women to psychiatry requires exploration. Overall, women receive a psychiatric diagnosis more often than men. However, diagnosis is gendered as is the site in which it tends to take place. For example, in tertiary services, such as medium- and maximum-security hospitals, men, not women, are over-represented. In secondary services (acute psychiatric units in local general hospitals) gender differences are not significant. The bulk of the diagnostic practices leading to overall female representation are accounted for by 'common mental disorders'. The latter are mainly diagnosed and responded to in primary care settings. The majority of those diagnosed are not referred to specialist mental health services.

Turning from overall numbers to type of diagnosis, a gendered pattern is evident:

1   Some diagnoses are not gendered, such as those of schizophrenia and bi-polar disorder (Mitchell *et al.* 2004), though in the former case it is diagnosed on average 5 years earlier in young men (Gelder *et al.* 2001).

2   Some diagnoses are inevitably limited to women, such as post-natal depression and post-partum psychosis. Some of these referring to the emotional concomitants of

menstruation and the menopause are contentious and some groups of women reject medical labelling around menopause in its entirety (Edge and Rogers 2005).

3   Some diagnoses are overwhelmingly female, such as anorexia nervosa and bulimia nervosa (Van Hoecken *et al.* 1998).

4   Some diagnoses are overwhelmingly male, such as anti-social personality disorder (Tyrer 2000). The great majority of sex offenders (whether or not their conduct is classified as a psychiatric condition) are men.

5   Some diagnoses are more likely in men than women, such as substance misuse (Meltzer *et al.* 1994).

6   Some diagnoses are more likely in women than men, such as anxiety states, depression and post-traumatic stress disorder (Fryers *et al.* 2004). Because women live longer than men higher female prevalence rates for both dementia and depression in old age also make a contribution to female over-representation.

Thus, female patients in points 2 and 3, and especially 6, account for the overall over-representation of women in psychiatric statistics. The above list summarizes the picture in North America and Europe. However, there are substantial international differences, which highlight the problem of taking psychiatric positivism at face value. For example, eating disorders are virtually unknown in developing countries (where the main challenge regarding food is not its refusal but its availability). In another example, in China (contra the Western picture) women are diagnosed as suffering from mental illness more often than men but in a different way. The prevalence of depression and neurotic disorders is lower in Chinese than Western women. However, the prevalence of the diagnosis of schizophrenia is significantly higher for women than men in China, which might be accounted for by the cultural tendency in that country for women to be disvalued and coercively controlled (Pearson 1995).

In a Western context community surveys since the 1970s have consistently confirmed point 6 on the list above. For example, Walter Gove and his colleagues, focusing on higher rates among married women than men, claim that women experience psychological distress more than men (Gove and Tudor 1972). Blaxter (1990) also found that, throughout the life-span, women report greater psycho-social malaise than men, and the gap between the sexes increases in older people. Blaxter's self-reported factors included depression, worry, sleep disturbances and feelings of strain. A large international study using the World Health Organization (WHO) Composite International Diagnostic Interview assessed the lifetime prevalence and age at onset of mental health problems, including anxiety, mood and substance disorders. It found gendered differences in mental health in all countries. Women had more diagnoses of anxiety and mood disorders than men, and men had more 'externalizing' and substance disorders than women. However, the researchers also found a narrowing in recent cohorts of rates of diagnosed major depression and substance misuse (Seedat *et al.* 2009).

How, then, can this apparent excess of female over male 'mental illness' be explained? The reasons for the over-representation of women in mental health statistics are highly contested, with a number of competing explanations being evident in the literature. These explanations can be broadly categorized into three main perspectives:

- Social causation – does society cause excessive female mental illness?
- Artefact – is female over-representation a measurement artefact?
- Social labelling – are women labelled more often than men?

These three questions will now be explored.

Does society cause excessive female mental illness?

That mental illness is rooted in women's life experiences has been expounded by a number of commentators. Most of these explanations have focused on the link between the 'stress' of women's lives and mental disorder. Gove (1984) and his colleagues (Gove and Geerken 1977), who have written and researched extensively in the area of women's mental health, claim that the amount and particular type of stress experienced by women results in higher rates of female psychiatric morbidity. In particular, they look at two aspects of women's societal role to explain why women experience more psychological distress than men. First, the lack of structure in women's roles (which tend to be more domestic than for men) makes them more vulnerable to mental distress because they have time to 'brood' over their problems. In contrast, men have relatively 'fixed' roles. According to Gove, this means that the necessity of responding to the immediate and highly structured demands of the workplace distracts men from their personal problems and this offers a degree of protection that is not available to women.

Citing community studies, Gove points to evidence that poorer mental health is found in situations where women are more likely to occupy nurturant roles (e.g. divorced women who care for children have a higher incidence of mental distress than divorced men and women without children). It is hypothesized that the social demands and lack of privacy associated with this role may be a causal factor.

Evidence of social aetiology and depression among women comes from the research of Brown and Harris (1978), who identified different factors which together point to the social origins of depression. This picture of aetiology is sometimes referred to as a multi-factorial social model, where a wide selection of factors interacting with each other may be necessary preconditions for developing a psychiatric condition.

Brown and Harris (1978) draw attention to three groups of aetiological factors that need to be understood as interacting with one another to produce depression.

Vulnerability factors

Such factors might make women more susceptible to depression during a time of loss or in the face of another major negative life event. These biographical events include loss of mother before 11 years of age. Subsequent research linked this to the quality of care that followed this loss. Those with poor subsequent care were particularly vulnerable to depression (Brown *et al.* 1986). The absence of a confiding relationship with a partner also makes women more susceptible to depression, as does lack of employment (full- or part-time) outside of the home. The presence at home of three or more children is also a vulnerability factor. When the opposites of these factors were found to be present, for example high intimacy with a partner and the presence of a mother after the age of 11, they acted to 'protect' women against depression.

Provoking agents

These are factors operating in women's contemporary everyday lives that may lead to depression, and include detrimental 'life events', such as loss through bereavement or marriage breakdown, or episodes of serious illness. Chronic difficulties as well as specific stressors are included here. The occurrence of these events determines when the depression will arise.

Symptom-formation factors

These factors determine the severity and form of depression. In Brown and Harris's (1978) research, depression was found to be more severe if there had been previous depressive episodes and the woman was aged over 50. These social factors were linked together in Brown and Harris's research with psychological variables (cognitive sets). Women whose personalities were characterized by low self-esteem were more likely to experience the onset of depression than those who had high self-esteem.

The work of Brown and Harris in the 1970s has been extended in the interim. More data has been collected and, recently, more theoretical issues have been raised by Brown and his colleagues.

Brown *et al.* (1995) compared clinical and non-clinical populations in Islington, north London. Drawing upon the work of Gilbert (1992) and Unger (1984), they elaborate their position about depression and the experience of life events. They conclude that the probability of depression increases not necessarily with loss or threatened loss *per se* but with the coexistence of humiliation and/or entrapment.

Gilbert and Unger note that depression is commonly associated with feeling defeated, humiliated and entrapped. The latter may then make the difference between a depressive and a non-depressive trajectory. For example, Brown *et al.* (1995) suggest that a woman being told that the paralysed husband she is caring for will not recover might become depressed, but another, able to leave her violent or feckless partner, may feel liberated. Thus, being able to 'leave the field' may head off depression or reverse it in those already distressed.

The Islington study also highlighted more details about the risk factors associated with adverse childhood experiences. A third of the depressed women studied had experienced neglect or physical or sexual abuse in their childhoods. This subgroup had twice the chances of becoming depressed in one year, compared to those without such adverse antecedents (Bifulco *et al.* 1992). These childhood events also increase the probability of anxiety symptoms. Brown (1996) suggests that this might account for the common coexistence of anxiety and depression in adult patients.

Rigorous research, such as that of Brown and his colleagues, can tell us a great deal about the possible direct and indirect influence of social factors in the cause of female mental illness. However, the extent to which we can accept the conclusions of research that suggests that women experience more mental disorder than men rests on the way in which both mental health and gender are measured. The epidemiological work of this type rests on medical constructs (Brown and Harris accepted 'depression' and other diagnoses measured by the Present State Examination). Likewise, work on prevention of mental health problems, in the wake of Brown and Harris's study, does not question psychiatric knowledge (e.g. Newton 1988). This is not the case with the next and subsequent positions, which consider that psychiatric labelling is part of wider processes of social negotiation.

Gendered power relations, and constructions of masculinities and femininities during adolescence, are important for understanding social identity and processes that might be implicated in the generation of mental health problems. Negative and positive aspects of three social processes: social interactions, performance and responsibility appear to be highly gendered. Girls typically experience these processes more negatively, which arguably places them at greater risk of developing mental health problems. By contrast boys' greater positive mental health appears to be linked to a lower degree of responsibility-taking and the easier negotiation of cultural norms of masculinity (Landstedt *et al.* 2009).

Is female over-representation a measurement artefact?

The artefact explanation suggests that epidemiological measurement and its interpretation are faulty. From this point of view, some or all of the excess in psychiatric morbidity is not 'real', rather it is created by the design, assumptions and interpretations operating in social psychiatric research (using, for instance, the Present State Examination and the General Health Questionnaire).

As an example of a traditional causation study subjected to an artefact critique, we can take the work of Gove (1984) and his colleagues, which has been the centre of considerable debate. This research focused on female psychiatric morbidity and marital status and claimed to demonstrate that married women have greater levels of mental distress than married men.

Gove and his co-workers take marital status as an accurate indicator for identifying differences in mental health between men and women. However, there are variations in marital relationships and the ways in which particular features of the relationship, such as the degree of role differentiation and shared power, act as a risk or a protective factor. Marital status does not lead to a unitary role outcome for men and women. For example, the notion of nurturant role assumes the presence of children in the marital relationship, yet it is also the case that 25 per cent of children in the UK are now born outside of wedlock. Similarly, a childless woman in full-time employment may have little in common in terms of role with another woman, without employment outside of the home, who is also a mother.

The evidence of a link between gender and mental illness based on marital status may also be challenged if other comparisons are made. For example, single status makes men, not women, more vulnerable to mental health problems. With regards to the explanatory links of different stressors associated with role, Gove does not explore why the same marital female roles seem to act as protective factors in physical illnesses. While married women have higher rates of hospitalization for psychiatric illnesses, married men have higher rates of admission for non-psychiatric illness than married women.

Finally, the definition of mental illness used by Gove to support his hypothesis that women suffer from problems more than men has been subjected to the criticism that he focuses exclusively on certain types of mental disorder, such as depression and phobias. He excludes other types such as organic conditions and personality disorders (Dohrenwend and Dohrenwend 1977). A review of community studies carried out during the 1980s showed that although rates for the most common types of disorder are generally higher for women than men, rates reported by one epidemiological study (Regier *et al.* 1988) showed an almost equal sex ratio by including drug dependency and personality disorders. Similarly, in the Seedat *et al.* (2009) study mentioned above, the authors suggested that a narrowing of the gap over time in relation to key disorders might be explained with reference to the greater blurring of gender roles in wider society.

These critiques seem to point to the possibility that an apparent excess of female mental disorder may be an artefact of the construction of epidemiological research. However, subsequent research provides convincing evidence that undermines the artefact explanation and further supports the likelihood that women's greater risk of depression is a result of differences in roles and in their experience of life events. Nazroo *et al.* (1998) compared men's and women's experience of severe life events. Women were found to be at greater risk of depression than men when the event experienced involved children, housing and reproduction and where there was a clear distinction within households in roles between men and women. This suggests that women's increased risk of depression is a result of gendered role differences which are associated with differences in the type and experience of life events.

Similarly, in relation to marital violence, gender differences in rates of anxiety (which are higher among women) have been attributed to the nature and meaning of physical abuse experienced by women (Nazroo 1995). Female perpetrators of domestic violence are now nearly as common as males (Rogers and Pilgrim 2003) but on average the severity of violence is greater when women are victims. And the latter are more likely to present with post-traumatic symptoms following victimization. Research such as this, which focuses on the meaning and context of events, provides us with a deeper understanding of the relationship between key variables identified by traditional social psychiatric epidemiology.

A more nuanced look at the nature of roles and events at particular points in the life course also indicates the complex relationship with mental health problems and the limitations in generalizing about men, women and mental health. Some of the findings of research are counterintuitive, or context- or time-dependent. Some events one might think are stressful do not have an impact but others do. For example, contra the researchers' presumptions, unintended childlessness and unplanned births were *not* found to be associated with psychological distress for women (Maximova and Quesniel-Vallee 2009).

Other complexity can be found in the particular circumstances of distress. For example, between those caring for disabled children compared to parents of non-disabled children, parents of disabled children experience higher levels of negative emotions, poorer psychological well-being, and more somatic symptoms. However, mothers were not found to differ from fathers in levels of well-being, and older parents were significantly less likely to experience the negative effect of having a disabled child than younger parents (Ha *et al.* 2008). Also, multiple identities draw upon layers of vulnerability which are both individually and structurally shaped. Collins *et al.* (2008) suggest that inner-city Mexican women (living in New York) with severe mental health problems carry multiple stigmatized statuses, including having a mental health problem, being a member of an ethnic minority group, having an immigrant status, being poor and not conforming to gendered expectations. In examining the interlocking domains of women's lives, the researchers found that respondents sought identities that defined themselves in opposition to the stigmatizing label of 'loca' (Spanish for crazy; e.g. as religious church-goers).

When studies ask questions about male mental health in traditionally female areas, such as pregnancy, then the male percentage of those suffering high levels of psychological distress peri-natally are revealed. The same pattern emerges as with women in relation to the risk of emotional, behavioural and social problems in raising young children (Kvalevaag *et al.* 2013).

Specific contexts of adversity where hyper-masculinity is culturally evident (such as in farming communities) has been linked to raised levels of male suicidal action. The usual recourse to hegemonic masculinity in rural areas, serves men well in terms of power and privilege in times of plenty. But it has the reverse effect in contributing to stress in difficult times, such as drought, flooding, crop failure or market downturns. This effect may be compounded by the stoicism typical of rural masculinity, which inhibits help-seeking (Alston and Kent 2008). So it seems that a failure to investigate the nuances of mental health among men may go some way to explaining the disparities in the taken-for-granted assumption about mental health.

Gendered differences in help-seeking behaviour

Because women report higher levels of mental distress (as well as somatic morbidity), this may result in a greater utilization of general health care. However, the relationship is more complex than this statement suggests; utilization is not a direct result of greater pathology alone. Koopmans and Lamers (2007) found that there is not necessarily a direct relationship between experiencing symptoms and the decision to seek help. Symptoms are experienced more frequently than rates of medical consultation and admission to hospital suggest. Patterns and processes of help-seeking are influenced by people's experience of illness, the way in which services and professionals have responded to people in the past, and the levels of social support and alternative health care resources available to them in the community (Rogers *et al.* 1998).

In the case of psychological symptoms, it is likely that the 'clinical iceberg' is larger than is the case with physical illness, because of the stigma of mental illness, the perceived ineffectiveness of medical interventions and a greater tendency to deny symptoms. Scambler *et al.* (1981) interviewed 74 working-class women and found that only 1 in 74 subjects who suffered 'nervous depression' or irritability consulted their GP, compared with 1 in 9 for sore throats. There is also some evidence to suggest that people with psychological symptoms delay seeking formal help for a long time. Rogers *et al.* (1993) found that the time-lag between experiencing psychological symptoms and seeking professional help was more than 1 year for 20 per cent in their survey of 516 post-discharge psychiatric patients.

The relationship between experiencing symptoms and getting help is further complicated in psychological distress because of the high rates of formal referral by other people. Thus, a decision to seek formal help in the case of psychological distress is a complex process dependent on both the incipient patient's and others' notions of mental health problems and the translation of the experience of these problems (e.g. tiredness, hallucinations and so on) into a willingness to contact formal agencies.

Overall, women are more likely than men to access health care, when they face minor or moderate mental health problems. As with the incidence of mental health problems discussed above, help-seeking actions may reflect not only the cultural values and expectations associated with a specific gender but also those associated with specific social roles adopted by women and men. Reported rates of symptoms in community studies may not be due to a greater incidence of mental disorder as measured by 'clinical symptoms', but a reflection of women's greater propensity to be disclosing about their symptoms.

Self-reported morbidity is determined not only by the presence or absence of clinical symptoms but also by the perception and interpretation of symptoms by the person, together with their willingness to report illness in an interview situation. This entails a willingness to label/view problems in psychological terms and to seek help once a problem has been defined. Both these interlinked processes may be influenced by differences in attitudes, norms, values and expectations between men and women. Debating this issue in the 1970s, Dohrenwend and Dohrenwend (1977: 1338) commented that:

> Sex differences in the seeking of help correspond to attitudinal differences: women are more likely to admit distress . . . to define their problems in mental-health terms . . . and to have favourable attitudes towards psychiatric treatment.

Women, then, may be more likely to recognize and label mental illness than men or, put another way, men may be less likely to view their problems as psychiatric ones. There certainly appears to have been an assumption on the part of researchers that women are more likely to be able and willing to talk about their mental health than men. This may, in turn, account for the female focus of much of mental health research, which we will discuss later. An example of how researchers operated such an assumption is in the cited community survey of Brown and Harris (1978: 22), who are quite explicit that their choice of a female-only sample stemmed from a gender assumption:

> It also seemed likely that women, who are more often at home during the day, would be more willing to agree to see us for several hours . . . most of the women we approached were willing to talk to us at length about their lives and appeared to enjoy doing so.

Women may also be more likely to act on their mental health symptoms than men by seeking professional help. Women are approximately twice as likely as men to refer themselves for psychiatric treatment. Men, on the other hand, have been found more frequently to seek help on the advice of others. Community studies suggest that, for those considered to be suffering from severe psychological distress (measured by the General Health Questionnaire), sex ratios for primary health care consultations are almost identical. However, in terms of overall rates of consultation with a GP, women appear to consult more than men (Williams *et al.* 1986; Rickwood and Braithwaite 1994).

It seems unlikely that this higher propensity to seek help is due to women having more spare time to visit the doctor than men. Women who combine maternal, domestic and employment roles have less time on their hands than employed men or housewives, and housewives work longer hours than employed men. There is some evidence that being in a professional or employed working role is an important influence on the decision of women and men to seek or not to seek medical care for mental health problems. Holding the role of worker tends to foster the use of psychological services in women, especially in married women (Drapeau *et al.* 2009). However, Verbrugge and Wingard (1987) argued that women's roles, as part-time workers or housewives, may allow them greater flexibility (not time *per se*) to visit the doctor.

Because of gendered assumptions about caring, women also make contact with GPs when taking their children to be seen for minor ailments. There is also some evidence to suggest that women with young children may put their children's health needs before their own, which inhibits them entering the sick role (Brown and Harris 1978; Rogers *et al.* 1999). Additionally, it may be that higher rates of consultation are not due only, or mainly, to the active help-seeking actions of women. Women's own accounts of stress, anxiety and depression seem to suggest that women normalize the mental health problems they report (Walters 1993), which is not commensurate with problem recognition associated with help-seeking from formal services.

Moreover, a study of women's pathways to care in post-natal depression suggests that only one-third of women considered to be depressed by primary care professionals believed they were suffering from the condition. Over 80 per cent had not reported their symptoms to any health professional (Whitton et al. 1996). This suggests that contact with health services for other reasons, such as the seeking of health care for children, may allow for increased detection of problems which may contribute to seemingly higher consultation rates for female mental health problems.

Are women labelled as mentally ill more often than men?

A different explanation for female over-representation in mental health statistics is proposed by some feminist researchers, influenced both by labelling theory and constructivist frameworks. From this viewpoint, patriarchal authority, which seeks out and labels women as mad, is responsible for the over-representation. Women become vulnerable to being labelled mentally disordered, when they fail to conform to stereotypical gender roles as mothers, housewives and so on or if they are too submissive, too aggressive or hostile to men. During the 1970s, feminist writers began to argue that there is both a general cultural sexism that renders women vulnerable to psychiatric labelling, and a specific sexism from professionals. For example, Chesler (1972: 115) asserted: 'Women, by definition [sic], are viewed as psychiatrically impaired – whether they accept or reject the female role – simply because they are women'.

There was evidence at the time of Chesler's writing that these patriarchal assumptions were not confined to psychiatry but operated in other parts of health services. Barrett and Roberts (1978) found that male GPs construed their middle-aged female patients to be overly neurotic and requiring minor tranquillizers more than male patients. The doctors also often thought that the distressed women who worked would be better off resigning and they expressed a greater sympathy for male counterparts. Goldberg and Huxley (1980) also found that GPs were less likely to identify psychological problems in male patients. Milliren (1977) studied older patients and found that male GPs diagnosed women as suffering from anxiety symptoms more often than men. When the latter were diagnosed they were offered minor tranquillizers less often than women by the GPs.

Subsequently, Sheppard (1991) provided further evidence that GPs discriminate against women. Doctors were found to be more likely to refer women as candidates for compulsory admission than men. According to Sheppard, this reflects the sexist practices of GPs, because their decisions were not always confirmed. That is, many of the female referrals were not subsequently deemed suitable for compulsory admission by social workers, and social work is a predominantly female profession. This was considered by Sheppard to be evidence of women workers being able to counteract the sexist practices of the predominantly male group of GPs.

However, others found evidence of sexist stereotyping of female roles among social workers in relation to women with severe mental health problems (Davis et al. 1985). This suggests that having a predominantly female profession might still not eliminate sexist practices. Similarly, Chesler's theoretical position rests on the premise that the psychiatric profession is numerically dominated by men, but this is not true (Parkhouse 1991).

It is likely that sexism in psychiatry has its roots in, and can be transmitted in, the type of knowledge, diagnostic categories and practices followed by the profession as well, which can still be called 'patriarchal' even when used by women doctors. Another dimension of feminist analysis has drawn attention to the assumptions inherent in the ideology of psychiatry. Disordered behaviour is defined according to what is considered normal or 'ordered' mental health.

Research by Broverman *et al.* (1970) provided evidence of bias in the construction of notions of mental health and illness. This research showed that behaviour defined as 'male' was viewed by psychiatrists to be congruent with healthy behaviour, while behaviour defined as 'female' was not. Healthy women were in comparative terms considered to be more submissive, less independent and adventurous, more easily influenced, less aggressive, less competitive, more excitable in minor crises, seen as having their feelings more easily hurt, being more emotional, more narcissistic about their appearance and less objective than healthy men. Women were couched in primarily negative terms, with even images of healthy women perceived as less healthy than men. Fabrikant (1974) reported that male therapists rated 70 per cent of 'female' positive.

Those interested in gendered labelling emphasize that it is shaped by new technologies (not just psychiatric diagnosis *per se*). For example, the new selective serotonin re-uptake inhibitor (SSRI) antidepressants have played a role in expanding existing categories of mental ill-health among women. Metzl and Angell (2004) studied the impact of these new drugs on popular notions of women's depressive illness. What were previously seen as ordinary life events now had become categories, such as 'premenstrual dysphoric disorder'. The enlarged notion of gender-specific mental health problems was also found to be disseminated in the mass media. Examples of negative stereotyping can be found even in biographical forms of psychiatric knowledge, such as psychoanalysis. Masson's (1985; 1988a) historical investigations of psychoanalysis reveal psychotherapists disbelieving reports from female patients of incestuous assaults on them, and compounding their distress through new abuse during treatment.

Gendered notions of mental health and illness seem to be prevalent among lay people as well as mental health professionals. Jones and Cochrane (1981) found from responses to a series of scales made up of terms depicting opposite personal characteristic (e.g. 'outgoing' versus 'withdrawn', 'sensitive' versus 'insensitive') that respondents clearly differentiated in the adjectives they chose to describe the differences between mentally ill men and women. In contrast, the terms used to describe normal women and mentally ill women were similar.

So far, a picture has been presented of how others have sought to define mental illness in a feminized way. As well as professionals and lay people constructing problems in this manner, there are also indications that patients conceptualize their problems in a sex-specific way. Women may be more likely to identify marital stress as the source of their difficulties. By contrast, men tend to report work stress to be of relevance more than women. This suggests that relationships in the domestic arena seem to take on a greater meaning for women than men. Women are more likely to share their difficulties with others more readily than men and to choose their lay network of friends and neighbours as their first attempt to seek help (Rogers *et al.* 1993). There is some evidence to suggest that this willingness to disclose is reversed once contact has been made with professionals. A Dutch study (de Boer 1991) noted that problem formulation in therapeutic encounters is a product of the interaction of two different discourses – that of the therapist and that of the patient. Sex differences in 'problem formulation' were found in so far as men appeared to be more able to account for their problem in a therapeutic situation than women, who appeared to be more diffident. As a result, male influence on the definition and formulation of a problem at this stage may be greater than the influence of women.

A caution needs to be introduced about generalizing the willingness of women to disclose and seek voluntary primary care or outpatient contact compared to men. This picture seems to hold true for white patients in European and North American clinical settings. However, the literature on ethnic minority women suggests a tendency for them to under-utilize such voluntary service contact opportunities (Padgett *et al.* 1994). The latter US study found that black and Hispanic women had a lower probability of accessing outpatient services than white women from similar class backgrounds. Overall, if race and class differences are ignored, women use outpatient mental health services more than men (Rhodes and Goering 1994) but within the female picture are racialized subgroups which are treated differently. For example, when young black women do have service contact they are offered less psychological treatment than white women (Cuffe *et al.* 1995).

There has been a tendency to view the social causation and the labelling explanation as contradictory; in other words, the over-representation of women is caused by either women's social situation making them sick or the pathologizing of women by a male-dominated mental health service. However, to argue that the phenomena which have historically come to be constituted as mental illness have their roots in the difficulties of women's lives is not inconsistent with the view that the social nature and social consequences of defining a woman as mentally ill are implicated.

The effects of labelling secondary deviance – women and minor tranquillizers

We introduced the notions of primary and secondary deviance in Chapter 2 when discussing labelling theory. Whatever the reasons why and how women enter the sick role in a psychiatric sense, a consequence is that they are subjected to more frequent medical and professional attention than men. They also tend to seek help and are diagnosed more frequently than men when suffering from problems that are dealt with by GPs. It is here that a controversy arose over the way in which women's problems are viewed and treated. In particular, attention has been directed towards the prescription of minor tranquillizers because of their dependency-inducing properties. Women consume psychotropic drugs in far greater quantities than men (Olson and Pincus 1994a). This is despite evidence which suggests that women express a strong antipathy to using drugs to solve their problems (Gabe and Lipshitsz-Phillips 1982).

By 1980, the excess of the female rate of consumption was estimated as 2:1, with four-fifths of this consumption being attributed to minor tranquillizers and sedative hypnotics (both types of benzodiazepine) (Cooperstock 1978). Although the dangers of benzodiazepines were well known by 1980, by the end of that decade the prescription rate was still over two-thirds of that a decade earlier, despite both litigation/campaigning from addicted users and cautions from professional bodies such as the Royal College of Psychiatrists (Medawar 1992).

The prescription of minor tranquillizers and antidepressants can be seen as a medicalized response to personal troubles. From this vantage point the benefits of a medical response are to remove personal responsibility from the individual for their problems. For example, the guilt and unhappiness associated with depression can be dealt with simplistically if it is framed as an illness, which can be relieved by mood-altering drugs, rather than the responsibility of the individual's actions and their social circumstances.

However, from a different perspective, the prescription and use of such drugs can be viewed as a means of 'social control' because they transform social problems into medical ones. The social effects of treating personal problems by medical sedation were highlighted by Waldron (1977), who pointed out that the treatment of individual 'pathology' disguises its social causes and deflects attention from the need for political change to ameliorate the oppression of women.

Gabe and Thorogood (1986) found that women were most likely to find benzodiazepines to be a 'prop' in the absence of other means of support, such as paid work, adequate housing, leisure activities, and so on. This was particularly so in the case of middle-aged women, who were less likely than other women to have access to resources with which to manage their everyday lives. Women tended to express ambivalent views about taking minor tranquillizers: on the one hand, they expressed the view that they gave them 'peace of mind', and on the other, they emphasized the dangers and dependency-inducing aspects of taking these drugs.

Paradoxically, perhaps, in publicizing the dangers of addiction, women who have been prescribed such drugs have been subject to what labelling theorists refer to as 'deviance amplification'. The media, in taking up the problem of minor tranquillizer dependency, has tended to reinforce images of women as helpless, dependent and passive victims of addictive drugs (Bury and Gabe 1990). Not only did their original behaviour or primary deviance expose women more frequently to an addictive prescribed drug but the consequent addiction then became associated with their gender.

Does this additional labelling of women imply that they are subjected to medical control more frequently than men? Their greater contact with services and the minor tranquillizer problem being labelled as a 'women's problem' might imply that this is the case. Certainly feminist scholarship has been instrumental in gaining a wider recognition of the ways in which women have been oppressed by being labelled as mentally ill. This in turn has led to the setting up of alternative services for women. According to Scambler (1998), these women's services retained a collective notion and awareness of the social by providing group support aimed at re-socializing women to reject a subordinate position within domestic and social life. However, as Scambler points out, their being outside of state-provided services means that access to the voluntary women-only mental health services may be denied to those in most need.

As we noted in our introduction, generalized claims about the *overall* predominance of mental disorder being an essentially male or female phenomenon are risky. The nature and construction of mental health problems differ according to diagnostic category and cultural context. However, the discussion of male mental disorder is, compared with the feminist literature on women and mental health, rare. This corresponds to a more generalized tendency in the sociology of health and illness to focus on female rather than male health disadvantage (Cameron and Bernardes 1998).

Men, distress dangerousness and mental health services

Men's behaviour is more frequently recognized as being dangerous than women's. It seems that being the recipient of intimate partner violence, sexual violence and peer/school violence has a much larger psychological impact on women than men (Romito and Grassi 2007). Thus men who are victims of violence speak from that experience less than women. However, overall it is not in doubt that men are violent more often than women in society. As a consequence, though, all men (including non-violent ones) may be subjected to stereotypical expectations, just as all women are at risk of being stereotyped as weak and ill, all men may be stereotyped as being violent.

Comparisons are sometimes made between the statistics, which show women to be over-represented in mental health populations and men in prison populations. This may be related to the type of social judgement made about 'rule breaking'. The recognition both of mental disorder and of criminality involve judgements being made about a person's state of mind and their conduct. In conditions such as depression, the judgement being made is more about a person's anguished and irrational state of mind, judged by their social withdrawal and 'motor retardation'. By contrast, a criminal act is more about a person's self-interested motivation, judged by the manifest gain made from their offence. However, both entail judgements about the relationship between mind and conduct – and weighing up the nature of this relationship decides whether the deviance ascribed is of a criminal or psychiatric type. As we noted in Chapter 2, these distinctions between rational or goal-directed, and irrational or incomprehensible, rule breaking are not always clear cut in the minds of either professionals or of lay people.

The connection between these considerations and gender is that men's conduct has been more associated with public antisocial acts, violent and sexual offences, drunken aggressive behaviour and so on. In contrast, women's behaviour has been associated more with private, self-damaging acts, where aggression is directed at the self rather than others; depression, parasuicide, eating disorders and self-mutilation together summarize this tendency. Men are more likely to indulge in behaviour that is antisocial, and to be labelled as criminally deviant more than women. This is then reflected within psychiatry, in that men are more likely to have labels which refer to and incorporate the threat of their behaviour.

The notion of 'danger to others' is more frequently ascribed to male than female patients. The question of 'danger to self' is more complicated. Although women attempt suicide more frequently then men, the figures for actual suicide are consistently higher for men than women. However, a Finnish study of parasuicidal behaviour suggested that men make more gestures of suicide, as well as committing suicide more often (Ostamo and Lonnqvist 1992). Of course, suicidal and parasuicidal behaviours are ambiguous – they may be adjudged to be either self-injurious or antisocial or both. This may account for the prevalence being split between the two sexes and the contradictory findings about the ratio of such a split. Female problems are more likely to be dealt with at the 'soft' end of psychiatry since, as we have already seen, they tend to be labelled with the type of problem that is usually dealt with in primary health care settings. Although such management is by no means always benign, as demonstrated by the negative effects of the reliance on minor tranquillizers discussed earlier, it more rarely requires compulsory admission. By contrast, men are more likely to be dealt with at the 'harsh' end of psychiatry as mentally disordered offenders in secure facilities.

Thus, once a label has been affixed, overall as a group, men are dealt with more harshly than women. This is especially the case at the interface between psychiatry and the criminal justice system. It is mainly men who are over-represented in the most stigmatized and policed part of the mental health system, the 'special hospitals'. Though many in these institutions are there for sex offences and other violent crime, and their behaviour or threat to society might have warranted such a response, many have not been convicted of a criminal offence. The effect of such management can be seen not only in the negative media stereotypes portraying the inmates of such hospitals as 'animals' and 'monsters' but also in recurrent government inquiries into the mistreatment of special hospital patients. With regard to psychiatric referrals from the police, under section 136 of the Mental Health Act 1983 there is evidence to suggest that men are subject to arrest more frequently than women. Moreover, the police use handcuffs and detention cells more frequently for men than women (Rogers 1990). Even where the differences in the rate at which a diagnostic label is attached are not great, the negative consequences of a label may be greater for men than women. This can be seen in the case of schizophrenia in Western countries, where, overall, there is little difference in incidence between men and women. There are, however, wide differences between the sexes in the incidence of the illness at different ages. It has been estimated that the occurrence is twice as great for men aged 15–24 than for women of the same age. For women the peak age is between 25 and 34 (Warner 1985: 231). This may reflect career- and work-related stress upon men at this stage in their lives. Because men are diagnosed younger, when they are physically at their strongest, this may induce more coercive actions from professionals during an inpatient crisis.

The course of 'schizophrenia' is also, in some ways, more benign for women than men. Warner (1985: 142) reports that, historically, the proportion of patients discharged as recovered is consistently higher for women. Differences in prognosis have also been noted. In the WHO (1979) international study of schizophrenia, proportionally fewer women were in the worst outcome group at follow-up, and more were in the best outcome category. In industrialized countries women tend to have shorter episodes of schizophrenia.

If we look at other disease categories, then the male/female distinction drawn by feminist analysis above is only applicable to a Western social context. In other places, men do worse than women. For example, some cross-cultural studies of depression have shown a slightly higher proportion of men than women suffering from depression (Carstairs and Kapur 1976). While women take sick leave for minor psychiatric problems more often than men, the latter tend to be off work for longer periods (Hensing *et al.* 1996). These studies suggest that it is the *context* of people's experiences that influence the type and rate of mental distress, rather than anything intrinsic or constant about being a man or woman. In some contexts, work outside the home can be a threat to mental health, just as the domestic environment can.

Masculinity meets femininity

The specific examples we have just discussed point to the way in which mental health related social practices are also a means of expressing gender identity within everyday interactions. In this respect we can see how the construct of depression for example is inconsistent with a notion of hyper-masculinity that places an emphasis on being 'strong' and 'tough', for example. Thus men displaying signs and symptoms of depression (such as fatigue) may be ignored or treated less emphatically than women displaying similar behaviour. This in turn may feed into and re-enforce hegemonic masculinities which marginalize attitudes and mental health risks, which in turn may affect treatment-seeking recommendations. Gender differences in what is termed 'mental health literacy' illuminates the point. Swami (2012) found that when given vignettes of men and women reporting a set of symptoms and behaviours synonymous with depression respondents were more likely to indicate that the male vignette did not suffer from a disorder compared to the female vignette. The close link with masculine and feminine identity is flagged by the fact that male participants were *more* likely than women to indicate that the male representative in the vignette did not suffer from a mental health disorder. Correspondingly male respondents were very likely to rate the case of the female vignette as very much more distressing, problematic to treat and deserving of sympathy than they did in the case of the male vignette.

Gender and sexuality

Both gay men and lesbians present with more mental health problems than do heterosexuals and are more likely to abuse substances (King *et al.* 2003). Gay and bi-sexual men are four times more likely to commit suicide than their heterosexual equivalents (McAndrew and Warne 2004). This may reflect the stress created by homophobic reactions, and the discrimination and violence that ensues in hate crimes (Huebner *et al.* 2004). It may also reflect developmental challenges. Girls and boys growing up with an emerging realization about their homosexuality may struggle with a particular identity problem, over and above the general one when shifting from childhood to adulthood. In Britain the demonization of a gay identity in schools has sometimes been an explicit educational policy. This was evident with the introduction of Section 28 in the 1980s in the UK, which made it illegal for teachers to discuss homosexuality. A similar policy has recently been adopted in Russia.

Thus the ascription of a form of devalued sense of self or 'otherness' to young gay people can operate at both lay and 'official' levels. The rates of depression, anxiety and suicidal ideas among gay people compared to heterosexuals are not only higher but they vary significantly across place and country. Epidemiological data suggest that while there are high rates of poor mental health outcomes in the UK and large gay–heterosexual variations in the Netherlands, in Canada (Vermont and British Columbia) there are lower and improving rates of risk and outcomes. Such disparities in recorded mental health can be accounted for by local policy-making, mental health programme responses, and the ways in which sexual minorities are discussed and responded to in different localities (Lewis 2009).

The psychiatric response to homosexuality in one sense has differed from responses to other types of 'problem' behaviour. During the mid-twentieth century homosexuality was designated as problematic by psychiatrists (it was a form of mental disorder under DSM). During the nineteenth century its assumed biological determination led not to active physical intervention (as was the case with madness) but with a fatalism, which prompted little therapeutic interest (Bullough 1987). It was only when psychoanalytical and then behavioural therapeutic methods were introduced during the twentieth century that psychiatrists began to interfere with homosexuality and aspire to 'cure' the condition. At the end of the century, the gay liberation movement opposed and undermined this pathologization but did not eliminate it. The very optimism encouraged by these environmental/psychological theories of mental disorder prompted professionals to be more interventionist with homosexuals. Moreover, both male and female homosexuality were problematized by psychiatry because they were problematized more widely in Western society. As Al-Issa (1987: 155) noted: 'Deviation from gender role expectations is traditionally considered abnormal'.

Leaving aside psychiatry's response to homosexuality, have gay men and lesbians been treated equitably? Certainly differences in society are discernible. Since the nineteenth century, male not female homosexuality has been designated as criminal. In Great Britain it is no longer criminal, but until 2001 when the age of homosexual consent was reduced to 16 it had a higher age of consent than heterosexuality (21 not 16 years). Once more, as with dangerousness, differential legal and cultural assumptions about homosexuality seem to associate maleness and antisocial behaviour. This is also reflected in the therapeutic discourse on homosexuality. While most therapeutic schools have clinical reports, and even research on treatment outcomes, for both gay men and lesbians, male problems are alluded to more frequently or given a greater priority.

This prioritization of men as 'suitable cases for treatment' was at its most exaggerated in the late 1960s and early 1970s, when behaviour therapists attempted to 'cure' male homosexuals using electric shock aversion therapy. More benign behavioural methods were used for lesbian patients requesting reorientation (such as desensitization and assertiveness training) but men were singled out for the aversion treatment. The latter failed to induce a shift of sexual orientation in gay men; it merely induced phobic anxiety and impotence in some of its recipients (Diamont 1987). However, subsequently, some psychiatrists still pursued a form of 'therapeutic optimism' about reorientating homosexual desire and identity (Spitzer 2003).

Another way in which homosexual men suffer especially restrictive or punitive attention from the mental health system relates to the point made earlier about secure environments. Because there are more men than women in secure psychiatric provision, this means that there are more gay men than lesbians living in closed systems. In such systems, homosexual behaviour is constrained by the lack of privacy permitted for sexual contact. Thus, advocates of women's rights in secure provision understandably complain of the plight of those lesbians who are incarcerated at the 'harsh' end of psychiatry (Stevenson 1992). However, it is logical to deduce that the infringement of homosexual rights must occur with a greater regularity for men than women, as the latter are under-represented in secure provision.

However, the more frequent constraints on male, rather than female, homosexual rights in secure provision need to be considered alongside the greater vulnerability of women, once they are in such environments. Those women who do find themselves in secure provision are more vulnerable than male patients to sexual harassment and assault, from both patients and staff. Such predatory attention from men is particularly relevant given the type of women appearing in conditions of maximum security. For instance, Potier (1992) reported that 34 out of the 40 female patients with a diagnosis of psychopathic disorder at Ashworth Special Hospital had been sexually abused in childhood or adolescence. Outside of secure services there is evidence that the mental health needs of gay people, which extend into mainstream health and social care, are marginalized or under-acknowledged due to discrimination (Addis et al. 2009).

There has been recent interest in mental health outcomes, which are linked to the daily lives of lesbian and gay couples. This moves the onus away from a focus on contact with mental health services to one of dealing with emotions and intimacy in everyday life. Within this research orientation, attention has been paid to the personal strategies which are adopted and enacted to maintain a sense of well-being during transitions to parenthood, which involve same-sex couples having to construct novel understandings of relatedness to establish new parental authority (Nordqvist 2012). As a pathway into parenthood, assisted conception, involving donor insemination, raises questions less prevalent but not absent in heterosexual couples about sex and sexuality.

Lesbian couples increasingly negotiate access to medicalized donor insemination. They also conceive in informal arrangements with donors, which involves intimate negotiations; these also raise particular dilemmas of intimacy, and this is potentially stressful for lesbian couples. The term 'sperm donation choreographies' has been used to refer to the personal strategies and resources that enable couples to negotiate the personal, private, sexual and intimate tensions surrounding sperm donations, and also takes into account the subjectivity of the sperm donor.

In relation to growing older, the influence on risk and protective factors of depression among lesbian, gay men and bi-sexual older adults has been investigated. Lifetime victimization and internalized stigma have been found to be a predictor of disability, depression and vulnerability in later life (Fredriksen-Goldsen *et al.* 2013).

Discussion

The concentration on women and mental disorder is a relatively new phenomenon, arising in the late twentieth century. Gove and Geerken (1977) found that of the 11 studies reviewed from before the Second World War, three showed higher rates of mental disorder for women, while eight showed higher rates for men. Following the Second World War, studies showed higher rates for women while none showed higher rates for men. Recent research also points to the volatility of this finding, which may be related to changing and overlapping roles between men and women, social identity and structural changes such as employment and the impact of legislative change.

How might these changes be accounted for? They may be a result of changes in women's social situation and psychiatric practices. A further possibility is that feminist scholarship itself may be a factor in constructing women and mental health as an object of study. Put another way, the shift towards identifying higher rates of mental disorder in women may be the result of a change in discourse. As the discourse changes, so too do the objects of attention.

Identifying women as an object of study, in itself, may accentuate the 'female character' of mental ill health, establishing it as an essentially women's problem. For example, the work of Brown and Harris is often cited in texts as evidence that depression is a female problem. From this it may be inferred that the same problems are not experienced by men. However, Brown and Harris did not set out to study men, who were excluded from the research design at the outset. Therefore, from this study we do not know anything about the nature of *male* depression. If research is directed at women, to the exclusion of men, it is likely to produce evidence that links depression to women's experiences and social roles. Also, in attempting to make women more visible, some feminist scholars may have made men relatively invisible.

Feminists make much of the social disadvantage under which women suffer. Indeed, socio-economic indicators do demonstrate unequivocally that, overall, women suffer greater material deprivation than men. Notwithstanding such evidence, it is clear that particular groups of men are also subject to social disadvantage. There may be substantial evidence that men make women mentally sick, by stressing and labelling them more often than women do men. However, the existence of a large number of men who are mentally disordered and particularly disadvantaged means that an exclusive focus on women and mental health precludes a full picture of the relationship between gender and psychiatry.

Having addressed the question of dangerousness and sexuality, we can now see why men are treated more harshly than women by psychiatry more often, though the small ratio of women at the secure end of psychiatric services may suffer individually more than men. Thus the focus on the over-representation of women in psychiatric statistics and the relative absence of men from the sociological discourse may gloss over important questions of gender, which are about *both* women *and* men. Women may be over-represented in psychiatric populations as a function of their longevity and greater primary care contact, but it is men who are exposed to the greater threat of State coercion and involuntary iatrogenesis.

Rather than focusing on men or women and psychiatry, comparative analyses of men and women along a range of dimensions, including treatment, behaviour and portrayal of images of abnormality, are needed. In addition to gender, other variables need to be taken into consideration in understanding the mental health of women and men. What is clear in understanding gender and mental disorder is the need to focus more on the context and meaning of the cause and experience of mental health problems.

As we have argued elsewhere, a close relationship with social psychiatry had created one form of sociological analysis, following Durkheim, of treating mental health problems as social facts. Useful as this may be at showing the social origins of mental health problems, an understanding of the relationship between agency and structure, when considering the gendered nature of mental health problems, is also required. Recognition of meaning and context is also relevant to responding to the differing needs of men and women using mental health services. We return to this issue in the chapter on treatment. As will be seen in the next two chapters, gender as a variable in mental health is overlain by age and race.

Gender and mental health have been considered extensively by sociologists. However, there has been an overwhelming focus on women. Paradoxically, this may have contributed to a discourse linking women and psychological vulnerability. It also runs the risk of understating those underlying social processes, which make some men particularly vulnerable to coercive psychiatric treatment. Despite the continuing interest in gender and mental health, there is still not a clear sociological account of why women are over-represented the way they are in psychiatric populations. This chapter has rehearsed some factors which can be seen as additive or competing in this regard.

Questions

1 Which factors might explain why women are over-represented in mental health statistics?
2 How are psychiatric diagnoses gendered?
3 Provide a socio-historical account of psychiatry's response to homosexuality.
4 What has the *Social Origins of Depression* (Brown and Harris 1978) taught us about gender and mental health?
5 Why do women take more psychiatric drugs than men?
6 Why might men be overlooked in sociological studies of mental health?

For discussion

Consider arguments for and against the notion that women are less mentally healthy than men.

4   Race and ethnicity

Chapter overview

This chapter will examine investigations into the relationship between mental ill-health, ethnicity and race. We will focus on the psychiatric response to black and ethnic minority (BME) groups in Britain but also draw on research undertaken elsewhere. The large-scale migration of people as a result of war, political persecution, famine, natural disasters and poverty has created a sociological interest into the post-traumatic impact and the adversity that stems from the experience of being a refugee or asylum seeker. Epidemiological studies undertaken in the 1960s and 1970s tended to draw out fairly 'rough and ready' differences about ethnic groups. A poverty of data, as much as theorizing, particularly about the way in which ethnicity was classified in the British national census, produced forms of analysis based upon crude distinctions.

The inadequate measurement of ethnicity, the lack of good data on socio-economic position, and life-course variables and the neglect of social disadvantage, particularly experiences of racism, meant a lack of rich detailed and contextualized investigations (Nazroo 2003). More recently, more informed epidemiological work has displaced some old assumptions (including ones available when writing the first edition of this book in the early 1990s). Now we are faced with a more complex picture in relation to the relative impact of racism and social exclusion, with socio-economic factors predominating in the latter.

The chapter will cover the following topics:

- theoretical presuppositions about race;
- race and health;
- the epidemiology of mental health, race and ethnicity;
- South Asian women and the somatization thesis;
- Migration and mental health

Theoretical presuppositions and approaches to race and ethnicity

In the past, many social scientists rejected the use of the concept of race because of its association with a dubious anthropological tradition left over from the nineteenth century. The latter used the concept of race to make biological distinctions between groups, and assumed white supremacy. This can be seen in relation to eugenics, the 'science' of racial improvement, which was a backdrop to the development of both anthropology and psychiatry at the turn of the twentieth century (Pilgrim 2008a).

In its most extreme form eugenics culminated in the mass extermination of 'racially inferior' groups in Nazi Germany, along with physically and mentally disabled people of any race (Meyer 1988). The sterilization of mental patients and the eventual killings were instigated by the German medical profession and endorsed by the Nazi Government. Thus, social policies influenced by eugenic principles have intertwined considerations of both race and mental illness. Medically supported initiatives about sexual segregation and sterilization for all disabled groups were also found in the rest of Europe and North America. Nazi social policy extended this general trend. It took the exclusion of purported eugenic threat to its ultimate conclusion (hence the notion of the 'final solution').

Fernando (1988) pointed out that there has also been a long and strong medical tradition which has operated on the basis that the brains of black people are inferior to those of white people. So, the link between race and mental illness has historically been a close one and medical–scientific knowledge has been far from neutral about the assumed relationship. It has played a significant role in the perpetuation of pejorative theories and oppressive practices about certain racial groups.

Some empirical studies find little support for notions of singular or primary identities, such as having a psychiatric diagnosis or being black. Instead they point to identities being multiple, complex and contingent (Ahmad *et al.* 2002). For example, Nazroo and Karlsen (2003) used survey data of ethnic minorities to identify five main dimensions along which people defined their ethnicity. Two of these related to self-descriptions. In addition people alluded to traditional identity, community participation and membership of a racialized group. Diversity exists about the balance of these multiple descriptions across and within ethnic minority populations in Britain.

Much of the debate about minority ethnic groups and health has centred on cultural difference as a way of explaining the differential experience of groups within the community (differences in language, values, norms and beliefs). This type of analysis focuses on the individual, or their culture, and is concerned mainly with examining the role of prejudice and discrimination in determining differences in health behaviour and the use of services.

Within these debates, 'prejudice' implies a psychological concept in that it refers to a set of personal attitudes. Transcultural or cross-cultural psychiatry, for example, is concerned with how different ethnic groups are treated by mental health workers socialized in the ways of the 'dominant' culture (Kleinman 1986). This position advocates initiatives aimed at challenging and changing prejudices through 'race awareness' training. This works on the premise of challenging the stereotypical and negative views about minority ethnic groups held by powerful individuals, including professionals.

Cross-cultural psychiatry began by focusing on the differing manifestations of mental disorders among diverse societies. More recently, it has broadened its focus as a means of incorporating social and cultural aspects of 'illness' into a clinical framework. This has meant that transcultural psychiatry focuses more than it did in the past on illness experience than on bio-medical notions of mental disorders viewed from the health practitioner's perspective. But what still tends to be missing from analyses based on prejudice is a consideration of the impact of inequality – how the latter is manifested in rates of psychiatric diagnosis, service contact and variable professional responses to black and other minority groups.

Race and health

Before we start our examination of race and mental ill-health, a more general note will be made about race and health. An account which respects multi-factorial causality extends beyond a focus on racism alone. A fuller account would need to take into consideration the following:

- *Genetics* Because of their eugenic associations social scientists may have a tendency to avoid genetic explanations. While most (75 per cent) of the genetic material of human beings is identical and most (85 per cent) of the genetic variation occurs between individuals not races, the latter do show some differences (about 7 per cent of variance). The upshot of this is that some racial groups are more genetically susceptible to certain disorders. For example, there are differential incidence rates of sickle cell disease and phenylketonuria in Africans and North Europeans.
- *Migration* This is a complex topic in itself. Migrants may encounter new health threats in their host country. Also the circumstances of migration may be traumatic both physically and psychologically (as in warfare). Alternatively, it may be linked to high expectations,

achieved or dashed, when a migrant wants to move in order to make a new life. Economic motives for migration may lead to racialized patterns of living in the host country, when people of the same origin move to the same area to work in the same employment context. Low-paid work in poor areas of inner cities, for example, may lead to health outcomes that affect not just the migrants but subsequent generations.

- *Material disadvantage* While migrants may enhance their wealth by moving, they may at the same time be relatively deprived within their host country. Low pay, housing disadvantage and unemployment make migrants susceptible to the direct health impact of poverty.
- *Cultural factors* Lifestyle, social networks and kinship differences from the host culture may lead to health losses and gains.
- *Racism* The health impact of racism is twofold. First, the direct effect is that racially victimized people are prone to stress, injury and death. Second, the indirect effect is that racial discrimination in the housing and labour markets produces lowered health outcomes.

A more specific anti-racist approach to studying aspects of health and illness, including mental health, has encouraged a greater consideration of discrimination, exclusion and the consequent socio-economic disadvantaged position of minority ethnic groups' experiences (Ahmad and Bradby 2007). We extend this point in the next section.

The epidemiology of mental health, race and ethnicity

A number of studies have compared the prevalence of 'common mental disorders' (i.e. diagnoses of neurotic symptom presentation) between ethnic groups. Compared to their white counterparts, African-Caribbean people have lower rates of diagnosed anxiety but higher rates of depression (Nazroo, 1997; Sproston and Nazroo 2002). This general finding also seems to hold true for gender-specific constructs, such as post-natal depression (Edge *et al.* 2004). However, as Nazroo and Iley (2011) note, there is a tension between this data from community studies of depression in African-Caribbean people and *treatment rates*. As far as the latter is concerned these are actually *lower* for depression than in white counterparts. One explanation for this relates to the lesser uptake of primary care services. Depression is typically diagnosed and treated in that service setting. We discuss types of service contact below.

In the past, low prevalence levels of anxiety were reported among Bangladeshi, Pakistani and Indian groups compared to their white British counterparts with a slightly different pattern for depression. Compared with the white British group, the rates of depression were similar in the Pakistanis and lower in the Indian and much lower in the Bangladeshi groups. Given that women have high prevalence rates of common mental disorders generally, the relative differences between white and South Asian groups are more marked for women than men.

These findings were consistent across a number of surveys. However, the confidence we might have in the pattern is affected by the nature of psychiatric epidemiology, which has traditionally been tied closely in to service utilization. This is because the profession has been committed to the validity of diagnosis and assumed need for service contact, rather than being interested in the prevalence of forms of distress and dysfunction in wider society (Rogers and Pilgrim 2003). By contrast, social epidemiology links the genesis of mental health problems with broader social and economic influences, which may differ. For example, job security for black rather than white men appears to be a more important factor in preventing 'depressive symptoms' (Zimmerman *et al.* 2004).

Since the early 1960s some very general trends in racialized service contact were identified. Cochrane (1983) analysed 1971 psychiatric admissions and found that rates for Irish, Polish and

Scottish immigrants to England and Wales were higher than for native-born people. Rates for those born in the Indian sub-continent were lower, while the rate for Caribbean immigrants was virtually the same as for the English-born. This contrasts with the findings of two other studies carried out in the 1970s and 1980s. Dean *et al.* (1981), examining first admissions to hospital in south-east England for 1976, found one and a half times the expected numbers for Caribbean-born people than for British-born people. Carpenter and Brockington (1980) recorded two and half times the rate of admission for Asian-born people and one and a half times the rate for African-Caribbean groups than for white British-born people.

Looking at the cumulative findings over a period of 30 years, there seems to have been more consistent evidence for the over-representation of African-Caribbean groups in admissions than Asian groups (Cochrane 1983; cf. Hemsi 1967; Rwegellera 1977; Carpenter and Brockington 1980; Koffman *et al.* 1997). Although Carpenter and Brockington found higher rates for Asians overall, Hitch (1981) found higher rates for Pakistani-born people and lower rates for people born in India than native-born.

Even many years after these original studies Tolmac and Hodes (2004) found that black adolescents were still over-represented in mental health services, especially if they were born outside of the UK and had refugee status. However, some earlier studies had indicated that British-born blacks were *more* over-represented than migrants. This may reflect a change in forms of data collection shaped by changes in migration patterns, which now include particular stressors associated with refugee status. By contrast, in the early 1990s the children of voluntary Caribbean migrants raised in Britain were studied. What is clearer are the rates of difference and cause of differences.

The elevation of incidence and prevalence rates of African-Caribbean people, in the treated populations of statutory services, is largely accounted for by them having higher rates of diagnosed psychosis (typically the diagnosis of 'schizophrenia'). This continuing pattern, according to studies since the mid-2000s, is evident not just in the UK but in other countries as well (Bresnahan *et al.* 2007; Cantor-Grae *et al.* 2005; Veling *et al.* 2006).

Thus, in this area of research, methodological factors may shape the conclusions we draw. More recent studies using different methodologies have shown smaller differences and attributed causes to social factors. While prevalence rates of psychotic symptoms are still higher, they are not consistent with the much higher first-contact rates for psychotic disorder reported previously, particularly in African-Caribbean people (i.e. twice the rate of reporting of psychotic symptoms) (King *et al.* 2005). More importantly, these increased rates are explained not by reference to cultural factors. Rather, the higher prevalence of psychotic-like experiences in Black Caribbean people is explained by high levels of social disadvantage over the life-span (Morgan *et al.* 2009).

For people from South Asian groups the picture has been much more variable over time. This relates to significant differences between different cultural groups in terms of place of origin, social and status differentials, at both a group and individual level. Research carried out in the 1970s tended to simplify or disregard the significant national, regional, cultural, religious, linguistic and political differences between the communities often studied under the umbrella term 'South Asian'. The latter implicitly presumed the existence of homogeneity. More recent research in the health and social science field pays greater attention to heterogeneous identities and concerns (Ahmad and Bradby 2005).

As well as providing a rather inconsistent picture, many of these studies, particularly the older ones, suffer from a further methodological weakness. Although in the past they told us something about the rates of admissions among people entering Britain, they tell us little about admissions for different racial and ethnic groups *within* Britain as a whole. When place of birth as an indicator of racial and ethnic origin is used, black people born in Britain are not counted with people entering the country from Africa and the Caribbean. There have been attempts to deal with this shortcoming by recording ethnicity independently of place of birth. McGovern and Cope (1987) using this method found that more African-Caribbeans than expected, as measured against numbers in the general population, enter the inpatient system.

A further methodological caution relates to accuracy of records. Hospital admission records are often incomplete and inaccurate. Consequently, they may be a poor indicator of the incidence and prevalence of mental disorder in the community. Hospital admission has traditionally been used as a measure of the incidence of mental illness among different racial and ethnic groups. However, this method may be misleading as admission is shaped in part by the supply side and demand-management policies. It is not only determined by community incidence. For example, a study conducted in the USA explored why there seemed to be higher admission levels in areas with higher concentrations of poverty and African-American residents. It found that the admission trends were more likely to result from changes in hospital management and funding affecting access to hospital services than the socio-demographic make-up of the local population (Almog *et al.* 2004).

A study carried out in Nottingham did not confine itself to hospital admissions (Harrison *et al.* 1988) but included all patients in contact with psychiatric services over a two-year period. The researchers estimated that the incidence rate of schizophrenia for African-Caribbean people was 12 to 13 times higher than that of the general population. In *community* studies of hallucinations, African-Caribbean people are found to experience them at around twice the rate of comparable white groups (King *et al.* 2005). However, only a quarter of the hallucinating black group fulfilled psychiatric criteria for a diagnosis of psychosis. Thus not only are there cultural differences in the reporting of hallucinations, these differences are not accounted for in most cases by a psychotic context (Johns *et al.* 2002).

In the psychiatric literature, two types of explanation predominate in attempting to explain the apparent over-representation of African-Caribbean people with a diagnosis of schizophrenia and the overall under-representation of Asian groups. The first tends to look for reasons at the level of 'cultural difference'. For example, it has been suggested that the relatively low number of admissions for Asian groups is an accurate reflection of low rates of distress because of psychological robustness or fatalistic attitudes to suffering. It has also been suggested that there may be a tendency to avoid service contact in the Asian community because of the stigma attached to psychiatric conditions or because of the inappropriateness of existing services, which results in low uptake. A particular controversy that surrounds the discussion of Asian mental health relates to the adequacy of Western psychiatric research to respect diverse meanings of distress (see later discussion on somatization).

The second type of explanation, in addition to this cultural consideration, suggests a vulnerability to distress related to an adverse environment – in other words, social deprivation and unfavourable conditions, such as poverty, racial harassment and discrimination over housing. However, since few studies have systematically investigated the impact of external stressors on the mental health of black people, the consequences of racism in employment, housing and education have not been assessed adequately. Also, if the stressors of racism are the main explanation for poor mental health, and both African-Caribbean and Asian people are affected by it, why is the former group over-represented in service contact but the latter is not? Compared to that carried out in North America, there has been little substantial British public health research on health and race to answer this question (Karlsen and Nazroo 2004). This is not to argue that white racism is absent from British society (it is clearly present). The argument here is that from the studies available there is not clear evidence that it has a powerful direct causal impact on mental health status. The data on Asian groups, with their lower rates of admission but high exposure more widely to racism makes this point strongly.

Black mental health groups themselves describe diverse forms of stress derived from racism, which affect their mental health. In one study, African-Caribbean users identified a variety of factors to explain their mental health problems. These included: problems of coping with adolescence and the education system, which builds up and then dashes expectations; growing up in a hostile environment with few positive images of black people; and parental and British white cultural input leading to confusion and conflict over identity (Frederick 1991). Another study has illuminated how Asian women tended to identify isolation and cultural differences as the root of their problems (Fenton and Sadiq 1991) while Asian men identified feelings of powerlessness as a result of unemployment or racism (Beliappa 1991).

Thus the groups involved place a construction upon the sources of their problems, which include views about both race and culture. However, aggregate comparative data leads to the confusing picture we need to re-emphasize. It would seem that a simple social stress hypothesis, with racism predominating as a causal variable, cannot be sufficient to account for the data available on psychiatric morbidity. After all, in poor inner city areas, Asian people as well as African-Caribbean people suffer recurrent racism. And yet, overall, the evidence seems to point to only the latter being over-represented in psychiatric records, not the former. This is not to argue that different racial and ethnic groups do not experience peculiar stressors, which lead to mental health problems emerging in *particular individuals*. But it would seem that such external stress is not a strong enough unitary explanation to account for the *aggregate* data on over-representation among African-Caribbeans (or the Irish, as we will see later).

Methodological cautions about findings

Community studies, as well as those that have examined admissions to hospital, have been criticized on methodological grounds, casting some doubt on the validity of their conclusions. Such criticisms include the unreliability and lack of conceptual validity of the diagnosis of schizophrenia, which means that data about ethnic groups is subject to a large margin of error (Sashidharan 1993). In the case of the Harrison study above, for example, critics have noted that:

> If one case was misclassified a 4 per cent change in incidence would be recorded. Likewise, if they [the researchers] had under-counted the number of people in the population deemed at risk by 200 the incidence recorded would be reduced by 40 per cent.
>
> (Francis *et al.* 1989: 161)

Fernando (1988) has also pointed out that because these studies tend to be suffused with cultural stereotypes, it is difficult to make accurate estimates about 'true rates' of mental illness among different groups. He cites the example of a study by Bebbington *et al.* (1981), which attempted to explain the lower levels of minor psychiatric disorders, such as depression among Caribbean-born people, by their tendency to respond to adversity with 'cheery denial'.

In the US context, Brown (2003) applies critical race theory to the social complexity surrounding race and mental health. He notes that this theory operates five main assumptions of relevance to this complexity.

1   Racial stratification is ubiquitous in white-dominated developed societies and is constantly reproduced in ordinary and sometimes extraordinary ways.
2   The privileges of the dominant group are protected by research claims of objectivity which obscure underlying racist processes.
3   Racial categories are invented not natural and are manipulated and reproduced for political and ideological ends.
4   Racially oppressed groups can account for these processes directly, if we listen to their lived accounts (an epistemological privilege should be extended to BME respondents).
5   Critical race theory is predicated primarily on the aim of social justice not claims of scientific disinterest (common in Western positivism).

When applied to mental health problems, Brown contends that these principles create advantages for researchers of race and mental health, because a consideration of social constructs and social causes together might explain the kind of complexity of findings we discuss in this chapter. The list also sensitizes researchers to the *particular experiences* of BME research subjects. Thus Brown is not arguing that social stressors are irrelevant and that racial differences are merely a matter of social construction. This is both/and not either/or reasoning; it is a version of social realism discussed in Chapter 1. One social process of particular importance in this framework is the differential way in which service contact is sought and impacts upon BME groups, which we consider now.

Type of service contact

In addition to explanations which focus on 'cultural' differences, or vulnerability to mental distress according to ethnicity, another explanation for over-representation lies with the way in which others involved with psychiatric practice respond to black people. This issue will be considered in relation to initial service contact and subsequent treatment.

African-Caribbean people are much more likely than white people to make contact with psychiatry via the police, courts and prison. These African-Caribbean patients are also more likely to be young and male (Bean *et al.* 1991). Young black men are much more likely to come into contact with forensic psychiatry than their white peers. During the 1980s, migrant and British-born second-generation black men were found to be referred 29 times more frequently than their white counterparts (Cope 1989). Also, the 'non-white' group had committed less serious offences prior to admission. Patients in forensic medium secure psychiatric units are significantly more likely to be of African and African-Caribbean origin (Thomas *et al.* 2009).

At each point of the processing of the criminal justice and mental health systems there appears to be a staged increase in discrimination. For example, Browne (1990) found that black defendants, deemed to be mentally vulnerable, were less likely than white defendants to be given bail and more likely to receive court orders involving compulsory psychiatric treatment. At the other end of the spectrum from coercive psychiatry, there is evidence to suggest that black people are under-represented in outpatient and self-referred services (Littlewood and Cross 1980) and are less likely than other groups to be referred by GPs (Hitch and Clegg 1980).

While psychiatric epidemiology has enumerated differences in sources of referral and rates of admission to hospital, it has provided fewer insights into why black people come into contact with specialist services in this way. Studies undertaken in the early 1980s identified a number of inter-related factors. They focused on factors that were viewed as characteristics of black people themselves. It was suggested that the culture of black people made them more susceptible to being identified by lay people and the police. The crux of this argument was that black people express their distress in a culturally idiosyncratic way (Littlewood and Lipsedge 1982). It has been suggested, for example, that the manifestation of 'mental illness' predisposes African-Caribbean people towards police arrest because they present in a particularly disturbed or violent way (Hitch and Clegg 1980; Harrison *et al.* 1988).

There is a relative low level of registration with primary care services on the part of African-Caribbean people who are subsequently admitted to hospital (Koffman *et al.* 1997) and lower rates of treatment for depression compared to other ethnic groups when they are in contact with these services (Nazroo 1997). The place where behaviour takes place may also be significant. According to Bean (1986) if a greater part of young African-Caribbean social life takes place in public, then deviant conduct is more likely to be detected and dealt with by agents of the State, such as the police and psychiatrists, than is the case of white people, who have more of an indoor culture. As was mentioned earlier, explanations which emphasize cultural difference have been criticized because they tend to make stereotypical generalizations about behaviour, which may be erroneous. They also incline towards identifying the problem as being situated in the person's own culture, thereby viewing it as pathological. One of the logical conclusions of this approach is that to avoid detection as being mentally ill, black people should adopt white ways of behaving, such as staying off the streets.

While a research focus on black culture runs the risk of contributing to a form of victim-blaming, a focus on the part played by other people in reacting to ethnic difference reframes the problem. It is not the conduct of black people in itself that is at issue but the way others react to it. Horwitz (1983) has noted that the tendency to label a person mentally ill increases with the cultural distance between the labeller and labelled. In other words, members of minority ethnic groups are more likely to be labelled mentally ill than dominant indigenous groups. This may lead to a pre-disposition on the part of white people in Britain to interpret black people's behaviour as signs of insanity and danger. One study found that lay people were more responsible for initiating police action than police officers themselves. African-Caribbean people were also found to be less frequently referred by their relatives or neighbours and more frequently by strangers and passers-by than other ethnic groups (Rogers 1990). Thus, perhaps the conduct of black people is interpreted in a more negative light by the lay (white) public than is white conduct.

The way in which black people's behaviour is viewed, together with the high number of black police referrals, has suggested a process of 'transmitted discrimination' (Reiner 1986). This entails the police acting as a conveyor belt or conduit for community prejudices about black people's behaviour constituting a threat to public law and order. This transmitted discrimination could then be compounded by other factors, such as a general conflictual relationship between young black men and the police and intensive policing strategies on inner-city housing estates with large numbers of black residents. These factors contribute to higher levels of police detention of all forms of deviance, including mental disorder.

The pathways by which black people come to the attention of mental health services have led some commentators to view psychiatry as part of a larger social control apparatus that regulates and oversees the lives of black people (Francis 1989). That black people, and in particular young black men, are also over-represented in all parts of the criminal justice system suggests indeed that both the 'criminalization' and the 'medicalization' of black people are closely connected processes. According to Francis, higher rates of entering the psychiatric system via the criminal justice system indicate a coalescence of the criminalization and medicalization of black people. He argues for a much wider definition of what constitutes the psychiatric system to be adopted, which views it as an extended network of scientific expertise and professional practice.

Admission to hospital and service use could serve the function of responding to mental health need, but this is a common but contestable psychiatric assumption (see earlier discussion). A complementary theoretical position to that provided by Francis has been suggested by Smaje (1996) and Nazroo (1998), when explaining ethnic inequalities in mental and physical health. Their analysis involves abandoning an emphasis on ahistorical and decontextualized genetic and cultural factors, which has found favour in previous epidemiological work, and replacing it with a structural approach, which considers the fine-grain aspects of disadvantage faced by black people in society. The latter includes the experience of racism, ethnic identity and the relevance of 'group affiliation and culture while acknowledging the contingent and contextual nature of ethnicity' (Nazroo 1998: 710).

Disproportionate coercion

During the 1980s, when only around 8 per cent of all admissions to hospital were compulsory, 20–30 per cent of African-Caribbean patients were detained involuntarily (Cope 1989). The rate was even higher for young Caribbean migrants. One study monitored detention rates over a 4-year period and found this group to be compulsorily admitted at 17 times the rate for compulsory admissions made from the community and, under admissions via the criminal justice system, 25 times more frequently (Cope 1989). This pattern was confirmed by studies in the 1990s, which found that black people were over-represented in admissions to psychiatric hospitals (Bhui *et al.* 2003). They were more likely to be admitted compulsorily and to be placed in locked wards (Koffman *et al.* 1997) and were more likely to have been in conflict with the police (Commander *et al.* 1999).

Black people have had a history of generally being treated in a more coercive way within the psychiatric system. Black patients have been over-represented in the statistics relating to locked wards, secure units and the Special Hospitals (Commander *et al.* 1999; Lelliott *et al.* 2001). They are more likely to receive physical treatments than whites. Two studies have indicated the over-use of ECT for Asian and African-Caribbean patients (Littlewood and Cross 1980; Shaikh 1985).

The study by Littlewood and Cross also found that black patients were more likely to receive major tranquillizers and intramuscular medication, and were more likely to be seen by junior medical staff. Chen, Harrison and Standen (1991) confirmed these findings, noting that while no differences between black and white patients in medication levels were evident at admission, over time the black group received higher levels and were more likely to be prescribed depot medication. Littlewood and Lipsedge (1982), found excessive Caribbean detention to be independent of diagnosis, while Bolton (1984) found that black patients identified by staff as uncooperative, but not aggressive, were much more likely to be transferred to locked wards than white patients.

Likewise, Noble and Rodger (1989), who reported a longitudinal record of violent incidents in the Bethlem Royal and Maudsley hospitals in London, found that in their control group of non-violent patients, 50 per cent of African-Caribbean patients in the sample were detained formally or on a locked ward, whereas only 15 per cent of non-violent whites were managed in the same way. Black patients were also recorded to be violent more often than white patients, raising the question (for us but not the investigators) about a 'spiral' of expectations, similar to that found in authoritarian penal regimes. That is, staff treat black people more coercively than they do whites and so black people react to a discriminatory regime in a more aggressive way. This then prompts staff to behave coercively more often to incidents involving black patients, and the spiral continues.

Despite the widespread evidence of continuing over-representation of black people in compulsory admissions and in coercive interventions, these findings have been slow to influence policy and strategies to ensure that services appropriately meet the needs of the culturally diverse population in this country (Morgan *et al.* 2004). Coercion experienced in the community prior to contact with services also impacts on help-seeking from services. In a study investigating ethnic differences in the relationships between partner violence victimization, psychiatric symptoms and the use of mental health services, a significant relationship was found between past coercion, violence and the use of mental health services. This suggests that coercion has a different impact on those from minority groups, which may influence their decision-making to seek out professional mental health services (Prospero and Kim 2009).

The shift towards taking into account users' views of services now has produced additional evidence that black patients experience their contact with services as being unsatisfactory and characterized by racism (Parkman *et al.* 1997; Secker and Harding 2002). This trend is also apparent in the USA. There, Diala *et al.* (2000) found that African-American patients prior to service contact had more positive views than whites. After contact this was reversed. Studies which take wider accounts of the black community's perception of psychiatric services confirm that early service contact is avoided because it is associated with racism and mistreatment (McLean *et al.* 2004).

Black people's conduct and attributions of madness – some summary points

While it is clear from the evidence summarized earlier that black people are over-represented in inpatient settings and are disproportionately coerced, how is this trend explained? Three explanations can be gleaned from the literature on the subject, some of which has been touched on earlier: black people are mentally ill more often than whites; black people may be mentally ill more often but they are given the wrong diagnosis; psychiatric theory and practice is part of wider racism in society. Let us now look at these three accounts in a little more detail.

Labelling merely reflects actual incidence of mental disorder

High rates of schizophrenia have been cited as an explanatory factor for the high rates of civil compulsory detention of psychotic black patients (Cope 1989). In other words, it is argued, black people become 'schizophrenic' more often than whites and therefore warrant more aggressive treatment in services. However, methodological uncertainties about the data on ethnic monitoring mentioned earlier, together with uncertainties over the diagnosis and aetiology of schizophrenia in general, and among black people in particular, cast doubt on this as an adequate explanation. The uncertainty over the aetiology of this disease category is indicated at the end of a study on the subject by Harrison *et al.* (1988) who identified a multiplicity of possibilities: potential biological differences in terms of genetic factors, neurochemistry, pre-natal and perinatal trauma, virology and immunology, as well as possible effects of living in decaying areas with high unemployment and poor housing.

Misdiagnosis

An alternative viewpoint is that admission rates for 'schizophrenia' and other psychoses do not necessarily reflect the incidence of these disorders in community populations. Instead, records may reflect biases in diagnostic practices. Fernando (1988) has suggested that it is the ethnocentric view of psychiatrists that has resulted in this misattribution of labels, such as 'schizophrenia', by imposing Western concepts with little regard for the cultures of non-Western people. According to Littlewood and Lipsedge (1982), terms such as 'schizophrenia' and 'cannabis psychosis' are used when black people display disturbed behaviour. Evidence for the difficulties that psychiatrists have in affixing appropriate labels is derived from the observation that many more black than white patients had their diagnosis changed over time.

The misdiagnosis hypothesis tends to leave unchallenged the fundamental assumption that high rates of psychopathology actually exist among black people. What is claimed instead is merely that the wrong label is being applied. For instance, from studying patients with 'religious delusions' Littlewood and Lipsedge suggest that patients with 'acute psychotic reactions' may be misdiagnosed as schizophrenic. This viewpoint does not challenge the validity of diagnostic categories themselves, or the scientific status of psychiatric knowledge or practices – it actually confirms their basic legitimacy. Transcultural psychiatry, of which the Littlewood and Lispsedge study is an example, has also been criticized on the grounds that it provides a simplistic notion of 'culture', which has been adopted by predominantly white psychiatrists about black client groups (Sashidharan 1986).

Fernando *et al.* (1998) argue that the misdiagnosis hypothesis needs to be accepted only as a partial account of the data on African-Caribbean over-representation. In their view, in addition to the misdiagnosis hypothesis, other concurrent explanatory factors need to be taken into account, which include institutional racism and the conceptual inadequacy of psychiatric knowledge in its totality. Within such a wider critique of psychiatric theory and practice lies an account of why psychiatry is unjust and unscientific, to an extent, not just about black patients but also about its whole client group.

Racialized psychiatric constructs reflect and reinforce wider racism

Earlier we noted that police referrals to psychiatry reflected 'transmitted racism'. This starts with lay judgements about the meaning and perceived threat of black conduct by white onlookers. The police are called and refer on to psychiatrists. Both the police and psychiatrists are embedded in the same societal context as the public. A number of commentators have noted the tendency of psychiatric constructs to be shaped by this context. From this perspective, the notion of psychiatry as a scientific discipline, which remains unaffected by social forces, is rejected. The way in which race and culture are inextricably bound up in the construction of disease categories is illustrated by a number of past and current examples. For example, 'drapetomania' was defined by an American psychiatrist, Cartwright, in 1851, as a disease which made slaves run away: 'The cause in the most of cases, that induces the Negro to run away from service, is as much a disease of the mind as any other species of mental alienation, and much more curable, as a general rule' (quoted in Ranger 1989: 354).

Fernando (1988) points out that the rise in racist categories is bound up with the institution of slavery and social control. Examples which have more relevance to contemporary psychiatry and the social control of black people are the constructs of 'cannabis psychosis' and 'schizophrenia'. Cannabis psychosis is a label which has been attached selectively to African-Caribbean people when British psychiatrists are perplexed by their behaviour (Ranger 1989). Psychosis is defined by the Royal College of Psychiatrists as a mental illness which 'cannot be understood as an exaggeration of ordinary expression'. As discussed in the previous chapter, on gender, the notion of 'ordinary' here is based on dominant groups in society in terms of numbers, status and power. Thus, in Britain, 'ordinary' implies having a white skin.

Others have pointed to the racist assumptions underlying the theoretical tradition of Kraepelin, the German psychiatrist responsible for the development of the category and classification of schizophrenia (which he dubbed 'dementia praecox'). Kraepelinian theorizing has dominated Western psychiatry since the 1970s and it points to a 'tainted' gene pool as a causal factor in schizophrenia. This pool is associated with other forms of disruptive and dangerous conduct. These suggestions neatly fit racist stereotypes held about black people (Francis 1989).

Certainly it is well documented that German eugenic medicine, which underpinned the Nazi programme of racial hygiene and evinced the degeneracy theory of disability and dangerousness, also gives Western psychiatry many of its presuppositions. Indeed, most standard psychiatric textbooks documenting the evidence for the heritability of 'schizophrenia' (e.g. Gottesman and Shields 1972) report uncritically the early influential genetic research of Rudin and Kallman during the Nazi period in Germany (Marshall 1990; Pilgrim 2008a). Thus, assumptions about genetic inferiority and race are deeply ingrained in psychiatric theory.

The question of racist constructs relates to the wider question, about the capacity of Western psychiatric knowledge to respond adequately to cross-cultural differences. Thus, even when psychiatric knowledge is not implicitly or explicitly racist, it is inevitably a product of its time and place. At present this means the dominance of ideas derived from nineteenth-century Europe, particularly the work of Kraepelin and Bleuler, which has been modified by later Anglo-American psychiatrists.

Even when less biologically and diagnostically orientated mental health workers have developed therapeutic rationales – such as Sigmund Freud in Europe, or Carl Rogers in the USA – they are clearly Western in their assumptions (for example about individualism and mind). Despite this, these psychotherapeutic systems are offered as being trans-historically and transculturally valid by their founders and followers (Pilgrim 1997a). In this sense they are not different to the biomedical rationales offered by their competing colleagues in the mental health industry. Despite a much greater sensitivity to the racial biases of psychiatric constructs, they remain implicit in most epidemiological studies (Bhui and Bhugra 2001).

In summary, the picture drawn above about mode of referral, diagnosis, compulsory admission and psychiatric management indicates that black people (particularly young black men) are subjected more to the harsh end of mental health services than white people. One of the challenges to psychiatric constructs about ethnicity and mental health is research exploring the way in which different ethnic groups construct and experience different types of psychological distress. For example, lay concepts of distress explored by researchers from Anglo-Australian, Ethiopian and Somali communities in Australia, suggest both commonalities and differences in lay understandings of 'depression'. While Anglo-Australian accounts predominantly portrayed 'depression' as an individual experience framed as narratives of social isolation and personal misfortune, accounts from the Somali and Ethiopian refugees identified family and broader socio-political events and circumstances more frequently. In the latter group 'depression' was framed as an affliction that was collectively derived and experienced (Kokanovic *et al.* 2008). Now we turn to another ethnic group in a British context.

South Asian women and the somatization thesis

The focus within the psychiatric literature on the 'madness' of young African-Caribbean men masks an important, but until recently less explored, question related to the misery of South Asian women. Studies of consultations in primary care show that South Asians consult with physical problems more frequently compared to white/British subjects (Goldberg *et al.* 1997). In particular, the rates and consultations for widespread musculoskeletal pain are higher among South Asian groups than white groups (Allison *et al.* 2002).

The discourse from psychiatric researchers about this topic suggests that South Asian women present their mental distress as bodily symptoms – the 'somatization thesis' (Currer 1986). This provides a case for an apparently legitimate form of medical management; in other words, doctors need to diagnose and treat an underlying mental illness (depression) despite the patient's somatic presentation. However, there are problems with this somatization thesis. Fenton and Sadiq-Sangster (1996: 69) point out that the presentation of bodily symptoms by South Asian women is ambiguous for a number of reasons:

> It could mean several things: (a) a non-recognition of mental illness, so that ailments are always presented as somatic, (b) a non-recognition of the link between physical ailments and emotional states, (c) a presentation of ailments as somatic despite some recognition of mental distress, and (d) simply a non-presentation of mental symptoms to bio-medical doctors.

The assumption that physical distress is 'really' a mental illness may reflect a form of Western cultural imperialism on the part of the psychiatric profession (look at our discussion of 'global mental health' in Chapter 1). For example, according to Skultans (2003) psychiatric language in Latvia has been taken over recently by the diagnostic category of 'depression' and 'masked depression', which has replaced the more established language of somatic distress that was central to previous lay conceptualizations under Soviet psychiatry.

Skultans raises the argument that it might be assumed that a psychiatric rather than physical diagnosis raises the probability of a patient-centred approach to care. However, the language of depression does not in itself lead to a greater appreciation of, or engagement with, patients' subjective narratives. Indeed, conversely, doctors who begin by addressing their patients' physical discomfort and presentation keep an open mind about a range of narrative possibilities. By contrast, a point diagnosis of depression leads usually to the prescription of antidepressants. The diagnosis and treatment then close down the need for further exploration.

Given this unexplored ambiguity, the psychiatric assumption of somatization in Asian women is a pre-emptive construction. The latter has a tendency to stereotype whole groups of people. Another example of this is in relation to the investigation itself of 'Asian' health. The attempt by medicine to seek a pattern of health in a variegated group of people from a large land mass (say, the Indian subcontinent) containing several countries, religions and nationalities reflects a homogenization stereotype. Also, as Watters (1996) has pointed out, Asian people may encounter different styles and qualities of mental health services in various parts of Britain. Despite this, the psychiatric literature studying differences in hospitalization rates in Asian people assumes that these exist as a result of patient variables.

Watters (1996) criticizes researchers for a number of rash generalizations about Asian mental health. He includes the following examples: an uncritical acceptance of the somatization thesis, an assumption that Islam is a protective mental health factor but Hinduism is not, and the assumption that Indians have an easier migration experience than Pakistanis. Another example of pre-emptive stereotyping is the assumption that Asian culture fails to have a notion of psychological causation (Ineichen 1987).

A final point which the literature on Asian mental health highlights is the vulnerability of Western medical knowledge. The somatization thesis implies that physical symptoms disguise a true mental illness. However, given the centrality of the heart in south Asian culture (Krause 1989; Fenton and Sadiq 1991), sadness is articulated readily as being in that area of the chest – the heart 'sinking' or 'falling' (*dil ghirda hai*). The sufferer is not 'disguising' depression but is simply experiencing their distress in that way. One analysis which seems to bridge the gap between cultural determinism and medical positivism can be found in a study of South Asian women's lay knowledge. Fenton and Sadiq-Sangster (1996), in a follow-up to their earlier research, found that women describe and express mental distress in a culturally specific way but their descriptions did correspond with a number of the features associated with the Western psychiatric category of depression.

A problem with Western psychiatric positivism is that it assumes a neat division between mental and physical illness. It also assumes that the linguistic expression of emotions is transculturally stable (Pilgrim and Bentall 1999). However, cross-cultural comparisons reveal large variations in the use of words to describe subjective states. For example, some cultures have no word for 'anxiety'. The current Western notion of 'depression' is a contemporary convention, which may change in the future and was certainly different in the past. In the nineteenth century it was not used. Instead lethargy, weakness and low mood were labelled as 'neurasthenia' and extreme sadness dubbed 'melancholia' by psychiatrists. In China, the former term is still favoured over 'depression' by lay people and doctors (Kleinman 1986).

A study exploring widespread pain among ethnic minority groups highlighted the relevance of physical imagery and 'somatic metaphors' to represent physical and mental health problems. For South Asian women in particular somatization or the notion of bodily pain was merely a starting point to providing a more wide-ranging narrative of pain and distress related to psychological distress and external social events (Rogers and Allison 2004). Somatization may also reflect the way in which the family and the group are more important than individual autonomy in the expression and management of distress. In the study of widespread pain, the apparent lack of reference to individual coping strategies among the South Asian respondents was accompanied by an importance attributed to family members in dealing with pain and distress and an emphasis on a transfer of domestic and everyday duties to others.

In this context, mental health treatments which foster individualism (say through psychotherapy) may result in dissonance with family members, which might undermine, rather than engender, social support and the patient's sense of self-worth. As a result, as Kirmayer and Young (1998) point out, solutions that make sense from the perspective of Euro-American psychiatry may not be embraced by many Eastern cultures. For example, the Western assumption that disclosure and emotional catharsis lead to healing may not have a global application. This somatization thesis about South Asian women may reveal more about the epistemological weakness and de-contextualized approach of Western psychiatry than the subjective weakness of its diagnostic targets.

A final note about this topic comes from Nazroo and Iley (2011). They suggest that more recently stereotyping about South Asian women has focused on people who are Muslims. However, the empirical evidence on distress in the latter (largely from family origins in Pakistan and Bangladesh) suggests that reported rates of distress are lower not higher in this group than those from Indian or East African origins, who are more likely to be Hindus. As the authors note: 'the significance of a particular ethnic identity can change dramatically over a short period of time' (Nazroo and Iley 2011: 87). This reminds us of the point from Brown (2003) earlier that racial stratification is a complex process in flux, implicating forces that both shape social constructs and generate particular and contingent social stressors.

Migration and mental health

In previous editions of this book we noted that Irish people in mainland Britain have had high rates of diagnosed mental health problems, despite being English speaking and Caucasian in appearance (Sproston and Nazroo 2002; Fitzpatrick and Newton 2005).

Thus when we come to consider the vulnerability of ethnic minorities to mental health problems, the direct social stress of racism elicited by skin colour cannot be the sole variable of explanation. For example, South Asian groups in Britain are all exposed to, and sometimes are individually subjected to, racism in their lives but not all of them have elevated rates of psychiatric diagnosis.

The Irish in Britain were treated prejudicially for a range of historical reasons, and social rejection and stereotyping of them from the English came in a variety of forms. Moreover, like the Caribbean migrants appearing in England in the 1950s they were forced into poor housing. In addition, their employment patterns typically involved low pay and this could be an important associated variable to account for raised rates of mental disorder. Earnings were often sent back home creating immediate poverty despite being in employment.

While some migrants are rich, this is rare. Economic migrants by definition are seeking to escape from absolute or relative poverty. Economic migration involves more 'choice' than some other social conditions (see below) but it still might reflect psycho-social pressure to escape from native poverty. In the case of the Irish, that pressure was at its most evident in the mass migrations to the UK and the USA during the nineteenth century, because of starvation. The depopulation of Ireland continued until the mid-twentieth century.

And if migration is forced, for example by starvation, warfare or torture, then subsistence existence is typically experienced by those fleeing. Asylum-seeking in these circumstances has become an important social policy question for governments of developed countries in recent decades. It has particular implications for the mental health status of those seeking refuge (Tribe and Patel 2007). More generally we know that stressful life events impact on mental health. Consequently, forced migration implicates general additive vulnerability factors following the experience of a traumatic event. The latter include the magnitude of the event, its personal meaning to the victim, lack of control over the event, its predictability, its impact on physical welfare, and its diversionary impact on expressed needs or normal expectations in the life course (Dohrenwend 2006).

It is easy to see from this list the cumulative vulnerability for people living in conditions of forced migration. Under conditions of intensifying entrapment in life all people (and other mammals) are more and more likely to 'give up' and experience 'learned helplessness' (Seligman 1975). Two common outcomes of this social-existential predicament are to become profoundly sad ('clinical depression') or nihilistic. Brown et al. (1995) discuss these outcomes in relation to self-harm and it can even extend to psychotic escape attempts, such as a black person denying that they are black. Also, especially in those subjected to trauma, there is a constant hyper-vigilance about new stressors, which can be construed as evidence of paranoia by onlookers.

The universal appeal to social causationist arguments just outlined can be tempered by evidence of cultural differences. For example, Obeyesekere (1985) notes that in Buddhist cultures suffering and its acceptance are both expected. This could account for why in conditions of extreme population level trauma (such as genocidal wars in Sri Lanka and Cambodia) depression does not have the same meaning as it does, say, in the USA. For this reason, comparative studies of migration and depression imply the need for careful ethnographic consideration (Kokanovic 2011).

Also note the different norms of indigenous adaptation cited in Buddhist Sri Lanka or Cambodia and compare them to different norms in receiving countries during asylum-seeking. That clash of norms might itself generate personal confusion, especially when receiving mental health professionals deploy assumptions about universal criteria of psychological abnormality. (We discussed this contention in relation to current arguments about 'global mental health' and Watters' thesis about 'the globalization of the American psyche' in Chapter 1.)

And where social causationist arguments are developed about migration and culture then this introduces another factor of amalgam social stress: fear and dislocation *combined with* poverty. With this subjectively experienced amalgam vulnerability, there comes a form of structural division, as migrants become identified by others in class terms because of their typical poverty: a process of social construction then which is economically driven (Miles 1996). We can see then that the process and outcome of migration and its health impacts have both subjective and objective aspects.

When migrants finds themselves in a new setting it will be culturally unfamiliar. They may seek social support in areas containing those of a similar background. This is a familiar scenario in most developed countries that have had spates of immigration, such as the UK, Australia and the USA. If those localities are poor then this increases the risk of all forms of mental disorder. To complicate matters, if people with pre-existing mental health problems live in unfamiliar areas with low ethnic density then this increases the chances of relapse (Karlsen *et al.* 2005). Thus direct environmental risks to migrants come in more than one guise.

The children of migrants may retain levels of disadvantage in a number of ways including continuing prejudice, poverty and identity confusion. In the latter regard problems of the 'post-colonial identity' can affect those now being born and living at home in the land that historically colonized that of their ancestors (DelVecchio *et al.* 2008). Racial harassment and these post-colonial impacts may persist for several generations after migration, which can translate into psychological distress (Karlsen and Nazroo 2002).

Discussion

There is an alternative way of viewing the debate on race and mental health, which goes beyond attempting to identify causal factors in the high incidence of mental illness among BME groups or pinpointing prejudicial labelling practices. This focuses on the discourse of race and psychiatry.

As Foucault (1965) has argued, we live with an ingrained predisposition to view madness as essentially 'other'. The use of the Victorian asylums for warehousing the insane was a mechanism for bringing about a break in the dialogue between reason and unreason on the one hand, and society and the disturbed on the other. In our contemporary era, where large mental hospitals are now extinct, the narrative of loss and difference is preserved in the status of becoming a patient. This is clearly expressed by Barham and Hayward (1991: 2), who note that people who receive a diagnosis of schizophrenia tend to be viewed as 'lost to the disorder'. They become a stranger to themselves and others. They become alien:

> Schizophrenia is more than an illness that one has; it is something a person is or may become. The person who has suffered a schizophrenic illness is someone in which a drastic rupture has been effected in the continuity of his or her biography . . . some schools of thought, we discover, do not accept there is an 'after' with schizophrenia, only a 'before'.

The use of the English word 'alien' to describe an outsider or foreigner resonates with the early nineteenth-century use of the term 'alienist' to describe an expert on madness. This notion of 'otherness', which characterizes the discourse on psychosis, fits well with a new type of racism. The latter is preoccupied with who should be included or excluded from the mainstream of society:

> The new racism is primarily concerned with mechanisms of inclusion and exclusion. It specifies who may legitimately belong to the national community and simultaneously advances reasons for the segregation or banishment of those whose 'origin, sentiment or citizenship' assigns them elsewhere.
>
> (Gilroy 1987: 45)

Within this discourse, people from black and ethnic minorities are identified as an alien force responsible for national decline and social disorder. While the old racism, underpinned by eugenics, proposed sterilization and extermination, the new racism suggests banishment and exclusion. In the context of the British historical legacy of colonialism, the debate on race and madness may be seen as central to the inner workings of this 'new racism'. This chapter has reviewed the evidence on the mental ill-health of groups of people, who are the legacy of British colonialism as ex-slaves, servants, imported service labour and, in the case of the Irish, have been implicated in a post-colonial armed struggle.

Academic and psychiatric literature alluding to race accentuates those mental illnesses which imply a threatening and hostile alien presence. Professional and academic texts then become part of a wider discourse about a threat to a traditional social order. This threat includes terrorism, non-Christian faiths, alien diet, arcane cultural norms, violent street crime, illicit drug use and so on. These images may then reinforce, or even be used to justify, English racism and endorse processes of segregation, exclusion or banishment.

Mental health and anti-terrorist legislation may be conceptualized as being part of what Althusser (1971) called the 'repressive state apparatus', which allows for preventive detention without trial, and the segregation or exclusion of threatening or undesirable 'others'. Banishment and exclusion can be reinforced by powers under mental health law to repatriate mentally ill aliens. Entry to the country on psychiatric grounds can also be banned under immigration legislation (Rogers and Pilgrim 1989).

However, the legitimacy of repatriation has declined in a context where a growing proportion of black people are British-born. It has become logically untenable. British-born black people have no identifiable nation state to which they can be banished (whether it be to the Indian subcontinent or the Caribbean of their parents, suggested only now by neo-Nazi groups in Britain). Likewise, Europeanization has ensured that rights of residence will be protected for people from any part of the British Isles.

Coercive psychiatry, as part of the wider repressive state apparatus, offers itself as a post-colonial, Europeanized alternative to repatriation. Ideas about banishment to another country can be replaced by the mechanisms of exclusion and control afforded by the mental hospital, prison and physical treatments. Not only are black and Irish people more likely to be incarcerated in locked facilities, and restrained using physical treatments, they are concomitantly represented as the 'other' in the texts and practices of academics and mental health professionals.

Most of what is summarized in this chapter is part of a discourse in which threat predominates, not distress. For example, compared with the extensive psychiatric literature on compulsorily detained African-Caribbean men, there is relatively little to be found on the sadness and despair of Asian women living in the community (Beliappa 1991; Fenton and Sadiq 1991). Ironically, this picture of differential attention is reinforced by some critiques that concur with our points here about repressive control in a post-colonial context. For example, Fernando *et al.* (1998) provide an elaborate and sophisticated critique of post-colonial psychiatry.

This chapter has summarized arguments and evidence about the mental health of African-Caribbean, Asian and Irish people in Britain. It has drawn attention to methodological problems of interpreting evidence about over-representation and discussed the errors of Anglo-American psychiatry using a diagnostic approach that is ill suited to people from black and ethnic minority populations. At the time of writing, the challenge of understanding the impact of post-colonial conditions upon formerly colonized groups of people, be they black or white, has become complicated by new migration patterns.

Asylum seekers and refugees are now coming to Britain often with experiences of recent trauma. Sociological accounts of this group of people are now invited to add to the literature on those once colonized by Britain. This is likely to produce different sorts of mental health profiles for these newcomers. In other words the mental health of migrants is determined both by their departed country of origin and by the conditions awaiting them in their 'host' country.

Questions

1 What factors need to be considered when understanding the relationship between race and health?
2 Discuss the evidence about the psychiatric treatment of African-Caribbean people in Britain.
3 What factors might account for the over-representation of Irish people in psychiatric admissions?
4 What problems are highlighted for psychiatric knowledge by the 'somatization thesis'?
5 Discuss ways in which psychiatric services could improve their response to Asian people.
6 Discuss the role of racism in the creation of mental health problems and the character of psychiatric services.

For discussion

Consider the ways in which your background has influenced your views about mental health in your own racial group and in that of others.

5　Age, ageing and mental health over the life course

Chapter overview

A life-course approach to mental health allows us to think about the importance of social context as a slice in time or across time. From conception onwards biological, psychological and social factors affect personal development. As life progresses for the individual, particular new influences upon mental health are encountered but the impact and legacy of earlier life remain pertinent. This is why a strong consensus exists in social science that the quality of life of children has particular life-long salience for mental health. Also normative expectations shift across the life course: what we expect to be psychologically normal in part takes into account 'age appropriateness'. Accordingly, in this chapter, we examine the mental health implications of phases of the life-span:

- age and the life course;
- childhood and mental health: a life-course perspective on mental health;
- childhood sexual abuse and mental health problems;
- social competence in adulthood;
- adolescence, social media and mental health;
- the 'Third Age' retirement and mental health.

Age and the life course

In previous chapters we have explored the way in which mental health and illness are socially patterned, with reference to race, class and gender. Age and ageing represent another dimension to social patterning. In exploring the age dimensions of mental health its different nuances in social context are revealed. An example of the latter is in relation to the epidemiology of suicide. This reveals year-on-year rises in the 1970s, 1980s and early 1990s of the rate in young men. However, since the early 2000s, rates in young men have declined to a 30-year low. This has led to the exploration of factors that might be responsible, such as changing employment patterns in young adulthood (Biddle *et al.* 2008). A sociological perspective allows the systematic examination of trajectories that arise out of understanding the social and psycho-social impact of social conditions in flux.

Life courses are studied in sociology as culturally shaped life stages, implicating variable social conditions and norms of expected conduct as people age. From this perspective people's lives can also be viewed as being linked dynamically over the life course. In this light, we can think in terms of:

1　the identification of structural and institutional influences that pattern early exposure to stress;
2　the stress universes for people at different ages;
3　identifying key aspects of the life course that set, or alter, trajectories of mental health in childhood and adolescence and their continuing implications for adulthood.

These patterns, which connect through time, are embedded within aspects of social life and institutions, such as our shifting domestic environments, workplaces and political and social organizations. Turning this point back on to the example of suicide, Shiner *et al.* (2009) suggest that the suicide rate in young men has been exaggerated as a social problem. Using an analysis of coroners' records they show how patterns of suicide coalesce with more conventional features of a socially structured life course. These include, for example, transitions and trajectories with young people in crisis about their identity and future prospects, mid-life gendered patterns of work and family, and older people in social and biological decline. Shiner *et al.* draw attention to less-publicized suicide patterns among those in middle age and to the role of 'social bonds' and attachment to significant others. This opens up wider social contextual features, beyond simply the psychological struggles of young men and instead illuminates the *life course as a whole*, linked to other social relationships, networks and positions.

Childhood and mental health

During childhood two factors become highly relevant to the question of mental health. The first is the emotional life of young people. The second is 'primary socialization': the ways in which newcomers learn how to become accepted and acceptable members of their parent society. Both of these factors are relevant for our purposes, because the field of mental health implicates distressed experiences and distressing conduct on the one hand and deviance from norms on the other.

As far as emotions are concerned, sociologists have drawn largely upon psychoanalysis. Freudianism has influenced a variety of social theories from structural functionalism to neo-Marxism (the 'Frankfurt School'). Psychoanalysis (see Chapter 1) offers a theory that connects the individual's inner life to their external social context. It provides an account of the emotional life of individuals, while at the same time offering an explanation of how mental ill-health is determined by society. For Freud, civilization puts limits on the free expression and experience of emotions, particularly the instincts of sexual desire and murderous aggression. These limits lead to the need of the child to repress their antisocial feelings in exchange for family and societal acceptance. This battle between emotions and social conformity leads to the development of neurosis. However, Freudianism is a limited social theory. Freud's emphasis is on civilization (Freud 1930) leading to repression and neurosis. According to Freud, we are all neurotic (to some extent) for more or less the same reasons to do with balancing our instinctual needs with the constraints of reality made clear to us by our parents. Consequently, differences between social groups were not addressed systematically by his theory, although later psychoanalytically orientated writers explored women's issues with the establishment of feminist therapy (Mitchell 1974; Eichenbaum and Orbach 1982).

Freud offered an explanation for neurotic behaviour arising from anxiety. Later psychoanalysts also tried to address the question of depression (Bowlby 1951) and psychosis (Winnicott 1958; Laing 1967) by looking at the impact of poor care and separation on the infant (from birth to 2 years). However, as an example of the divergent views within psychoanalysis, the influential work of Melanie Klein is distinctive because it focused on the pathogenic impact of the infant's inborn aggression (rather than poor care). By contrast, the work of Bowlby, Winnicott and Laing was heavily environmentally orientated; it emphasized parental privation and deprivation as the source of later mental health problems. Whereas Klein can be seen to blame the instincts for mental ill-health, the 'environmentalists' can be seen to point the finger at parents, particularly the mother.

Thus, variegated psychoanalytical accounts certainly emphasize a general social backdrop ('civilization') to emotional development, but the nuclear family then becomes its main frame of sociological reference. Mainstream clinical psychoanalysis tends to play down or ignore variables other than the family, such as the particular stresses associated with class, race, gender, age and sexuality. It also ignores the potentially powerful role of extra-familial social institutions, such as the school, in shaping the child's identity and their emotional life.

Turning to primary socialization, there is a strong consensus across theoretical positions in both sociology and psychology that childhood is a special part of the life-span. It is a time when most of the rules and mores associated with the society and particular class and culture which the child inhabits are learned. It is also a time when gender-specific conduct is acquired. The child learns what is expected of him or her both at their current age and in the future, through their exposure to adult models of conduct. They learn gradually to control their body and their emotions in order to perform competently and efficiently in the presence of others. They learn the importance of a shared view of reality with their fellows in gaining security and in meriting credibility. All these learned capacities are also bound up with an increasingly elaborate and defined sense of identity. Thus, socialization is about learning how to behave in a context-appropriate way in society and it is about a person gaining a confident sense of who they are.

The relevance of socialization for mental health is that children learn to behave confidently and appropriately, following rules and complying with norms. This competence can fail if the person lacks the intellectual capacity to grasp what to do (currently this is termed a 'learning difficulty' and used to be called 'mental handicap' or 'mental subnormality'). It can also fail if the person lacks confidence in their performance as a social actor (this might be a way of thinking about 'phobic anxiety') or if they are too sad to participate in everyday activities ('depression'). The competence can also be adjudged to have failed by others if the person fails to comply with everyday expectations of appropriate behaviour in context or they make idiosyncratic claims about reality. We will return to this later when discussing 'schizophrenia'.

A final aspect of socialization relevant to understanding mental health is that children learn to control their emotions. The strong emotional expressions tolerated in childhood become less and less acceptable as the person matures into adulthood. Consequently, if an adult becomes more exuberant or sad than is deemed appropriate for the context by others, they may acquire the label of 'manic depressive'. In modern industrial societies, which are regulated by versions of rationality, adult conduct is marked by a capacity to comply with both moral propriety and rational rules. By young adulthood, those of us who act either immorally, incompetently or irrationally will be deemed by others to be either bad or sick (Pilgrim *et al.* 2011).

Most psychologists assume that problems in childhood make the person susceptible to later mental health problems. Likewise, sociological models of depression in adulthood emphasize developmental vulnerability factors as well as current stressors (Brown and Harris 1978, discussed in Chapter 4). The social causationist model of depression from Brown and Harris involves a multi-factorial approach. As far as childhood is concerned, a strong case has been recently made for a uni-factorial causationist model, which links a variety of mental health problems to sexual abuse in childhood. Because of the strong evidence for this relationship, we will look at this in some detail below.

What is important to note here are the competing values underlying these approaches and an awareness of the socially negotiated ideas and theories about children and young people. The latter is important if knowledge about children and mental health is dominated by an adult-centric view of the world and the views of children are not taken into account. Those undertaking a corrective to this adult-centric position by using a participatory approach with children themselves, such as Liegghio and colleagues (2010), lay out the themes and qualities of a sociology of childhood perspective, as shown here in Table 5.1.

Sociology, childhood and adversity

The relationship between age and mental health has only occasionally been addressed directly by sociologists. This may, in part, reflect the relatively low status that children have had within mainstream sociology. As Mayall (1998) has pointed out, children have been 'regarded unproblematically,

Table 5.1 A participatory framework for studying childhood

Themes	Qualities
Values	Individual agency/social responsibility
Ontology/epistemology	Social constructionist
Views of child, development competence, differences	Models of children situated in socio-historical context and challenging deconstruction traditional models of mental health and distress
Agency and power in adult–child relationships	Children have unique roles and positions in relation to power
	Children have inherent rights
	Children need opportunities to develop competencies and access to valued resources, and opportunities to participate and have influence
Intervention/change focus	Need to focus on an expansion of contexts from individual and family to a broader social context and social policy where children play an active role in the intervention and change process

as socialization projects within the private domain'. It is only relatively recently that a sociology of childhood has begun to be established, which focuses on understanding children's social position as a minority group and as 'embodied' health care actors (see Table 5.1). This sociological inquiry explores inter-generational relationships and the ways in which children's identities are constituted in and through particular places and spaces. Adolescents and children identify more with, and make distinctions between, groups of people in relating back to their own sense of self and place in the world, rather than identifying with a particular locality or national identity (Scourfield *et al.* 2006).

Identity, which in the young is strongly bound up with peers, leads to an age-bound and highly specific view of mental health and help-seeking. For example, suicide and depression were not always conceptualized as a 'problem' for which help-seeking from formal or informal sources is required (Biddle *et al.* 2007). The use of the Internet and mobile phones has also increasingly become central to the latter (social networking sites, MSN communication, Facebook, etc.), with consequences for understanding the configuration, and expression, of mental health topics. For example, the Internet increasingly acts as a forum for suicidal identities to be tested out, authenticated and validated by individuals. The same is true of the Internet's support of anorexic tendencies in young people (Horne and Wiggins 2009).

There has been some interest in people's conception of health and illness through subjectively defined stages of the life course (Backett and Davison 1995) and in the impact of mental health risk at different points in childhood, adolescence and adulthood (Power *et al.* 2002). However, there has been little integration of the different dimensions of ageing within sociological thought (Arber and Ginn 1991). An exception is the work of Backett-Milburn and colleagues (2003), who explored the social and cultural processes in different accounts of childhood, health and inequalities provided by children. They found that children display considerable emotional resilience and tend to play down the effects of relationship and material factors. At the same time children highlight how familial and personal challenges, such as bullying, divorce or learning difficulties, constitute a set of commonly held childhood experiences which cut across differences of class and gender.

This type of study on childhood processes is important because of the emergence of roles and norms during primary socialization (both traditional topics of interest for sociology as well as social psychologists). For example, children, adolescents and adults who follow a certain sequencing of their social roles are assumed to be better adjusted than their counterparts who follow other life-course patterns. In early adulthood this normative order is defined as first entering the paid labour force, then getting married, and later having children. Both men and women seem to benefit from following the normative course of role transitions. However, there are differences for different population groups. For example a US study suggests that African-Americans who work first, then have children, and later get married report better mental health than their peers (Jackson 2004).

It is widely recognized that the point at which young people become adults is historically and socially constructed. Changing views about when a person is a child and when they become an adult has been evident in recent mental health research. For example, it has been found that early pubertal timing is associated with increased mental health problems (Kaltiala-Heino *et al.* 2003). Additionally, the point at which children are considered to become adults has implications for identifying mental health trends. A study found that malaise symptoms in the age group 11–16 seemed to have a similar pattern to young adults, suggesting that the boundary between childhood and youth might need to be set at an earlier age (West and Sweeting 2004).

Societal values also seem to define to an extent what is acceptable treatment and management of children and adolescents with mental health problems. For example, substantial media attention has been focused on the issue of psychiatric medication use and ECT for children. While the use of medication has increased dramatically since the early 1980s, for both children and adults, the vulnerability and special social status attributed to childhood means that this group receives more emotive and controversial coverage. This change has led to concerns about the long-term impact of medication on the immature brain (Carlezon and Konradi 2004) and the ethical implications of parents consenting to treatment on their children's behalf (Breeding and Bauman 2001).

Lay people express mixed views about the use of medication in childhood. In a study of the acceptable use of Prozac, specifically for children, a survey of US public opinion found that just over half of the adults interviewed considered it appropriate to use Prozac for children or adolescents expressing suicidal intentions, but there was growing opposition to the use of such medication for hyperactivity and other behavioural problems (McLeod *et al.* 2004).

Among lay people, strong and consistent correlates of willingness to give psychiatric medications to children include trust in doctors and the respondents' own expressed willingness to take psychiatric medications. However, it seems that most people consider that psychiatric medications affect child development, give children a flat, 'zombie'-like affect, and delay resolving 'real' behaviour-related problems. The view that physicians overmedicate children for common behavioural problems is also widespread. Women and those with more education tend to report more negative views on medication (Pescosolido *et al.* 2007).

Finally in this section, a methodological challenge about studying adversity is highlighted by mental health research about young people. Measuring a *cumulative* effect is seen as the most meaningful way of measuring the impact of adversity, rather than the sum of the number of occurrences of *distinctly* experienced events. For example, a recent US study found that total cumulative childhood adversity is related to depressive symptoms, drug use and antisocial behaviour; there is thus an incremental impact on mental health which increases as a range of adversities accumulate over time (Schilling *et al.* 2008).

A cycle of disadvantage is also apparent with evidence of the effects of childhood social adversity impacting on developing parent/child attachments and on learnt parenting styles. Symptoms of depression in parents who had themselves suffered adversities in childhood were associated with an 'insecure' attachment style in relation to their own children. Both material and emotional deprivation are associated with low levels of expressed parental warmth. By contrast, high parental warmth is associated with decreased risk of insecure attachment styles (Stansfeld *et al.* 2008). Similarly Kiernan and Huerta (2008) found that economic deprivation and maternal depression separately and together diminish the cognitive and emotional well-being of children. Part of this impact arises from the less nurturing and engaged parenting style of those with fewer economic and emotional resources.

This interaction of (lower) class position and emotional resources highlights that models of mental health causation based either on material or psychological explanations are less persuasive than 'both/and' models. Poverty increases the risk of mental health problems but not all poor people develop the latter; mediating psychological factors are therefore important to consider. This links with the next section, which starts with the point that the psychological construction from victims about their adverse conditions in childhood is variable. Moreover, the presence of the adversity of abuse can happen in all classes, which highlights the need to consider family peculiarities not just social group membership.

Childhood sexual abuse and mental health problems

While the connection between sexual abuse and distress can be viewed as a unilinear relationship, this does not imply that there is a consistent outcome for all victims. Individuals do vary in their responses to similar abusive acts, and the severity of the abuse, its duration and the relation of the perpetrator to the victim have all been linked to variable outcomes (Finkelhor 1984). Another caution is that sexual victimization may be part of a wider picture of family disturbance, which could be pathogenic. As Briere and Runtz (1987: 371) point out:

> Although symptomatology in adulthood may co-vary with early sexual abuse, in the absence of further data it is not clear whether the former is caused by the latter or whether both are actually a function of some third variable, such as dysfunctional family dynamics.

The risk of childhood sexual abuse seems to be enhanced by a number of factors, such as troubled inter-generational attachment relationships in families. These include problems in maternal adult functioning, a negative relationship between the grandmother and mother, and a disrupted pattern of care-giving during the mother's childhood (Leifer *et al.* 2004).

Reviews of the literature on the immediate and long-term effects of sexual abuse on child victims come to the conclusion that there is strong evidence that they are significantly more prone to mental distress than non-abused children (Wyatt and Powell 1988; Cahill *et al.* 1991). Moreover, the offspring of survivors of childhood sexual abuse are at greater risk of mental health problems than others (Roberts *et al.* 2004). Not only is this evidence compelling but it points to a wide range of effects, which may account, in part at least, for the higher rate of reported mental health problems in women than men. Overall, girls are at greater risk than boys of sexual victimization. This is certainly true of intra-familial abuse (Rogers and Terry 1984) although there is some evidence that boys may be at greater risk from stranger-perpetrators (Abel *et al.* 1987).

The large gap between male and female victims in terms of rates of abuse and rates of distressing consequences may be accounted for in part by the greater readiness of female victims to disclose on both counts (Finkelhor 1979). Also, as we pointed out in Chapter 3, the discourse on females has been more wide-reaching than that on males, with the bulk of the research on prevalence of abuse and its effects being focused on women, not men (Becker 1988; Dimock 1988).

Sexual abuse makes child victims more likely than non-abused children to demonstrate:

- aggression;
- sexually inappropriate behaviour;
- sexual aggression.

'Sexually inappropriate behaviour' refers to the tendency of victims to become sexually interested in peers and adults in a way that is unusual for their age group. 'Sexual aggression' refers to this process when it is associated with anger or violence. This trio of symptoms characterizing child victims of sexual abuse does not mean that they have only these problems. Other forms of distress reported include those suffered by non-abused psychiatric referrals (anxiety, depression, night terrors, language delay, hyperactivity, stealing, peer relationship difficulties, eating disorders and so on). However, the trio does seem to mark sexual abuse victims off from non-abused children with emotional problems.

A number of epidemiological studies now indicate that these immediate externalizing effects in childhood translate into adult problems both of 'acting out' and of experienced distress. Studies of long-term effects have been on both clinical and community populations. Here we will give an example from each. Briere and Runtz (1987) examined the records of 152 consecutive women requesting appointments at the counselling department of an urban Canadian community health centre. Table 5.2 summarizes their results.

The significant results in the far right column alert us to the symptom profile of the abused group. Notice the suicidal behaviour and the substance abuse, as well as the battered adult picture. This phenomenon of 'revictimization' is common in adult survivors of childhood abuse. There is some evidence that disproportionate numbers of victims are found working as prostitutes (Browne and Finklehor 1986).

Table 5.2 Differences between sexually abused (AB) and non-abused (NAB) female attenders at a Canadian community health centre for crisis counselling ($n = 152$)

	% NAB	% AB	Sig. level
Current psychotropic medication	14.0	31.3	0.01
History of hospitalization	22.1	19.4	ns
History of attempted suicide	33.7	50.7	0.03
Battered as adult	17.6	48.9	0.0003
History of rape	8.3	17.7	ns
History of drug addiction	2.3	20.9	0.0005
History of alcoholism	10.5	26.9	0.02
Restless sleep	54.7	71.6	0.03
Nightmares	23.3	53.7	0.0001
Anxiety attacks	27.9	53.7	0.001
Trouble controlling temper	18.6	38.8	0.006
Desire to hurt self	18.6	31.3	0.07
Sexual problems	15.1	44.8	0.0001
Fear of men	15.1	47.8	0.0001
Fear of women	3.5	11.9	0.09
Derealization	10.5	32.8	0.0001
Out-of-body experiences	8.1	20.9	0.04
Chronic muscle tension	44.2	65.7	0.008

Source: Modified from Briere and Runtz (1987).

Other studies indicate that some victims also become perpetrators. Estimates of this vary. Longo (1982) reported that 47 per cent of male adolescent sexual offenders had been victims themselves. Becker (1988) reports a figure of 19 per cent in her adolescent sexual offenders' clinic.

The focus of the clinical discourse on sexual abuse is on male perpetrators and, with the exceptions just quoted, female victims. Recently, a minority interest in female perpetrators has emerged suggesting that they constitute between 1 per cent and 10 per cent of offenders. Women are much less likely to act alone than male abusers (though paedophile rings of men working together also exist). The infamous cases of Myra Hindley and Rose West illustrate this type of male–female collusion in a dramatic way because they culminated in several murders. Less dramatic cases, stopping short of death, receive less publicity, though in 2009 in England, the case of a female nursery nurse as part of a paedophile pornography ring was discovered and prosecuted, with extensive coverage in the mass media.

Given that the data reflect a preponderance of female victims and only a small minority of female perpetrators, it alerts us to the problems of accounting for sexual abuse, simply in terms of adults repeating abusive relationships from childhood. The switching from victim to perpetrator is not inevitable, nor can it be invoked as a strong causal explanation of most abusive acts, as most victims of both sexes do not go on to become perpetrators.

Turning to an example of a community survey, Stein et al. (1988) interviewed 3132 adults in two Los Angeles areas – one predominantly white, the other Hispanic (Table 5.3). The symptom profile of victims is confirmed again in this study. Drug and alcohol abuse is evident, as are anxiety and depression. Significant differences do not appear in the groups in relation to diagnoses of schizophrenia, mania and obsessive-compulsive problems. The final row shows the consistent pattern of victims being more likely overall to receive a psychiatric diagnosis than non-victims. Elements in this range of adult personal difficulties seem to be more amplified in victims of intra-familial abuse than for those abused by non-relatives. Not only do they suffer the psychological impact of assault common to all victims, they also struggle with a particular sense of betrayal and stigma.

Finally in this section it is worth noting the likely underestimate of childhood sexual abuse as a social problem. The actual rate of childhood sexual abuse is difficult to ascertain because of a reluctance to disclose a traumatic and stigmatized event. A study conducted in 2004 indicates the pervasiveness of a reluctance to disclose with 78 per cent of women interviewed about their experiences indicating that they had not told anyone about the sexual abuse when it happened. The most common reason for this was fear of not being believed (Lundqvist et al. 2004).

Table 5.3 Lifetime prevalence of psychiatric problems in those sexually abused (AB) and those not (NA) in childhood ($n = 3132$)

	Men		Women	
	% NA	% AB	% NA	% AB
Alcohol abuse	23.2	35.7	4.1	20.8*
Drug abuse	7.8	44.9*	3.1	13.7*
Severe depression	3.9	13.8	5.5	21.9*
Phobic anxiety	7.0	6.5	12.5	34.2*
Any psychiatric diagnosis	34.0	71.2*	24.0	58.6*

*Significance level of 0.05.
Source: Figures summarized from Stein et al. (1988).

The stigma of the abused victim and the shame and criminality of the perpetrator make accurate empirical estimates of child sexual abuse particularly difficult, but logically suggest underestimation. Baker and Duncan (1985) suggest child sexual abuse rates of 0.25 per cent for relative and 10 per cent (12 per cent female and 8 per cent male) for non-relative abuse in Britain. If these are accurate estimates, around 4.5 million British adults are victims of earlier sexual abuse. In the USA, Russell (1983) reported much higher rates in her community survey of women – 38 per cent reporting one experience of sexual abuse before 18 with 4.5 per cent of the sample reporting abuse by their biological fathers or stepfathers.

Prevalence rates of abuse victims of around 30 per cent are quoted by studies of psychiatric outpatient records (Gelinas 1983). This range of estimates poses a problem of interpretation. If Russell's estimates are correct, then it would appear that while the rates in the community of reported sexual abuse are high, this is not translating into a proportionate number of victims becoming psychiatric patients. What is implied instead, as with the Brown and Harris (1978) study of female depression in the community, is that there is a 'clinical iceberg' (see Chapter 1), with only some of the abuse victims presenting for professional help. By contrast, if the Baker and Duncan data are more accurate, then it would appear that sexual abuse during childhood is being reflected more closely in prevalence rates of psychiatric disorder.

Social competence in adulthood

All mental disorders manifest, or attributed, in adulthood reflect failures of social competence because rule transgressions and role failures are the features that come to be medically codified (psychiatric symptoms). The most dramatic forms of failure are present in those described as suffering from schizophrenia and the diagnosis demonstrates the inherent tautology of psychiatric diagnosis. A person is deemed to be schizophrenic because of their oddity and they are deemed to be odd because they are suffering from schizophrenia.

The questions begged for sociologists about 'schizophrenia' are thus mainly about how such a diagnosis is negotiated or ascribed. This tack has been taken most systematically by Coulter (1973). He argues that focusing on debates about aetiology obscures the ways in which madness emerges, first through social negotiation in the lay area and then in professional confirmation (a diagnosis). Coulter focuses on everyday expectations of normality and competence. For instance, in relation to hallucinations he argues that to maintain our credibility in a social group there has to be a consensus about what our senses detect around us. In most contexts, if a person sees or hears something that others do not, then their credibility, and therefore their social group membership, is jeopardized. However, it is possible in certain contexts that such idiosyncratic capacities might strengthen rather than weaken their credibility and group status. The Christian mystic and some African medicine men are expected to have extraordinary visions. Indeed, their social credibility may rest on having these abnormal experiences.

In some cultures where hallucinations are valued positively, the bodily circumstances which increase the probability of their occurrence (fasting, fatigue, drug taking and so on) are often contrived deliberately. Al-Issa (1977) notes that, in Western society, hallucinations offend rationality. Most of us suppress idiosyncratic perceptions because we learn that they are valued negatively. The 'schizophrenic' in contrast makes the mistake of, or is driven to, acting upon their idiosyncratic experiences. Community surveys indeed point to estimates of between 10 per cent and 50 per cent of the 'normal' population who hallucinate (Bentall and Slade 1985).

Thus, atypical idiosyncratic perceptions are not intrinsically pathological (although most Western psychiatrists may insist that this is the case). Whether hallucinations are deemed to indicate a gift or a defect depends on the roles people occupy in particular cultures. Likewise, weird speech patterns are highly valued in those Christian sects which respect the ability to 'speak in tongues' (or 'glossolalia') (Szasz 1992; Bentall and Pilgrim 1993). Outside of these sects, in everyday Western life, they may be taken to be an offence to rational discourse and so encourage attributions of mad talk from their fellows. Later these may be reframed as evidence of schizophrenic thought disorder by a psychiatrist.

Some recent sociological accounts of madness have gone beyond Coulter's point about the attribution of unintelligibility and explored the meaning of patient narratives as a pathway to understanding how people live with a psychiatric diagnosis. Once a young person receives a diagnosis of 'schizophrenia' then they reflect on their pre-existing sense of self. These reflections on identity are not always negative (Dinos *et al.* 2005). This ambiguity can be contrasted with the tendency of significant others to see the patient as being 'lost' to the illness (Barham and Hayward 1991). All of these ambiguities generated by contextualized approaches to narratives or the meaning of specific unusual experiences ('symptoms' in Western medical terms) can be contrasted with a traditional view from medical naturalism or positivism. Generally, psychiatrists have tended to conceive of thought disorder as a stable set of cognitive idiosyncrasies or failures: woolly thinking, vagueness, bizarre content, neologisms (invented new words), poverty of thought, fixed and rigid or repetitive expressions. Similarly they have simply assumed that hearing voices is inherently pathological. However, these medical attributions are extracted from the contexts in which judgements are made about social competence.

Coulter emphasizes that, in fact, people may be judged sane by their fellows and yet often manifest such cognitive failures. Following Coulter, what matters are the circumstances in which in one social setting such speech oddities are judged or are valued to indicate madness (by lay people) and confirmed subsequently as schizophrenic illness by psychiatrists.

For Coulter, there are no abstract defining qualities of schizophrenic thought, but there are social settings in which the thoughts of some people are judged to be meaningless or illegitimate. These settings, and the decisions associated with them, involve family members and neighbours at home, or strangers in public places, who appeal for the attendance of psychiatric professionals to deal with a discomforting situation. In other words, madness, like the sanity with which it is contrasted, is socially negotiated. Consequently, the best that sociologists can do is to describe the particular contexts in particular cultures in which ascriptions of madness are made. To do this, knowledge of norms and competence are vital for the investigator. The latter is really studying a moral order and the way in which social actors attempt to maintain its stability by correcting or removing offending group members.

While most cultures across time and place have some notion of oddity or madness, because norms of sanity vary, this notion is not constant. Nor is there a transcultural or trans-historical consensus on what causes oddity or how to respond to it when it emerges (Sedgwick 1982; Horwitz 1983). Each culture may have a notion of what it means to lose one's reason but these notions vary across time and place and so undermine the claims of modern Western psychiatry that 'schizophrenia' and its symptoms are a stable set of factors to be studied.

Adolescence, social media and mental health

The diagnosis of schizophrenia predominates in young adulthood because that is when role expectations based on rational rule following and goal orientation are highlighted. It is the age when the rationality of work and parenting are demanded of, and by, those involved. Adolescence is also a period of individuation and is seen in sociological terms as a transitional period between childhood and adulthood marking a change in status within society. A contextual perspective views development as being influenced by the everyday setting and contexts for an adolescent's life and this in turn has a positive or negative impact on mental health. This approach is important for understanding the emergence of trends in mental health impacting particularly on young adults.

Suicide, for example, is one of the three leading causes of death among adolescents, and is globally thought to be influenced by socio-cultural variables as well as personality and individual factors (Pritchard and Hansen 2005). The levels of anomic lifestyles, degree of cultural heterogeneity and extent of social competition have all been implicated in explaining differences around the world. In developing societies, African, Asian and Latin American adolescents appear to be less likely to think suicidal thoughts and commit suicide than their Western counterparts. In terms of social context, urban versus rural environments seem to be important in influencing mental health (as in the higher suicide rates among Chinese adolescents (Meng *et al.* 2013)). Less traditional contexts have also been influential. Within a relatively short period of time social media has revolutionized the way in which young people in particular interact with their peers and the social world. On the face of things sites such as Facebook are seen to provide opportunities for social interaction and thus potentially for social support. In some controlled settings there is some suggestion that online relationships for older people with a chronic condition may facilitate support in a way that is different from offline relationships, but also more beneficial to them. However, social media may in fact have a negative impact on and undermine mental health. An analysis of Facebook identified a decline in subjective well-being: how users feel and how satisfied they are with their lives. The more the young respondents used Facebook at one point in time the worse they seemed to feel. By contrast *direct* face-to-face social networking among the same respondents increased feelings of subjective well-being (Kross *et al.* 2013). The results were not a result of only using Facebook when young people felt bad. This research may indicate the emergence of a new form of isolation and loneliness among adolescents.

The 'Third Age', retirement and mental health

Particular dynamics of social position, inequalities and mental health coalesce at the individual level, as we approach retirement and become older adults. Older adults who are healthy, have an adequate source of income, educated beyond a basic level, active and retain extended social networks tend to adjust well to the challenge of retirement. Compared to people who retire voluntarily, those who are forced into retirement tend to be more depressed and unhealthy. A common cultural assumption has been that early retirement is inherently beneficial because it affords opportunities for more leisure and relief from the stress of job conditions and dissatisfaction. However, recent evidence suggests instead that it is associated with cognitive decline. This may be attributed in part to the shrinking of social networks (particularly at work) that keep people mentally agile (Borsch-Supan and Schuth 2013). This recognition of the importance of environmental and social networks is now translating into policies that also recognize their importance. In particular it has had an impact on new ways of thinking about primary and social care, which focus on the environmental and social settings of ageing. In relation to the increasingly recognized importance of the degree or lack of social connectivity, via social networks, two sociologically imbued terms have tended to be used interchangeably: 'loneliness' and 'social isolation'.

In research on older people, 'loneliness' generally refers to a negative evaluation of 'the nature, quality and quantity of an individual's overall level of social interaction and engagement' (Victor *et al.* 2006), whereas social isolation has been defined as the 'separation from social or familial contact, community involvement, or access to services' (AGE UK 2010). 'Solitude', a positive construct linked to mental states such as meditation and a precondition of a self-help tradition based on 'mindfulness', has been defined as something positive and productive, 'a constructive way of being separated from others in order to be by and with oneself' (Ettema *et al.* 2010: 142). Thus discussions of the psycho-social aspects of ageing and its relationship to being alone and being with others have to be considered in relationship to the nuances of these subjective and objective nuances of life (at any age), but have become particularly relevant to research on ageing.

Service provision for older people is skewed towards providing for dementia (discussed below). However, there has been some effort to provide for older people experiencing depression from within primary care. Treatment regimens for depression seem to mirror those being provided for other groups, which focus mainly on the use of antidepressants (Baldwin and Thompson 2003). More normalized activities might seem to offer better amelioration. For example, gardens have been identified as a 'therapeutic landscape': gardening activities have been found to offer comfort and the opportunity for emotional and spiritual renewal, and communal gardening activity on allotments has been found to contribute to psychological well-being, through the provision of a mutually supportive environment. This may enhance emotional well-being by combating social isolation (Milligan *et al.* 2004). However, social norms about depression and its management among health professionals are likely to have an impact on access to the means of prevention and management. Therapeutic nihilism (the feeling that nothing can be done for this group of patients) is a feature of primary care professionals' views, while older patients also seem to be characterized by passivity and limited expectations of treatment.

The Third Age, and focus on dementia and depression in older people

The emergence of the notion of the 'Third Age' is defined and explained by Chatzitheochari and Arber (2012: 455) thus:

> the decrease in the retirement age and the increase of healthy years people were expected to enjoy after retirement laid the foundations for a different experience of mature age after the relinquishment of paid work and family roles. Combined with the increased opportunities for leisure participation and the more 'refined' needs and interests of newer generations as a result of different socialization experiences and resources, these changes would lead to an altered trajectory of individual ageing; the Third Age was thus conceptualized as a new life-course stage of extended and self-fulfilling leisure and community participation following retirement. Its emergence was understood as a uniquely modern phenomenon that constituted a key development in the transformation of later life and of the entire life-course structure in Western societies.

This discourse on the emergence of the Third Age as a period of relative fulfilment and ongoing engagement with active leisure seems on the face of things to coalesce with the evidence discussed above of the relatively better mental health that is experienced as we age (e.g. Blaxter 1990). However, the latter does not apply to all. Active ageing seems to coalesce with the 'habitus' and the cultural expression of those who are also culturally and materially already advantaged. Moreover, this perspective seems to bracket out the significance given to accounting for deterioration in social competence, and specific mental health conditions which is the more usual focus of mental health as we age. To illustrate the point:

- 60,000 deaths a year are directly attributable to dementia. Delaying the onset of dementia by 5 years would reduce deaths directly attributable to dementia by 30,000 a year.
- Family carers of people with dementia save the UK over £6 billion a year.
- 64 per cent of people living in care homes have a form of dementia.
- Two-thirds of people with dementia live in the community while one-third live in a care home.

The most recent estimates suggest that in 2013 there are around 670,000 people with dementia in the UK. Although rates of dementia are broadly set to rise (because of changes in longevity), there is evidence of a cohort effect. It seems that 'later born populations' have a lower risk of developing dementia than those born earlier in the twentieth century (Matthews *et al.* 2013). The latter effect seems to be a function of cohort differences in norms of diet and exercise.

Health economic analyses suggest that the financial cost of dementia to the UK is over £17 billion a year (Comas-Herrera *et al.* 2007). However, the salience of dementia in mental health services and its purported biological causes in older people may be exaggerated. As well as people with dementia needing social support to maximize their quality of life and avoid physical jeopardy, there are many more older people with cognitive problems who have no proven neurological condition. Kitwood (1988) points out that Alzheimer's dementia can only be properly diagnosed postmortem. Moreover, some people who are clearly confused and suffering impaired memory show no post-mortem neurological signs. The loss of personhood, which accompanies the progression of dementia, has also been linked to the notion of 'social death'; those who are close to the sufferer come to believe and sometimes act as if the person is already dead (Sweeting and Gilhooly 1997).

Another point to note about dementia is that while it is mainly a problem of old age, it can occur, albeit more rarely, in middle age ('pre-senile dementia'). An example, of an even younger population being affected is the small but increasing prevalence of Creutzfeldt-Jakob Disease (CJD) among younger adults, which appears to be causally related to eating products of cattle infected with Bovine Spongiform Encephalopathy (BSE) during the 1980s. Epidemiologists remain uncertain about the long-term impact of infection inherited from that time. (The WHO reports that 175 cases of CJD emerged in the UK and 49 cases emerged in other countries from October 1996 to March 2011: www.who.int/mediacentre/factsheets/fs180/en.)

There is a secondary mental health impact of dementia, which affects informal carers (Morris *et al.* 1988). Stress reactions are common in this group of carers, although some other studies highlight positive, as well as negative, psychological features of the caring role (Orbell *et al.* 1993). In Chapter 12 we examine the problematic status of the concept of 'carer'. However, here we will note that, in those with advanced dementia, direct physical care is demanded in a way that is usually not implied in younger patients with diagnoses such as 'schizophrenia'.

Dementia is also associated with contention between informal and formal health care workers about diagnosis and treatment. One study found that diagnosis may involve conflict between GPs, family members and the person with dementia. Compared to informal carers, GPs did not consider that diagnosing dementia early was particularly important and even thought it might be harmful, and so they were sceptical about the advantages of dementia medications (Hansen *et al.* 2008).

While dementia may have become a dominant image in modern culture of becoming elderly, depression is actually more prevalent among the older population. While the prevalence of dementia is about 5 per cent in the over 65s, rising to just below 20 per cent for those over 80, depression is much more common in the younger age band of older people. In Britain, community surveys indicate prevalence rates for depression of between 5 per cent in Edinburgh (Maule *et al.* 1984) and 26 per cent in Newcastle (Kay *et al.* 1964) for people over 65. Other studies more typically quote rates of 11 per cent to 15 per cent (Copeland *et al.* 1987).

About 2 per cent of the UK population of over-65s is in residential care. In this particular population, the prevalence of depression rises dramatically. A London survey of 12 old people's homes revealed that around 40 per cent of the residents were depressed (Mann *et al.* 1984). Surveys in Sydney, Australia (Snowden and Donnelly 1986) found one-third of the residents depressed, and a similar survey finding was reported from Milan, Italy (Spagnoli *et al.* 1986). Mild depression is more common in older women than men and it is also more prevalent in those suffering from physical illnesses (Brayne and Ames 1988).

The extent of the association of depression and physical ill-health was shown by a study of 100 patients referred with depression to a psychogeriatric service over a 30-month period (Dover and McWilliam 1992). The authors found that only 3 per cent of the men and 20 per cent of the women patients were physically well. The rest had a variety of serious complaints including cancer, cardiovascular disease, arthritis, deafness and respiratory problems. Sixty-five per cent of the sample had 'multiple illnesses'. Moreover, many of the drug treatments for some of these physical disorders are known to cause or amplify depressed mood, suggesting an iatrogenic component in this group of depressed physically ill patients. The association of depression with physical illness in old age is highlighted by a recent review of several studies of medical (i.e. not psychiatric) inpatients which concludes that only one in five recover from their lowered mood state before death (Cole and Bellavance 1997). Suicide rates also increase in the older age group, and this is mainly accounted for by the high rates of male deaths.

What are the social implications of the data from psychiatric epidemiology of depression in older people? Starting with the very high rates of depression in residential homes, there are three explanations for these prevalence rates, which are not mutually exclusive:

1   It could be that those selected to enter these homes have been adjudged by relatives or professionals already to be in poor mental health, or vulnerable because of their lonely and under-supported home conditions (hence their referral to the homes).
2   The under-stimulating environment of these homes may induce apathy and morbid introspection (in the jargon of psychiatry, 'dysphoria'). This has led some psychiatrists of old age to speculate that the homes may contain a number of people who are not 'clinically depressed' but who, instead, suffer from environmentally induced dysphoria, which may dissipate with a more stimulating care regime (Pitt 1988). Such a construction on the data of course assumes that there are clear demarcations to be made between clinical descriptions of 'true' depression and other experiences, such as apathy, anomie, listlessness, sad brooding and so on. Some other psychogeriatricians have pointed out that, in fact, it is not easy in the bulk of cases of sad old people to pigeonhole them as being 'ill' or 'not ill' (Murphy 1988).
3   Being moved to a residential facility is disruptive, entails a loss of previous surroundings and may mark a loss of personal control or autonomy. This imposed disruption and loss may have a depressing toll on the old person.

Turning to the community data on depression in older age, there are other explanations that could be offered for depression in old people who are not in residential care.

1   The probability of physical illness increases with age, and this in turn makes older people vulnerable to depression (Post 1969). However, Blaxter (1990), studying the self-reported physical and mental well-being of people across the life-span, found that overall psychosocial well-being improves relatively in old age. This could be partially accounted for by the lower expectations of life quality in old age leading to an under-reporting of distress. Another factor is the dramatic improvement in the self-reported psychosocial well-being of richer people living in more comfortable surroundings (see below). An implication of the association of physical illness and depression is that good and effective physical care of depressed, poorer older people may have an ameliorative impact. Murphy (1988) suggests that the provision of aids for associated disability and other practical help to lessen the dependency of older physically ill people on their relatives may raise morale in the family system and thereby help lift depression.
2   Relationships that have accumulated during the life-span are lost. Spouses, friends and siblings die off around a surviving older person, making that person prone to the aggregating effect of grief. Depression in old age may be understandable in whole or part as cumulative grief.
3   Another social vulnerability factor is that of material adversity. In a community study of life events preceding depression in old age, Murphy (1982) found that poorer people who had experienced housing and financial difficulties were more prone to depression (of

both mild and severe proportions) than better-off older people. Blaxter (1990) found that the psycho-social well-being of older people varied significantly with social class. Social classes 1 and 2 improved with age overall but those in social classes 4 and 5 deteriorated. (For a discussion of class and other variables affecting social support see Wenger (1989).)

4   Another consideration is the role of supportive and confiding relationships. Lowenthal (1965) found, like Brown and Harris (1978) in their study of younger women, that the presence of a stable confiding relationship was a protective factor against depression in old age. She also found that those most vulnerable are old people who try to form relationships and fail, rather than people who have coped throughout life alone. Murphy (1982) found in her community survey that 30 per cent of those reporting the lack of a confiding relationship were depressed. Given that 70 per cent of this group was *not* depressed, a multi-factorial model of vulnerability and protective factors seems to be indicated (as with Brown and Harris (1978)).

5   A final factor to consider is that of abuse in old age. Eastman (1994) suggested that estimates of abused older people in the USA vary from 600,000 to over a million. As with the abuse of children, prevalence and incidence are difficult to investigate accurately, given that abusers will typically deny the act. When the abuse occurs at the hands of paid carers, their job is at stake, as well as their reputation. Estimates of elder abuse rates in Scandinavia vary from 8 per cent to 17 per cent of older victims across Denmark, Sweden and Finland. In one of the Swedish samples 12 per cent of relatives admitted violence (Hydle 1993). Some authors extend the notion of elder abuse to medical neglect and iatrogenic disease in hospitalized older people (Gorbien *et al.* 1992). They include here: poor skin care, poor infection control, failure to make accurate physical diagnoses, leaving frail elders to risk falls and inadequate dietary provision (as a cost-cutting method). The immediate and long-term negative psychological effects of abuse are difficult to ascertain. It is self-evident that sexual or emotional abuse or physical violence against, or neglect of, old people will not enhance their mental health. A complicating factor is that confused older people who suffer from dementia are prone to violence themselves at times which may trigger reactive aggression in some of their care-givers. In one study (Paveza *et al.* 1992) it was found that in the year following a diagnosis of Alzheimer's disease, 15.8 per cent of patients and 5.4 per cent of their carers were violent. Usually, age as a perpetrator risk factor for violence is linked to youth, but dementia raises the probability of violent acts in (one group) of older people.

Much of the work above takes a psychological or neuro-degenerative view about dementia. From a sociological perspective dementia as an ontological state can be viewed as a form of violence and destruction of the self. Davis (2004) points to the difficulty of the honesty this poses for providing dignified care for people suffering from dementia, and the inevitable consequences of mourning for the social death of a lost person by those closely involved with them. Informed by Heidegger, from a philosophical standpoint Davis identified the experience of dementia as one of 'what aspects of being change, or even disintegrate, as the existence of a person become subsumed by the dementia disease?' (2004: 373). Seen in this way, from a phenomenological perspective, the state of dementia becomes one of the 'fraying' of the self. 'Dementia effects the dismantling of the self until there is nothing left' (Davis 2004: 374). This has practical implications for the dominant approach to diagnosis and management based principally on cognitions. In line with Kitwood and Bredin (1992), part of the project about caring for people with dementia becomes one of how social processes contribute to the functional decline of the affected person through a 'malignant social psychology'. The ill-treatment and neglect of those with dementia is testimony to these processes, as evidenced by care scandals. A commitment to 'unique personhood' by Kitwood and Bredin, reversing the exclusion of the patient, based on defensive reactions held at an unconscious level and the socially debilitating obstacles created, is considered important now by those with this person-centred ethos to care. This is now shaping an ideal type of what dementia care should be.

Discussion

The sociological consideration of life-span and mental health is clearly uneven. At the start of life, socialization is considered to be important and there is certainly no shortage of interest in this arena of social determinism. Indeed, the consensus is very strong within social science that upbringing, acculturation and rule learning are all necessary considerations about societal functioning and the relationship between the individual and the collective. Admittedly, some have complained that this theorizing has been exaggerated (Wrong 1961) but, generally, primary socialization is given a privileged position in a variety of sociological (and psychological) theories. We noted at the start, though, that the sociological connection between primary socialization and mental health has been relatively under-scrutinized.

Psychoanalysis, a form of socialization theory itself derived from the psychological treatment of people with mental health problems, seems to have had a pervasive influence on different types of sociology. As far as childhood is concerned, sociological interest thus far has been theory-dominated. Despite this wide-ranging theoretical discourse about socialization, few sociologists have done empirical work on childhood and its problems (although there is the work of Finkelhor and Russell 1984) in the area of child sexual abuse and James and Prout (1990), who have studied 'normal' children).

The evidence of child sexual abuse we reviewed has, ironically, posed particular problems for clinical psychoanalysis. This theoretical framework, which has appealed so strongly to so many sociologists, has found itself accused of a central cultural role in suppressing evidence of the sexual abuse of children. This is because of Freud's reversal of his theory in 1896. Prior to then, Freud tended to believe women patients' recollections of incest from childhood. After that time, Freud succumbed to the more comforting notion that these represented subjective fantasies on the part of patients. This then became the accepted 'wisdom' when dealing with patient-reported abuse by Freud's clinical followers (Masson 1985).

When we turn to the core of psychiatry, interventions in young adulthood and beyond sociology became enmeshed with a social movement in the 1960s to challenge or discredit clinical theory and practice. Scheff's labelling theory (Scheff 1966) and Goffman's critique of the asylum (Goffman 1961) from within symbolic interactionism were associated with 'anti-psychiatry'. The retreat from this association with political activism and 'counter-culture' was then reflected in the sociology of mental health. The latter became more theoretical with the emergence of post-structuralist appraisals of psychiatric discourse. This was, in part, a reaction against the humanism and civil libertarianism that had been associated with anti-psychiatry. These post-1960s sociological approaches can be contrasted again historically with the earlier epidemiological tradition of the social causationists. The latter did not disappear from the map of the sociology of mental health, given the community survey approaches of, for instance, Brown and Harris and Murphy in the 1970s and 1980s.

The main sociological deductions about mental health problems in older people have, mostly, to be made from clinical researchers (social psychiatrists like Murphy). Consequently, harder data is considered from epidemiological surveys at the expense of sociological theorizing. While sociologists have theorized childhood extensively, but done little empirical work, they have done little in either realm as far as old people and their mental health problems are concerned. What theory does exist about later life has come from depth psychologists and has been poorly tested empirically (e.g. Erik Erikson's life-stage theory) or is from a position that emphatically privileges the individual over society (e.g. that of Carl Jung).

This relative history of an absence of sociological work on the mental health of older people may reflect a lesser-valued group of people who are consequently as readily ignored by sociologists as they are by other people of employable age. This leaves older people being studied in the main by clinicians or by those who have taken a particular interest in social policy rather than social theory (e.g. Walker 1980; Townsend 1981; Wenger 1989). 'Gerontology' as a hybrid academic discipline overlaps with, but is not a sub-discipline of, sociology. While sociologists have contributed substantially to gerontology (Fennell *et al.* 1988; Jefferys 1989) the specific issue of mental health remains largely absent from their ambit of interest.

Thus, there are three main questions for sociologists given the above summary. First, should they immerse themselves more in empirical research about childhood and mental health? Given that so many articles of faith have been linked to the theoretical assumptions of this period, for instance that the events of the formative years are predictive of adult personal functioning, sociologists could test their theoretical assumptions against longitudinal investigations. Second, will psychiatric professionals and their diagnostic and treatment activities be the continued focus of interest for the examination of adult mental health or will sociologists seek out new topics and dimensions of inquiry? Third, will sociologists be able to apply their liking for theorizing to the grey topic of older people, or will the latter continue to be scrutinized mainly by clinicians and social policy researchers?

This chapter has taken three periods in the life-span (childhood, young adulthood and old age) and examined their implications for mental health. The importance of socialization has been emphasized, and disputes about its meaning and relevance discussed. Adulthood brings with it expectations of role-rule consistency which mentally ill people challenge in their functioning. The social factors discussed in old age draw our attention to the importance of depression, not just dementia. They also highlight that ageism is present in sociological interest in mental health.

Questions

1 Why has the concept of primary socialization been so important in social science?
2 What is the relevance of primary socialization for adult mental health?
3 Discuss the impact of childhood sexual abuse on adult mental health.
4 What does the diagnosis of schizophrenia tell us about social norms?
5 What social factors influence the mental health of older people?
6 The sociology of mental health and illness is ageist – discuss.

For discussion

Think about your own family and others you know and consider the link between age and mental health within their relationships.

6 The organization of mental health work

Chapter overview

The organizational aspects of mental health work, where it takes place, as well as where and how people with mental health problems reside, are of major sociological importance. Between the mid-nineteenth century and the 1980s, the mental hospital as a total institution defined specialist mental health care. Since then 'decarceration' has been accompanied by the demise of the hospital as a place for the organization and delivery of mental health work, although reduced elements of inpatient care (sometimes on the actual sites of the old asylums) have remained.

In community settings, new ideologies about the intended outcome of patient management have accompanied changes in the organization and delivery of mental health work. Coercion and compulsory treatment was associated with the lunatic asylum and mental hospital; now that emphasis on compulsion has been limited to secure services and acute admissions but with some legal powers being extended into the community controversially. The philosophy of recovery (see Chapter 11) has generated a different discourse about the organization of work in a post-asylum world based more on therapeutic optimism and support for community living. As Sheppard *et al.* (2007: 6) note: 'The development of recovery-based services emphasizes the personal qualities of staff as much as their formal qualifications. It seeks to cultivate their capacity for hope, creativity, care, compassion, realism and resilience'. As well as this focus on recovery, recently there has also been a shift to public mental health policies and well-being (see Chapter 13). Thus the mental hospital is no longer the focus of most mental health work. The latter has entailed both community and primary care, as well as the residue of inpatient care to be found in acute units (typically now in most localities in district general hospitals (DGHs)). Consequently those involved now in mental health care as care staff or managers tend to think increasingly about the inter-connectedness of types of care and about notions such as 'clinical pathways' and 'enhanced' or 'stepped' care. Nonetheless the hospital still provides a historical benchmark from which new configurations and the organization of work have followed. Moreover, a socio-historical perspective reminds us that older tensions about the functioning of mental health care and the controversies surrounding it have not disappeared simply because large buildings have been destroyed and replaced by a range of smaller dispersed alternatives. Thus, this chapter will explore the changing organizational form of mental health work under the main headings signalled below.

This chapter will examine:

- the rise of the asylum and its legacy;
- the crisis of the asylum;
- responses to the crisis;
- community care and re-institutionalization
- primary care, open settings, ehealth and psychological therapies.

The rise of the asylum and its legacy

The structure and organization of the large nineteenth-century mental hospital did not fit the ideal type of the general hospital. Its architectural design and daily functions were organizationally incongruent in terms of therapy, structure and location. For example, while the general hospital was geographically located for easy access, many of the large Victorian asylums were deliberately built away from centres of populations. The lack of fit between institutional forms inspired by thinking in the nineteenth century and the 'new' twentieth-century norms regarding health care delivery led to a crisis within these organizations. This crisis formed the focus of a critique of the institution, which emanated from a number of sources.

The segregation of lunatics into large institutions took place over the final three centuries of the second millennium in Europe and North America. Psychiatric historians do not agree on the precise timing of this shift or on the exact explanation for its occurrence (Foucault 1965; Rothman 1971; Grob 1973; Scull 1979). Tracing the creation of large institutions can help us understand their demise but this involves the examination of competing historical claims.

A conventional and conservative account suggests that the asylum is viewed as part and parcel of medical progress and an increasingly humane way of dealing with 'mentally ill' people. For instance, Jones (1960) stresses the humanitarianism behind the reform movement leading to the Lunatics Act 1845. This Act compelled county authorities to establish asylums and enforced their regulation via a centralized Lunacy Commission and a system of medical records. Much of Jones's account centres around the official reports of Metropolitan Commissioners between 1828 and 1845 and the role of government-appointed bodies (such as Parliamentary Select Committees), which drew public attention to the poor state of workhouses and private madhouses. The establishment of early institutions modelled on the moral treatment regime of the York Retreat is described as arising from 'the consciousness felt by a small group of citizens of an overwhelming social evil in their midst' (Jones 1960: 40). In fact, moral treatment failed to transfer from the early charity hospitals like the Retreat to the state-run asylums, although its image dominated the rhetoric of asylum reformers (Donnelly 1983). Jones (1960: 149) sees the implementation of the 1845 Act in a humanitarian light: 'Ashley and his colleagues had roused the conscience of mid-Victorian society, and had set a new standard of public morality by which the care of the helpless and degraded classes of the community was to be seen as a social responsibility'.

Critical historians reject this more conventional account of events. The incarceration of mad people in asylums is seen as inextricably linked to the wider-scale containment of social deviancy: the poor in workhouses and criminals in prisons. The accounts of alternative histories vary. Scull (1979), a Marxist, suggested that mass confinement (of which the asylum system constituted an integral part) was a product of urbanization, industrialization and professional forces during the first half of the nineteenth century. The development of capitalism, with its demand for wage labour, meant that the existing means of poor relief was ill-equipped to deal with social deviance produced by the new market economy. Thus, the old outdoor system of relief in operation since the Elizabethan Poor Law was replaced by mass incarceration in institutions.

From the beginning of the nineteenth century a gradual process of segregation took place. Poor, able-bodied people (that is, those fit to work) were sent to workhouses, which were orientated towards instilling 'proper work habits'. These people were separated from those that could not work, which included those deemed insane and in need of incarceration in asylums. At the same time, ideas about madness were changing. It became recognized as a loss of self-control and not, as previously, a loss of humanity. These changing values were influenced by the exposure of the brutal treatment of those in madhouses. This encouraged the abandonment of mechanical restraints and it endorsed regimes such as the York Retreat.

These new social values permitted a greater willingness to accept a medical view of madness, the ascendance of which Scull attributes to the entrepreneurial leanings of medical practitioners, who were at the same time making efforts to professionalize and expand. Lucrative pickings were to be had by the profession trying to capture the madhouses previously run by laymen. Rather than having to attract patients to them, the asylum provided them with a ready-made and captive clientele.

Unlike Jones or Scull, Foucault (1965) does not concern himself with the specifics of the history of institutions. He views the Hôpital Générale at the end of the seventeenth century (where at one time 1 per cent of Paris's population who were 'incapable' of productive work was incarcerated) as symbolizing a new concept of madness. The spirit of capitalism, which Foucault traces from the Enlightenment onwards, promotes rationality, surveillance and discipline. Reason becomes separated from unreason. This separation out of unreason, whereby madness comes to be seen as the lack of the faculty of 'logos', is symbolized in the replacement of lepers by lunatics. The latter became the new 'race apart', and their confinement followed.

Critical histories therefore challenge self-congratulatory versions of history, which tend to mask the interests of powerful sections of society, such as the psychiatric profession and the central capitalist State. However, Rothman (1983) suggests that there are problems with critical, as well as conservative, histories because in both accounts 'conception triumphs over data'. According to Rothman, a focus on ideology, whether it is humanitarianism (Jones), capitalism (Scull) or surveillance (Foucault), can divert the historian's attention from the complex empirical reality of specific individual cases. For example Scull's emphasis on the economic, Rothman claims, is overstated. The early American system of asylums appeared in the absence of a market economy. Ideas about madness, he suggests, can be influenced by idiosyncratic factors other than those associated with a capitalist mode of production (for example ideals related to localized political activity and religious doctrine).

Sociologists in the 1960s were party to critical arguments about the dehumanizing effects of the asylum when the direction of mental health policy was clearly focused around whether or not to proceed with mass hospital closure. With the passage of time, when hospital closure and resettlement have become the norm, more recent sociologically informed commentary suggests that the history of the asylum is a contradictory one, particularly when seen in the context of the rise in new forms of surveillance, ways of dealing with psychiatric patients, and in a society which is arguably no more tolerant of psychiatric patients than previous generations.

Gittins's (1998) socio-historical analysis of a large psychiatric hospital in Essex, based on the biographical narratives of staff and patients who lived or worked in the hospital, suggests contradictions and paradoxes about the way the asylums were. In relation to women patients it is clear, for example, that the hospital, based as it was on men-only or women-only wards, constituted a 'women-only space' and true asylum in a social context in which there was little such space in external community life. Moreover, the hardships and restriction of asylum life need to be balanced against the external social, economic and political conditions during the heyday of the asylum, such as extreme poverty, unemployment and wars which affected people's abilities to cope with difficult material and personal situations. The ambiguous history of the asylum is captured by Gittins (1998), who argues that the asylum had some advantages of stability and patient protection, though its drawbacks were also not in doubt.

These different histories and interpretations point to the way in which accounts of psychiatric organizations are themselves socially constructed and influenced by the particular point in time in which they are written. We turn now to the processes underlying the dismantling of the asylum system. Again, competing explanations influenced by different perspectives and reading of events provides a complex and contested picture of the causes of hospital rundown and closure.

The asylum system was problematic from its inception. The ideals of 'moral treatment' were abandoned almost immediately. The system rapidly became overwhelmed by the numbers admitted with chronic conditions. Political pressures were encountered to keep costs down. Although the dominance of the institution began to wane from the 1930s onwards, with a gradual reduction in the number of asylum residents, it was not until the late 1950s and early 1960s that it was faced with a sustained analysis and critique. These criticisms will now be examined.

Ronald Laing, David Cooper, Franco Basaglia and Thomas Szasz were psychiatrists who challenged traditional professional theory and practice. (Collectively they were dubbed 'anti-psychiatrists', although only Cooper conceded the label.) They wanted to develop services for patients based on voluntary psychological approaches, and consequently they attacked current coercive, biological and institutional psychiatry. Goffman (1961), in his seminal work, *Asylums*, considered the mental hospital to be a 'total institution'. This he defined as a place of residence with a large number of people isolated from wider society, for lengthy periods of time, which runs according to an enclosed and formalized administrative regime. Goffman described four types of total institutions:

1   those which care for the incapable and 'harmless' (such as nursing homes and hospices);
2   those which provide for those who are perceived as an unwanted threat to the community (for example, sanatoriums for people who suffer from TB);
3   those which cater for the dangerous people where the welfare of the inmate is not paramount (for example prisons and prisoner of war camps);
4   those that are designed for people who voluntarily decide to retreat from the world, for instance for religious purposes (monasteries and convents).

The old asylums were examples of the second type of total institution. Secure psychiatric provision (medium-security units and high-security hospitals such as Ashworth and Broadmoor) are remaining examples. Model (or Weber's 'ideal type' of) total institutions possess a number of characteristics. All aspects of life are conducted in the same place. Activities always take place in the presence of others and are strictly timetabled and geared towards fulfilling the official aims of the institution rather than the needs of individuals. A strict demarcation exists between 'inmates' and staff.

The crisis of the asylum

On entering the mental hospital (the 'inpatient' phase of the patient's 'moral career') individuals underwent what Goffman called the 'mortification of self'. 'Self' is not used to refer to a personal attribute; instead it is conceptualized as being constructed by the pattern of social control which exists in an institution. The mortification of self occurred as a result of two stages. On entering the hospital a person was deprived of their previous identity through regimentation. This entailed stripping a person of their previous affirmation of self: movement was restricted, clothes worn on entry replaced with pyjamas or hospital-owned clothing, and personal belongings such as money and jewellery taken away. Goffman referred to this manner of entering the hospital as a 'degradation ceremony'. Once on the ward, inmates were invited to disown their former selves through a devaluing of past lives in 'confessionals' with staff and in-ward groups. Daily life on the ward was subjected to close and constant scrutiny, making privacy an impossibility.

Although Goffman's work was undertaken in an American context, similar analyses were being made of British mental hospitals. This British work was carried out by researchers who accepted psychiatric knowledge as being legitimate. Although their work was critical of custodial care, they need to be distinguished from the 'anti-psychiatrists' (whom Wing (1978) went on to attack). Moreover, their work is more empirical in its methodology than Goffman's study, whose work can be dismissed or queried as being theoretically elegant but weak on substantive evidence, beyond his own participant observations.

By contrast Wing (1962) drew attention to the social withdrawal and passivity of hospitalized patients, which could be correlated with length of stay and was independent of clinical condition (i.e. psychotic symptoms). Wing and Freudenberg (1961) demonstrated how such signs of institutionally induced apathy could be quite rapidly reversed if chronic patients were placed in a stimulating work environment. Brown (1959) and Brown and Wing (1962) demonstrated the severe effects of institutionalization and showed that sustained efforts by clinicians to reverse these effects could be demonstrated by comparing hospitals with custodial and more therapeutic policies. Nonetheless, the same pattern of withdrawal and apathy being correlated with length of stay was evident in all three hospitals. Brown and Wing cautioned that although enthusiastic medical leadership in the better hospitals could improve the functioning of chronic patients, these could be reversed by others later. Moreover, they commented: 'it is unlikely that the functions of an energetic reformer can be built in to the social structure of an institution' (1962: 169).

Scott (1973) highlighted the passivity and symptom-inducing effects of the mental hospital and its attendant illness model, which he viewed as forming a 'treatment barrier' between professional and client. Russell Barton's *Institutional Neurosis* (1959) is traceable to his observations of Nazi concentration camp inmates. Inmates surrounded by corpses and excreta refused to move from the huts they were living in. Their bizarre attachment was compounded by stereotypical pacing. Barton noted the similar stereotypical behaviour in the closed and unstimulating environment of 'backward' life in large mental hospitals after his return to civilian medicine in England.

This Anglo-American critique of the mental hospital from the 1960s was augmented by later work. Braginsky and colleagues (1973) found that acute patients wanted to leave hospital but that chronic patients took no interest in their clinical condition. Instead they found ways of remaining invisible to staff, while maximizing the comforts they could find in the hospital. These patients actively wanted to stay in hospital in preference to the uncertainties of poverty on the outside.

At the very time that the service-users' movement was emerging (see Chapter 12) and the large hospitals were on the brink of eventual collapse, Martin (1985) reviewed the failures of caring in British mental institutions between 1965 and 1983. During that period, ten inquiries of national significance took place into incidents and bad conditions within British mental illness and handicap hospitals. The problems forming the basis of complaints (which were often exposed by 'whistle-blowing' staff) ranged from inhumane, brutal and threatening behaviour by staff to lack of care through negligence and indifference.

Since the publication of Martin's work, mistreatment in large institutions continues to be exposed, for instance in Broadmoor and Ashworth Special Hospitals during the early 1990s. Thus his analysis is pertinent wherever the character of the total institution is retained. Recent accounts from Eastern Europe, where patients are sometimes kept in cages inside hospital wards indicate the contemporary relevance of critiques of hospital care from Goffman to Martin.

Two questions were posed by Martin: how do trained carers come to behave contrary to professional standards? And how have hospitals been arranged in such a way that abuse and neglect have not been prevented? Martin found that some other organizational goal (such as staff convenience or public safety) had implicitly usurped the goal of caring ('the subordination of care'). He also identified six types of isolation, which largely answered the second question. These were:

1   *Geographical isolation.* Most large institutions were situated out of main town centres, and even where they were not they were cut off from local communities.
2   *Immediate isolation.* Wards within hospitals were often isolated from one another and operated as little 'fiefdoms'. Martin found that it was only a small minority of wards within each hospital investigated which formed the basis of complaints.
3   *Personal isolation.* Individuals were left in charge of large numbers of difficult-to-manage patients. Untrained and isolated staff were often left to cope with unbearable conditions.

4   *Consultant isolation.* The worst wards were found to be those rarely visited by the responsible consultant, with everyday management being left to junior medical staff. Thus, professional abdication of responsibility and lack of leadership were important factors.

5   *Intellectual isolation.* There was a lack of professional stimulus, staff development and access to training opportunities.

6   *Privacy.* This was a prerequisite for abuse; patients who were regularly visited by relatives were not usually the focus of complaints.

The structural nature of this isolation led a number of social scientists to have a pessimistic stance towards the possibility of reforming the internal workings of large institutions. As we noted earlier, even those accepting the legitimacy of psychiatric theory and practice, such as Brown and Wing, questioned the reformability of psychiatric hospitals (even before the series of inquiries burgeoned after the mid-1960s). Whether or not all attempts at reform are futile is a moot point. However, what can be pointed out is that hospital scandals have continued where large hospitals exist – they are predictable sites of abuse and 'the corruption of care'.

Responses to the crisis

An early attempt to humanize the large impersonal isolated institutions was to introduce a more personal democratic approach to care. Therapeutic communities (TCs) – small units or wards designed to make the social environment the main therapeutic tool – were pioneered in Britain during the Second World War by psychotherapeutically orientated psychiatrists. The number of soldier patients suffering from the stress of warfare meant that the individual model of therapy became untenable because of scarce staff resources. These army psychiatrists were encouraged to experiment with a variety of group methods to increase staff cost-effectiveness. The twofold objectives looked for in therapeutic communities were identified by Main (1946) as the need to resocialize patients who had become dependent as a result of traditional hospital practices, and the use of the hospital environment as a therapeutic agent through establishing social participation. The latter was considered to be particularly valuable in treating people with neurotic conditions.

Later in civilian life, the TC approach was adapted more often to treat people with a diagnosis of personality disorder (Warren and Dolan 2001). The modification of the institution to form a TC has been reviewed sociologically by Manning (1989). These reviews focus on examples, such as the Henderson Hospital in Surrey, where the whole institution was involved. In other places a TC approach implemented piecemeal in a larger custodial setting tended to peter out. For example, the rapid turn-over of acute psychiatric units, with their 'revolving door' patients and bio-medical treatment regime, have tolerated the TC model poorly.

Inherent to the TC ideal was the belief that the social structure of the ward, group atmosphere and ward morale were important elements in the therapeutic endeavour of psychiatry. Central to these objectives was the need for rapid change in the organization of the hospital in order to make it more flexible and egalitarian. Attempts were made to break down the traditionally rigid and hierarchical role divisions between staff and patients, and decisions on the running of the TC were to be decided through group discussion. The latter measure was designed to promote communication between staff and patients.

Therapeutic communities developed rapidly during the 1960s, but soon after they became marginalized. Thus, their success in changing mainstream psychiatric theory and practice has been modest. The main weaknesses seem to stem from their organizational form. Perrow (1965) has pointed to the shortcomings of TCs as viable organizations. In particular he points to the failure to change fundamentally the social structure of the organization, which he traces to the failure of the TCs' 'technology' (or the means used for reaching the set goals).

The wider organization (the mental hospital), of which TCs formed only a small part, continued to operate custodial practices and the bureaucratic and professional structures remained relatively impervious to change. This limitation was clearly recognized in Italy, where TCs were seen as only a preliminary step towards the total dismantling of the asylum system, which came to be viewed as unreformable (Basaglia 1964).

The 'technology' for reaching the set goals of therapeutic communities was not enough to change a custodial culture and existing structures. In other words, the group work and social environment were not effective in changing sets of superordinate institutional relationships. Only one of Perrow's three conditions of organizational functioning was present and so the effectiveness and viability of TCs were undermined by the total institution. Certainly, the success of the TC, as an ideology or therapy, was limited in persuading British psychiatry to move away from a medical model, as indicated in an interview with Maxwell Jones, a pioneer of TCs, in 1984: 'For orthodox psychiatry it [the therapeutic community ideal] has provided a name to be wheeled out whenever it wants to defend Britain's reputation as the country which pioneered social psychiatry and to be conveniently forgotten otherwise' (*The Guardian*, August 1984).

A radical alternative to trying to humanize the institution was the run-down and ultimate closure of large mental hospitals. In the later part of the twentieth century many countries followed a policy of hospital run-down and closure, often referred to as 'deinstitutionalization'. The latter is also used interchangeably in some policy texts with the terms 'decarceration' or 'desegregation'. In 1954 there were 154,000 residents in British mental hospitals; by 1982 this had fallen to 100,000. In other countries the degree of deinstitutionalization has been even greater. For example, in Italy between 1968 and 1978 the asylum population fell from 100,000 to 50,000.

The various clinical and research critiques of institutional life may not have been influential in changing policy. Scull comments that the work of social scientists on the disabling and custodial function of the asylum was not accompanied by evidence of greater public tolerance towards emotional deviance. In some cases, as in the work of John Martin discussed earlier, social scientists were probably more witnesses to the crisis of the institution than participants in crisis resolution or policy reform.

The reasons thought to be responsible for deinstitutionalization are multiple and contested, and implicate a complex set of inter-relationships between the medical profession, public morality, the State and political economy. A number of different accounts have been offered for deinstitutionalization policies, which we will consider in turn.

The 'pharmacological revolution'

The 'pharmacological revolution' is a frequently cited explanation for hospital run-down. Simply put, it suggests that advances in medical treatment of mental illness permitted patients to be discharged from institutions en masse. According to this view of change, the introduction of major tranquillizers in particular enabled the alleviation of symptoms in psychotic patients, allowing large numbers of asylum residents to move into the community. Its explanatory power is still expressed in recent respectable psychiatric textbooks. For example:

> The introduction of chlorpromazine in 1952 made it easier to manage disturbed behaviour, and therefore easier to open wards that had been locked, to engage patients in social activities, and to discharge some of them into the community . . .
>
> (Gelder *et al.* 2001: 769)

This account of deinstitutionalization generates both theoretical and empirical difficulties. For example, it cannot explain why community care policies were applied to a range of care groups, such as people with learning disabilities and older people, who are not psychotic. They are not, therefore, the supposed target of 'antipsychotic' medication. However, in later years at times the

Table 6.1   Post-war growth of psychiatric beds in Europe

Country	Year	No. psychiatric beds
Belgium	1951	19,841
	1970	26,553
Austria	1950	9,868
	1975	14,314
Italy	1954	88,241
	1961	113,040
Spain	1949	25,571
	1974	42,493
Federal German Republic	1953	86,640
	1975	112,791

Source: Adapted from World Health Organization Statistics Annuals

true role of these drugs as tranquillizers to suppress difficult behaviour showed through in their (mis)use with non-psychiatric patients, such as agitated older people and difficult-to-manage people with learning disabilities.

More importantly, a number of studies demonstrate that an increased pattern of discharges occurred prior to the widespread use of major tranquillizers. Nor did the introduction of psychotropic drugs appear to accelerate the rate of discharges. The pattern of the fall remained consistent with that preceding their widespread use. In a few countries inpatient numbers actually rose after the introduction of chlorpromazine (see Table 6.1).

The notion that medical intervention was principally responsible for 'decarceration' may have been deduced from a reading of the official statistics produced on mental hospital inmates of the time. However, Scull (1977: 83) points out that a reading of these sources of data may have led to erroneous interpretations being made, since they mask 'earlier changes at the local level and obscure the degree to which the fall in overall numbers, when it did come, represents a continuation rather than a departure from pre-existing trends'.

Thus, according to Scull, while psychotropic medication has helped manage deviance following deinstitutionalization (through the control rather than permanent alleviation of symptoms), it was not responsible for the genesis of this policy. The retention of the unfounded claim of a 'pharmacological revolution' in later texts, such as Gelder and colleagues', points up professional interest work in the preferred depiction of mental health policy history.

Other analyses of data sources indicate that organizational factors and social policy initiatives are responsible for changes in the location of psychiatric practice. Table 6.1 shows the growth in the number of psychiatric beds in a number of European countries following the Second World War, which ran counter to run-down in the UK and the USA. While the type of increased bed use varied from one country to another (in some it was short-term beds, in others new specialist facilities) the point is that inpatient care increased during a time when the major tranquillizers were widely and increasingly utilized.

'Economic determinism'

This is an alternative explanation for 'decarceration', by Scull (1977). He uses the term to describe the 'state-sponsored policy of closing down asylums' (1977: 1), which he relates to changes in social control mechanisms. Scull contends that, with the emergence of the welfare state, segregative control mechanisms became too costly and difficult to justify. The cost inflation of mental hospitals prior to, and after, the Second World War was brought about by the elimination of unpaid patient labour and increased cost of employees as a result of the unionization of labour. The latter had the effect of contributing to the doubling of unit costs (because of the cost of a shorter working day and holiday entitlement).

Thus the maintenance of ex-patients on welfare payments and the 'neglecting' of community care becomes a more viable State policy. The reality of community habitation for ex-inmates, according to Scull, has been an unmitigated disaster for the majority. The inhumanity of the asylum has simply been replaced by the negligence of the community.

A problem with Scull's account is that it is more applicable to the 1980s, when fiscal savings were undoubtedly the driver for changes in social policy in relation to a range of patients with long-term conditions. The fiscal crisis of the State thesis fits less readily, though, with the immediate post-war period when he claims deinstitutionalization started. However, although the time frame is wrong, there is certainly evidence that the driver of fiscal savings eventually found its time, at least as a partial explanation for hospital run-down.

Changes in the organization of medicine: a shift to acute problems and primary care

The history of the large hospitals was bound up with the warehousing of chronic madness. However, during the twentieth century the ambit of psychiatry changed in a number of ways. By the end of that century mental health services also dealt with a range of other problems, such as neurosis, personality disorder and substance misuse. The shift had been occurring since the First World War when male neurosis (in the form of shellshock) entered centre stage. Also, a professional norm developed within psychiatry about the need to treat acute psychosis (with two-thirds of patients being deemed to recover permanently or have their symptoms eliminated until another acute episode).

The rhetoric of the 'pharmacological revolution' described earlier boosted this change in professional attention. Specious curative descriptions began to emerge in medicine such as 'antipsychotic' and 'antidepressant' medication. There was a focus on acute, not chronic, problems and the development of acute psychiatric units in DGHs, with a limited number of beds (Baruch and Treacher 1978). This move aligned psychiatry with other medical specialties. In other words the desegregation was primarily of psychiatrists, to boost their medical respectability.

At the same time, it was becoming evident that conditions such as 'depression' (the 'common cold of psychiatry at once familiar and mysterious' (Seligman 1975)) and 'anxiety' could be contained in primary care. The great majority of patients with these 'common mental disorders' either did not seek help or were treated only by GPs, an arrangement still applicable today (Goldberg and Huxley 1980). Thus the remaining picture is that the bulk of people deemed to have mental health problems never access specialist services.

This change in the character of the medical framing of emotional deviance has been emphasized by some social constructivist analysts such as Prior (1991), who avoids both economic and technological determinism. Rather than attempting to identify causal mechanisms, his aim is to describe the object, ideology and organizational arrangements which constitute contemporary psychiatry. Prior argues that the target of psychiatric practice changes over time. Each new object is accompanied by a different type of clinical practice and organizational setting. For example, the nineteenth-century view of madness took, as its focus, the brain and forms of degeneracy, which demanded exclusion and control in the asylum. In contrast, the concepts of 'psyche' and 'the unconscious' in Freudian theory centred around the concept of 'mind'. The rising popularity of psychoanalytically informed ideas also started to cloud the distinction between normal and pathological behaviour which, according to Ramon (1985), helped destigmatize mental illness.

These new ideas required a socio-medical organization conducive to intimate therapeutic encounters between individual client and therapist. Prior argues that the lack of fit between modern psychiatric theories of the mind and madness necessitated the organizational change described as 'deinstitutionalization'. Prior perceives the 'therapeutics of mental illness at the end of the asylum age' as being widely dispersed. There is dual responsibility for mental health between medical and social services. The latter focus on aspects of patients' lives, such as 'social networks', employment and family relationships, the former are subdivided between nursing and medical input. Medical input takes as its focus the physical characteristics of the patient, diagnosis and physical therapies such as ECT and psychotropic drugs. The object of focus, for nursing in particular, centres around improving patient behaviour. However, such a focus on behaviour is not compatible with a hospital milieu since, by definition, it necessitates the patient's contact with society, both to test the patient's behavioural competence and to extend their behavioural repertoire. The attendant therapeutic endeavours, which centre around such things as the 'normalization' of behaviour and the building of social networks, thus require a community environment rendering the hospital 'functionless'.

Prior's analysis avoids the assumptions inherent in the economic interest argument of Scull and the pharmacological revolution position of official accounts. However, a set of empirical questions which are important in assessing the merits of the different theoretical positions that have emerged around deinstitutionalization remain unanswered. For example, although there has been an expansion of psychodynamically informed therapies and a greater focus on the social relationships of patients, it is a moot point whether a bio-medical hospital-centred psychiatric practice has actually been replaced with extra-hospital activities. More recently the psychological approach to care has expanded but not by the extension of psychodynamic models; cognitive-behavioural approaches are the new orthodoxy (see Chapter 8).

Community care and re-institutionalization

With a number of years passing now since the decarceration of chronic patients, there is evidence that relocation has positive outcomes for individuals in some service settings. In Italy, for example, where there has been a careful tracking of post-institutional careers, a recent study has shown the way in which a population characterized by a long history of illness and severe disability underwent a radical change in care setting and living arrangements with favourable outcomes (Barbato *et al.* 2004). In particular, this has been indicated by the absence of adverse events or clinical deterioration and by some improvement in social behaviour. The results confirm that most patients with long-term mental health problems can successfully leave psychiatric hospitals and live in community residences.

There remains substantial confusion surrounding the meaning of the term 'community care', which reflects a lack of clarity over the ultimate goals of such a policy. In practice, community care currently refers to mentally disordered people receiving 'care' in non-asylum settings. For example, the district general hospital psychiatric units in Britain noted above are considered to be part of community care (a back-up facility when those in community settings develop acute difficulties).

While no country has created a mental health care system that can function without 'acute' psychiatric wards for the admission of people with mental health problems, some countries, such as Italy, show that it is possible to minimize their use. However, this remains the exception rather than the rule. Generally, the acute psychiatric ward environment does not generate mental health gain. A census of standards on these wards at the end of the 1990s indicated that most were 'non therapeutic' (Sainsbury 1998). MIND, Britain's largest mental health charity, had a 'Ward Watch' policy to track conditions on these wards. Indeed, there is an emerging picture similar to the one about the old Victorian asylums: it may be that acute hospital units are inherently unable to provide a therapeutic culture (Quirk and Lelliott 2001). The reasons for this are multiple and similar, but not identical, to why their large predecessors failed as care environments (though they succeeded as sites of permanent or semi-permanent segregation – a form of apartheid determined by mental state):

- Because acute units retained a bio-medical emphasis they maintained the spurious illusion, pointed out in Goffman's final essay in *Asylums* (1961) that they can act as a breakdown services, like a repair garage. (A problem is brought in, fixed and then sent out mended.) In fact, the technological emphasis on medication does not provide this repair service because, despite their curative titles, psychiatric medications only control symptoms in some people some of the time. They do not cure the conditions diagnosed by psychiatrists. Even if they did, psychiatric drugs logically should work independently of setting – after all, most community-based patients are already medicated. When admission is effected to enforce poor compliance with medication, then once more the aversive aspects of coercion are experienced by patients.
- Acute units are charged with a coercive control role. The majority of patients are detained compulsorily or are aware of compulsion being invoked. This culture of compulsion is a poor starting point for active collaboration in change for patients.
- The increased risk associated with 'co-morbidity', especially psychotic patients who abuse substances, means that the limited bed capacity in acute units has been increasingly reserved for patients who are mainly there because of their assessed risk to others. In other words, acute units implicitly serve the interests of third parties and so are not able to be 'patient centred'.
- The presence of raised levels of risky behaviour in small mixed ward environments has led to physical and sexual assaults (on both patients and staff). On-site substance misuse has brought with it an illicit cultural network of non-patients bringing alcohol and illegal drugs into the ward environment. The control of substance misuse on site has necessarily become an organizational priority for the staff. With this comes a distrustful surveillance role in relation to patients; an anti-therapeutic process.
- Staff tend to withdraw into their own space (the nursing office) and potential therapeutic staff–patient contact diminishes. The patient experience of this milieu is one of oscillating anxiety and boredom. These emotional states are not conducive to personal change or mental health gain.
- Like the old asylums the acute units are isolated from their community context. Baruch and Treacher (1978: 223) describe this in their early case study:

  > staff members were effectively 'institutionalized' – they rarely made domiciliary visits to their patients and they were not involved in the communities from which their patients came, so they could never develop an understanding of the patients' way of life or devise methods for using community resources to help the patients.

- Since these early comments from Baruch and Treacher, other studies have confirmed the problems for staff of creating a therapeutic milieu in acute units. Medication still predominates and psychological interventions remain scarce (Lelliott and Quirk 2004). Staff morale remains low and patient dissatisfaction high (Norton 2004). (Indeed, consultation exercises about mental health care tend to elicit user responses, which often focus narrowly on complaints about inpatient regimes, even though the latter are not the only form of care now on offer in our post-institutional context.)

If these 'non-therapeutic' acute units are the back-stop for non-hospital services, what are the latter? Community care is constituted by a variety of activities and services. The main initiatives evident since the early 1990s include psychiatric services in primary health care settings, the expanded use of community psychiatric nurses, the development of community mental health centres, the provision of domiciliary services, the development of residential and day care facilities, an increased emphasis of voluntary services and informal care by relatives and friends, and the relocation of mental health responsibilities from the secondary care sector to primary care.

There was a rapid development of certain community resources as the asylums were run down. For example, between 1977 and 1987 Community Mental Health Centres (CMHCs) in Britain expanded from 1 to 54 (Sayce 1989). Psychiatric services delivered via primary care were another area of expansion. However, it would be misleading to exaggerate the extent of re-provision from hospital-based services to the community. Mental health provision in Britain is no longer largely hospital-based. In the USA, where a longer period has elapsed since the Community Mental Health Act 1963 than since the British National Health Service (NHS) and Community Care Act of 1990, the old, large State asylums have simply been replaced by a network of smaller, private inpatient facilities. Even in the USA, Community Mental Health Centres were forced under fiscal pressure to shift to a custodial role (Samson 1992).

Samson insists that the USA has never had proper community care but that instead a variety of economic and professional pressures have ensured a policy of re-institutionalization. Consequently, he argues that those who attack the 'failure' of community care policies are actually attacking a straw man, given that what has actually happened is deinstitutionalization followed by re-institutionalization.

In Britain, the theory of community living has often been replaced by the practice of deinstitutionalization. The political objective of community care was first mentioned in the Mental Treatment Act 1930 and, by the 1970s, there was a bipartisan political goal of transferring people out of institutions. Yet, it was only in 1985 that the first British mental hospital actually closed.

By the late 1980s, 85 per cent of resources spent on mental health by the State were still bound up with hospitals (Sayce 1989). Data supplied by the Department of Health in 1992 showed both numerical losses and gains to hospital-based psychiatry. Although the number of psychiatric beds decreased from 193,000 in 1959 to 108,000 in 1985, by 1985 there had been a rise in the number of small psychiatric hospital facilities from 303 to 492. And even though hospital resident numbers dropped by 24 per cent between 1980 and 1990, psychiatric facilities still contained 36 per cent of all hospital beds by the latter year. In 1990 there were more than 50,000 psychiatric inpatients in England alone, at any one time. Moreover, despite a steady decline in the number of people occupying hospital beds since the 1960s, short-stay admissions rose dramatically, creating 'revolving-door' hospital care, rather than fully fledged care in the community.

By 2000 there were just over 100,000 admissions to English psychiatric units, and there was a continuation of this decline in the first decade of the twenty-first century. However, an indication of the rapid throughput was that only 3.2 per cent stayed for longer than 90 days. Less than 1 per cent stayed for more than 1 year (Thompson et al. 2004). At the same time, these quick turnover units nearly always operate at 100 per cent bed occupancy. They are unable to provide either the stable place of residence offered by the old asylums or the continuity span required for a therapeutic community approach to be effective.

Despite the growth in the popularity of CMHCs as ideals at a local level (Sayce (1989) found that even in localities where there were no centres, policy-makers thought they should have one), they have remained on the margins of community care and almost disappeared in the twenty-first century. They were often established in the face of opposition from conservative forces within the psychiatric profession (Goldie et al. 1989) and were not included in official government plans for replacing asylum beds, as they were, for example, in Italy. As new services they were subjected to greater scrutiny and evaluations than hospital-based services. New day places to replace hospital beds were not only slow in coming (between 1975 and 1985 only 9000 new places were made available (Audit Commission 1986)), they were overwhelmingly placed on hospital sites. Similarly, although there was a decrease in the number of inpatients, as outpatients they still attended hospital premises for their appointments. Domiciliary services – the visiting of people in their own homes by mental health professionals – today constitutes only a tiny proportion of this total.

A health economic review of spending on mental health services (Sainsbury 2003) indicated a strong inertia about resources being bound up with hospital-based activity. Government spending was increased after 2000, in order to expand mental health services, but the report concluded that this intention was unlikely to be successful. Although mental health is designated as a priority in health policy, proportionally the growth in expenditure on it, compared to other forms of State spending, has been slower. As a result, in proportional terms, the share allocated by the local State to mental health services continued to fall. Also there was slow progress in the timetable to implement the National Service Framework for Mental Health (Department of Health/Home Office 1999).

Another factor indicating that mental health services continue to have a 'Cinderella' status relates to the range of peculiar costs or budgetary pressures experienced by them. These include debt repayment, staff shortages (which lead to expensive short-term agency payments) and the increasing prescribing costs associated with the introduction of new and expensive psychotropic medications.

A look at the breakdown of spending on mental health services reveals socio-political priorities. For example, Table 6.2 indicates that there is a socio-political emphasis on social control (the combined items on acute facilities, secure provision and mentally disordered offenders). These

Table 6.2 Service expenditure 2002/03

	Per cent
Community mental health terms	17.2
Access and crisis services	6.6
Clinical services including acute inpatient care	24.6
Secure and high-dependency provision	12.3
Continuing care	12.2
Services for mentally disordered offenders	1.1
Other community and hospital professional teams/specialists	1.6
Psychological therapy services	4.6
Home support services	2.1
Day services	5.3
Support services	1.5
Services for carers	0.3
Accommodation	10.3
Mental health promotion	0.1
Direct payments	0.1
Total direct costs	100.0

Source: Sainsbury (2003)

items account for nearly 40 per cent of government spending on mental health services. This can be compared with the amount spent on mental health promotion – a mere 0.1 per cent. Psychological therapy services only received 4.6 per cent of spending (suggesting a bio-medical inertia in the mental health care system). Other non-hospital-based services, which are meant to signal a service reconfiguration towards community-based interventions, lagged behind the political rhetoric of the chapter on mental health in the NHS Plan (Department of Health 2000). Between them the items on new assertive outreach, crisis resolution, early intervention and services for carers accounted for less than 7 per cent of spending.

A final consideration about the problem of re-institutionalization and the inertia of hospital-oriented State funding is the interaction of political interests which have impeded shifts to ordinary living and fuller citizenship for people with mental health problems. The old asylums were a total solution for the social problems associated with mental abnormality. In particular, they provided three main functions:

- semi-permanent or permanent accommodation;
- treatment;
- social control.

All of these functions occurred concurrently in one institution. Whatever disadvantages the old asylum system had for their inmates (by creating a form of disabling apartheid) as well as advantages (see comments from Gittins (1998) earlier), the socio-political benefit for others was that a group of non-conformist, troublesome, worrisome and economically inefficient people was segregated. Mental abnormality was swept away or 'warehoused' out of the sight and mind of the majority of free citizens. The consequences of demolishing these warehouses were thus obvious. The three functions would still be required by society for both economic efficiency and the maintenance of a moral order, but now they would have to be reconfigured or reconstructed.

This political challenge had tempted cautious politicians to hold on to revised forms of institutional care and encouraged them with new forms of legal measures to ensure the coercive control of community-based patients (see Chapter 10). In addition, the new context of acute units acted to provide the psychiatric profession with an opportunity to retain its traditional preferred link between power and beds. Moreover, the shift to DGH inpatient units was also an opportunity to increase the professional standing of a low-status medical specialty. Families troubled by patients in their midst would also look to new forms of safe residential disposal. Thus, a confluence of interests emerged in the final quarter of the twentieth century to retain a hospital focus to mental health work, despite the run-down of the asylum system. However, this has placed unrealistic expectations upon DGH units.

The interest groups just described have become immediately aggrieved about the inefficiency of the units compared to the old asylums, as the shift in scale means that the new units cannot replicate all the functions of the old hospitals. This has led to diverse demands in response; some of these centred on requests for more beds (from psychiatrists and patient-relative pressure groups) or calls for a halt to the run-down of the old asylums. There were also demands for greater community support to reduce the need for admission (from user groups).

It can be seen then that the prioritizing of control, professional preferences to treat in inpatient settings and the continued need for people with mental health problems to be accommodated together place pressure upon smaller-scale hospital facilities. This pressure created such political anxiety in the mid-1990s that in the short term Britain ministers opted to slow asylum run-down and keep high investment levels in beds. In response, critics argued that the three functions noted above should be dealt with as separate policy questions: accommodation implies social housing not hospitalization; treatment needs to be cost-effective and its appropriate siting clarified; and risk management should be dealt with rationally, not prejudicially (Pilgrim and Rogers 1997).

The macro policy context together with the micro behaviour of professionals making and dealing with mental health referrals determine the pace and success of community care. A comparison of community-based care for those patients with a diagnosis of schizophrenia in Verona and South Manchester indicated that the organization of services in the former resulted in shorter hospital stays as a result of better integration between hospital and community services (Gater *et al.* 1995).

Primary care, open settings, ehealth and psychological therapies: a new focus of mental health work

With the fragmentation of old structures like the asylums there has been greater attention paid to considering the cause and solution of mental health problems within a public health context. Previously, psychiatric epidemiology and the treatment of mental disorders were separated conceptually. With the rise of a 'new' public health, which integrates lay with traditional epidemiology, and the emergence of a strong primary health care agenda, epidemiology and treatment have come closer together as the hospital disappears as the symbolic focus of treatment for mental health problems. Attention shifts instead to inequalities in mental health (discussed in Chapter 13 on public health), prevention and the notion of 'positive mental health'. Alongside this within mental health policy, problem management stretches beyond the structural and organizational arrangements of traditional health services.

The policy response to mental health problems here implicates local and central players, community resources, the environment and individual action. Thus, the focus has moved to incorporate aspects of employment, social, community and voluntary organizations in the prevention and management of mental health problems. Within this scheme where service contact is needed, primary care is privileged over specialist mental health services. That is, the optimal service response is cast in settings which are as close as possible to the place where the genesis of mental health problems originate and are expressed.

The picture above suggests gradually changing mental health services since the 1990s. We have had a 'hotch potch' of community services, some of which like the CMHCs have had a short life, and a cautious conservative approach of experimentation with various forms of re-institutionalization. This shift has been influenced by attempts to reverse the Cinderella status in mental health. The first relates to the burgeoning of research activity in the mental health field in the area particularly of primary care and health services research. The proliferation of the use of new forms of mental health services is likely to be reinforced by the cultural shift towards the acceptance of evidence-based health care (discussed in Chapter 8).

This has particularly been the case for the management of depression but has also extended into the management of 'severe and enduring mental health problems'. Research on services has resulted in greater attention being given to the efficiency of service organization and pointed up the fact that many patients receive less than optimal care because of organizational barriers to co-ordinated care between primary and secondary care professionals.

A review of organizational intervention studies (Gilbody *et al.* 2003) found that effective interventions were multi-faceted, involving a combination of screening, professional and patient education, consultation-liaison between primary and secondary care clinicians, and, of most importance, case management. Case management situated within what has been termed a 'collaborative care framework' became the basis of policy and practice promoted by the guidance issued by the National Institute for Clinical Excellence as 'enhanced care for depression' (ECD). A case manager is a mental health worker with a remit to provide care within a 'collaborative care' model, where they work directly with patients, but also with other professionals responsible for their care, such as a GP or community psychiatric nurse, to ensure co-ordinated and structured care. Collaborative care when in operation now involves three elements:

- planned, proactive, regular contact between a case manager and patient;
- advice and guidance about treatment modalities (e.g. medication, problem solving or CBT);
- regular feedback of information on the treatment process from mental health professionals involved in the care.

New technologies and information systems have enabled new modes of organizing mental health work to emerge. The widespread availability of information technology, together with the community location of the overwhelming majority of patients, has changed the face of how mental health services are organized and delivered. For example, telephone counselling from a primary care base for patients with 'minor depression' has been found to be both efficient and effective (Lynch *et al.* 1997), as has psychiatric assessment over the telephone (Kobak 1997). Remote treatment of depression by 'telepsychiatry' has been shown to be as effective as face-to-face therapy (Ruskin *et al.* 2004). This change, in turn, is likely to dramatically alter the power relationships between providers and recipients of mental health services. More recent interventions, such as integrating mobile-phone-based assessment for psychosis, requires the active involvement of users in operationalizing the technology and controlling what happens with data used for monitoring symptoms which were previously the preserve of mental health professionals (Palmier-Claus *et al.* 2013).

The ambiguous legitimacy that mental health care professionals hold in the eyes of users is reinforced by research that evaluates the outcomes of services organized along these new lines. A randomized controlled trial compared face-to-face meetings with professionals and another group who used an electronic self-help computer programme in the form of a 'voice bulletin board'. Clients were found to be eight times more likely to participate in the computerized programme and were more satisfied than the group receiving face-to-face contact (Alemi *et al.* 1996).

Professionals' use of computer packages and the fashion for 'stepped' and collaborative care takes mental health care out of any one organizational context and introduces new problems in terms of the surveillance and 'follow-up' of patients. An aspect of this challenge that has become the focus of professional and academic interest is the notion of 'continuity of care'. A combination of assertive community treatment, case management, community mental health teams and crisis intervention has been found to reduce the likelihood of patients dropping out of contact with services (Crawford *et al.* 2004).

The Internet and computer-based programmes, by simplifying communication and being readily accessible directly to people, have the potential to 'cut out' professionals altogether from the care process. This also overcomes the problems caused by geographical location and variable personal quality (mechanical responses can be standardized). It is likely that the use of the Internet directly empowers users of mental health services by allowing them to feel in control of their treatment and everyday life more generally. (The issue of users as providers of care is returned to in Chapter 11.) Equally, if not more, important is the rapid increase in mutual non-professional support. The social isolation and 'poverty' of social networks have been a recurrent theme in the literature on people with long-term health problems.

One of the most important consequences of the technologies is the rapid increase they allow in mutual non-professional support. The anonymous helper in an electronic conference, or the support group on the Internet, provides the basis of a radical shift in mental health support. This has emerged as an unpredicted and major force in the global organization of mental health care.

The increasing shift from secondary to primary care and then into open setting, which started with deinstitutionalization policies and has accelerated since then, has meant an alteration in the place of the administration of treatment. This changes the range, nature and extent of what is provided. The introduction of primary care administered treatment by mental health workers, for example, has led to a reduction in primary care consultations, the prescribing of psychotropic drugs, greater recognition of the psychological bases of 'medically unexplained symptoms' (Peters *et al.* 2009) and referrals for treatment elsewhere. It has also, increased psycho-social interventions to patients in primary care.

Beyond a recognition of the changing administration of treatments, the notion of 'therapeutic landscape' has implicitly assumed a more central place in the discourse of treatment of mental health and well-being. In a general sense the notion refers to 'places, settings, situations, locales, and milieus that encompass both the physical and psychological environments associated with treatment or healing, and the maintenance of health and well-being' (Williams 1998: 129). Therapeutic landscapes focus on the importance of places for maintaining physical, emotional, mental and spiritual health, and link with holistic and alternative therapies and ideologies. This conveys a positive sense of place and the intrinsic therapeutic value of activities and environments outside of traditional mental health services. For example, in many localities gardening may be an important source of psychological well-being. The humanistic ideology of the notion of the therapeutic landscape concept has been turned on its head by reference to the notion of the anti-therapeutic environment and treatment of people with mental health problems in prison settings (Bowen *et al.* 2009).

There has been a gradual diversification away from hospitals as the single site of delivery. Mental health trusts and newly emergent local forms of commissioning and governance have been responsible for facilitating centrally directed policy implementation designed to improve the quality of care and patients' experiences by developing the capacity and skills of local mental health services based more on a networked approach of providing services according to function, population group and severity (see Figure 6.1).

Quality improvement programmes have more recently aspired to include organizations that lie beyond the hospital: health education and social services together with the independent sector and community organizations. However, mental health service organizations are relatively intransigent, with evaluations showing little demonstrable improvements in the quality of the services delivered (Beecham *et al.* 2010).

Discussion

The old mental asylum system can be thought of as representing part of the modernist project, although other forms of total institution, like the monastery, stretch back to feudal times. But while the monastery was guided by theological considerations, the asylum was peculiarly modern because rationality was its guiding organizational principle. Reason, not faith, now permeated the total institution. The pursuit of rational scientific knowledge about lunacy became the aim of modern psychiatry, even when such an aim was rhetorical rather than real. Accordingly, the elimination of mental disease was seen as a possibility, through its systematic organization and treatment in purpose-built institutions designed to segregate embodied irrationality from everyday life. There was no longer what Foucault called a 'dialogue between reason and unreason'; rather, the latter was trapped and codified by the former.

This Victorian project is now largely over (save relics of the psychiatric total institution like the high-security hospitals). The crisis of the asylum emerged not only because of considerations of cost but also because of changes in the discourse about mental abnormality and its treatment, in both the lay and professional areas. Earlier we summarized the expansion of the ambit of psychiatry after the First World War, and Prior (1991) argues for a more recent flux in psychiatric theory

---

Organization of statutory mental health services in the UK

Mental health trusts: inpatient, community, rehabilitation, residential care services and drop-in centres.

Community mental health teams: day-to-day support with the aim of assisting a person to remain living in the community.

Crisis resolution teams: management of people experiencing acute mental health crisis (e.g. suicide attempt, psychotic episode) and prevention of hospitalization. These operate on a 24-hour basis, have close links to the accident and emergency department, and are responsible for planning after-care aimed at prevention of future crises.

Assertive outreach teams: work with people with a history of service use who are no longer in regular contact with mental health services. They also work with agencies to locate people thought to be at risk and will sometimes seek to use compulsory management (e.g. sectioning under the Mental Health Act).

Early intervention in psychosis teams: the early intervention in psychosis team (EIPT) is designed to work with people aged between 18 and 35 who have experienced, or are at risk of experiencing an episode of psychosis. The team undertakes detection, assessment support and counselling.

Forensic mental health services: focus on people who have mental health conditions and who have committed a criminal offence or are at high risk of committing an offence. This involves incarceration in secure provision hospitals and prisons.

Services for children and young people: organized around four tiers:

Tier 1 – brief treatment for 'minor' problems and assessment for eligibility to specialist services by GPs, school nurses, teachers, social workers, youth justice workers and voluntary agencies.

Tier 2 – assessment and interventions for children and young people with more severe or complex needs. Services provided by community mental health nurses, psychologists and counsellors.

Tier 3 – services for severe, complex and persistent mental health conditions, bi-polar disorder and schizophrenia.

Tier 4 – specialist services for children and young people with the most serious problems (violent behaviour, a serious and life-threatening eating disorder, or history of physical and/or sexual abuse).

Figure 6.1   Diversification of care: place and function.

and practice. The asylum could not adapt to these changes and so its therapeutic legitimacy edged more and more towards crisis – but what of the asylum's replacements?

We have discussed two British responses: CMHC and DGH units. This divided response suggests that both continuity with Victorian modernism and a post-modern break have taken place, as far as the organization of mental health work is concerned. The CMHC is consistent with a definition here by Clegg (1990: 53) of post-modern organizations: forms of emerging organization that bear little or no relation to modernist variations on the theme of bureaucracy. These organizations are 'dedifferentiated': flexible, niche marketed and with a multi-skilled workforce held together by information technology, networks and subcontracting.

The emergence of the CMHC seemed to confirm the notion that mental health care delivery is moving into a different era. In this organizational context, role-blurring removes the strict division of labour typical of the hospital. The key worker system and multi-disciplinary working brings with it genericism and an increased individual responsibility for practitioners.

Outreach work with clients decentralizes or diffuses the locus of power away from the professionals' organizational base. Even that base has lost its architectural salience compared with the hospital: the more successfully 'normalized' it is the more it looks like an ordinary house. The knowledge base used by the professionals is eclectic (incorporating biological, psychological and social notions).

This picture of diversity and eclecticism in the CMHC no longer squares with Perrow's model of the hospital outlined at the start of the chapter. However, what does square with such a model is the DGH psychiatric unit. This seems to represent a continuity with the modernist project of Victorian psychiatry. Its power is clearly focused and centralized. There is the retention of a division of labour within the clinical team, and between clinicians and managers. Consultants continue to lead a pyramid of clinical power – they head up multi-disciplinary teams, even if their authority is less evident than in the past. Their power has been subordinated to some extent now to the rules of general management (a bureaucratic process), and the modern hospital has been subjected to some extent to the non-bureaucratic principle of marketization. So, while the contemporary DGH units represent a strong continuity with the nineteenth-century asylum, the psychiatric profession is enduring peculiar new stresses.

Another difference between the old and new is literally visible. The architectural form of the DGH unit is actually more clear-cut than the old Victorian hospital, especially when it occurs in the post-war, high-rise, concrete block. In the Victorian asylum the expansive grounds might have been mistaken for a public park, whereas the modern hospital block containing cramped wards with low ceilings, and no internal or external exercise space, has become a caricature of an impersonal, modern, urban building.

As Samson (1992) notes about the US experience, new hospitals for old marks re-institutionalization (or it could be dubbed 'trans-hospitalization') not community care. Consequently, if the Victorian asylums were found lacking as therapeutic institutions, then it is likely that this will also be the case for the DGH psychiatric units. With a much smaller physical capacity for beds than the old asylums, these new units are increasingly becoming a focus for the expert coercive regulation of high-risk patients. Locked wards have returned ('Special Care Units'), and risk assessment and risk management have become the anxious daily preoccupation of staff. Substance misuse on site has added to this role and brought an illicit drug culture into psychiatric settings (to add to the official pre-existing one of prescribed medication routines). Despite their recent title of acute 'mental health services', these units, more than the Victorian hospitals, have now inherited the displaced function to restrain and segregate, albeit for shorter periods, those deemed to be a risk to themselves or others. They are not about mental health but are very much about mental pathology.

A further fragment of the post-modern condition of psychiatry lies with the rise of new technologies in managing mental disorder, where organizational arrangements are largely irrelevant. This is even more the case with the introduction of collaborative care with its focus on managing across organizational and professional boundaries discussed in the final part of the chapter. Directly accessible information to users, via the Internet, and to professionals, via telemedicine, also signals abandoning old organizational forms and the beginning of a new form of organization and delivery of mental health services.

This chapter has focused on the rise and fall of the asylum and the ambiguities which attend our current post-asylum world. A variety of factors have contributed to the demise of the old large mental hospitals, some of which have been economic and others ideological in influence. What the current social policy controversies surrounding care in the community highlight is that the old hospitals contained the three inter-weaving functions of care, control and accommodation. Any new arrangement about the organization of mental health work will also involve these functions, but their dilution is also the opportunity for new forms of management and response to emerge.

Controversies have tended to emerge and will continue to do so for the very reason that critics (serving a variety of interests) have complained that government has still not delivered the correct blend of care, control and accommodation.

Questions

1 Why were the large mental hospitals closed down?
2 Why were the large mental hospitals not closed sooner?
3 Do new arrangements such as collaborative care reflect our post-modern condition?
4 'The pharmacological revolution is a myth' – discuss.
5 'Scull's fiscal crisis of the State thesis was 20 years out of time' – discuss.
6 How might new technology shape help-seeking for mental health problems?

For discussion

If you, or a friend or relative, had a long-term mental health problem how would you like services to be organized in response? When discussing this question, think about the points raised in the chapter about care, control and accommodation.

7 Mental health work and professions

Chapter overview

The questionable legitimacy of categories of mental illness (discussed in Chapter 1) extends to the roles, identities and functions of mental health workers. The explicit control function of some mental health professionals, alongside their role as paid carers, has meant that they have often been scrutinized in a more critical light than many other groups of health professionals. Their legitimacy has also been hard to establish at times and open to challenge both from other mental health workers and increasingly from some lay people. This criticism has extended from the risk of the 'corruption of care', for example in sexual abuse by mental health professionals (Melville-Wiseman 2011), through to the campaigns of users of mental health services. Professional work has also been subjected to the constraints and criticisms of services managers and been the focus of contention about the re-distribution of work in health settings.

Self-help has become ever more popular in the mental health field, and access to knowledge, information and programmes of CBT on the World Wide Web now might threaten the traditional mental health professionals' jurisdiction over treatments and diagnosis. However, a countervailing trend is the strong need for people to seek out relationality in treatment regimes. Relationships with health care professionals seem to form a separate function from those provided exclusively in the lay domain on the one hand and by computerized packages of therapy or self-help on the other.

This chapter will cover:

- theoretical frameworks in the sociology of the professions;
- mental health professionals and other social actors;
- sociology and the mental health professions;
- legislative arrangements, service redesign and the social practice of diagnosis
- the survival of psychiatry?

Theoretical frameworks in the sociology of the professions

When sociologists first began to investigate professionals they provided a set of rather flattering descriptions. This was because, by and large, they were prepared to accept definitions provided by professionals themselves. These tended to emphasize that practitioners have unique skills, which are put altruistically at the service of the public. This early view has changed over time in the light of critical accounts of the professions. For example, Illich (1977a) talked of medicine being a 'threat to health' and of welfare professionals being 'disabling' (Illich 1977b). Others reviewing the rise of the new middle class have accused welfare professionals of manipulating both the rich and poor in society for their own interests, as both providers and users of services (Gould 1981). Gouldner (1979) goes as far as speculating that professionals are coming to dominate not just public services but industrial, and even military, life.

Despite these criticisms by and large from professional academics, for many ordinary people the word 'professional' still tends to imply both special skills and ethical propriety. It implies competence, efficiency, altruism and integrity. Hence, the converse of this is the everyday notion of what it means to be 'unprofessional' – to behave incompetently, inefficiently or unethically. As for sociologists, they largely agree on some basic characteristics of professionals:

1   Professionals have grown in importance over the past 200 years and expanded massively in number during the twentieth century.
2   Professionals are concerned with providing services to people rather than producing inanimate goods.
3   Whether salaried or self-employed, professionals have a higher social status than manual workers.
4   This status tends to increase as a function of length of training required to practice.
5   Generally, professionals claim a specialist knowledge about the service they provide and expect to define and control that knowledge.
6   Credentials give professionals a particular credibility in the eyes of public and government alike.

However, beyond this rough consensus, there is much debate about how professions might be understood sociologically. Here we look at some of the main frameworks used within sociology to understand professions.

The neo-Durkheimian framework

Overviewers of the field of the sociology of the professions (Saks 1983; Abel 1988) emphasize a certain version of the progression of events. At first, as has been mentioned, sociologists tended to simply categorize the professions and describe their work uncritically. Claims of special knowledge and altruism were taken at face value. This sociological depiction of positive qualities was dubbed the 'trait' approach to the professions. A parallel and equally uncritical approach to the professions was provided by the structural functionalist accounts, which saw the professions as a static or stable social stratum that offered a socially cohesive role (Parsons 1939; Goode 1957). Durkheim saw professions as providing a disinterested integrative social function. They were one of the social forces that counterbalanced the tendency of egotistical individuals to fragment society. For the Durkheimian tradition, professions are a source of community for one another and stability for the wider society they serve. They regulate their own practitioners, ensuring good practice by establishing codes of conduct and punishing errant colleagues. They regulate their clients in their interest and in the interest of their host society.

The neo-Weberian framework

Those in the Weberian tradition (Freidson 1970; Abel 1988) emphasize that the professions develop strategies to advance their own social status, persuade clients and potential clients about the need for the service they offer, and corner the market in that service and exclude competitors. Two notions in particular emerge from this picture for those following Weber.

Social closure

Collective social advancement rests upon social closure. By cornering the market, professionals offer a service that is closed off from others. A monopoly is gained to work in a specialized way with a particular group of clients (e.g. medical practitioners treating sick people) so that other occupational groups seeking a similar role are excluded. This closing off also means that only those inside the boundaries of the profession can scrutinize its practices – others are denied access and are kept in a state of ignorance. In order for professionals to maintain their social status they must convince those on the outside of their boundaries that they are offering a unique service and so they develop various rhetorical devices to persuade the world at large of their special qualities.

To do this they must justify a peculiar knowledge base that has a technical or scientific rationality on the one hand, but that, on the other, is not so easy to understand that anybody can use it. Medicine as a whole can be seen to provide such accounts to the world. However, this persuasion is precarious. The growth of alternative medicine (Saks 1992) is testimony to this, as are the doubts about the coherence and credibility of psychiatric knowledge that we examined in Chapter 1.

Professional dominance

The second main feature of this Weberian picture is that of professional dominance. Professionals exercise power over others in three senses:

1   They have power over their clients. The latter, convinced of the need for the service they are offered or seek, are dependent on professionals. An imbalance of specialized knowledge keeps the client in a state of ignorance, insecurity and vulnerability. This power imbalance is reinforced if the professional operates on their own territory rather than that of their client, for instance by treating people in hospital rather than their own home.
2   Professionals exercise power over their new recruits. Thus, a dominance hierarchy is common in professions, with senior practitioners and trainers exercising control and discipline over their juniors. Power enjoyed in the upper ranks of a profession can only be secured by submission and deference in earlier junior days, as trainees are dependent on their superiors for career progression.
3   Professionals seek to establish a dominant relationship over other occupational groups working with the same clients. Professionals may seek to exclude existing equal competitors or they may seek to usurp the role of existing superiors. In medicine, in addition to excluding competitors (e.g. orthopaedic specialists who have kept chiropractors and osteopaths out of official health service practice) they also subordinate them (obstetricians directing the work of midwives) or limit their therapeutic powers to one part of the body (e.g. dentistry and optometry).

Thus, power relationships are of central importance to neo-Weberians. These are about gaining and retaining power over clients, new entrants and other occupational groups working with those clients. One way of thinking about the neo-Weberian focus is in terms of horizontal relationships between professionals and those they work with, as colleagues or clients, in order to sustain or extend the material advantages, status and comforts of middle-class life in society.

The neo-Marxian framework

When we look to the Marxian tradition, power relationships are also important, but now the focus is on vertical structural relationships. The question to be answered by neo-Marxians is: 'where do professionals fit into a social structure which is characterized by two main groups: those who work to produce wealth (surplus value) in society (the working class or proletariat) and those who own the means of production and exploit these workers and expropriate surplus value as profits (capitalists, the ruling class or the bourgeoisie)?' Marx gave scant attention to the third group of interest to us: those functionaries or 'white collar' workers who were neither exploitative capitalists who owned the means of production nor workers who produced goods and profits for their bosses in exchange for wages. Consequently, those sociologists upholding a Marxian tradition of analysis have had a number of conceptual difficulties with the professions.

Three positions have been taken up by neo-Marxians about the professions. The latter are deemed either to be part of the ruling class or part of the proletariat, or to constitute a separate and new social class holding contradictory qualities. The first type of claim is made by Navarro (1979), who argues that, for instance, the medical profession actually constitutes a part of the ruling class in capitalist society.

By contrast, Oppenheimer (1975) has claimed that the 'knowledge-based' professions have had control over their work eroded by the state bureaucracies that employ them (they have been subjected to 'bureaucratic subordination'). As a result, their control over their specialized skills has diminished ('deskilling') and consequently they have become part of the working class ('proletarianization'). Oppenheimer understands the collectivist strategies of professions as being no different from traditional trade union defences of working-class terms and conditions of employment. This contrasts with the neo-Weberians, who point to such collective action as being about upward social mobility. Thus, the neo-Weberians are clearly much more critical of the professions than Oppenheimer, who treats them with the sympathy implied by their status as an exploited group of workers who are vulnerable to wage erosion and unemployment.

Clearly, Navarro and Oppenheimer cannot both be totally correct if they claim to operate within the same sociological tradition started by Marx. Their apparent opposition is rescued by a third group of neo-Marxians, who argue that they are both partially correct. This group, exemplified by the work of Carchedi (1975), Johnson (1977) and Gough (1979), emphasizes the contradictory position of professionals in capitalist society. They are not capitalists but they serve the interests of the latter. They are not full members of the proletariat (as they do not produce goods and surplus value) but they are employees and so they share similar vulnerabilities and interests of the working class. For instance, mental health workers would be seen in this contradictory position as being both agents of social control acting on behalf of the capitalist state and employees of that state and so vulnerable to the same problems of any other group of workers.

Eclecticism and post-structuralism

The above picture of competing views is complicated further by many analysts of the professions drawing liberally on more than one tradition. For instance, Parry and Parry (1977), when discussing the rise of militant trade unionism within the junior ranks of the British medical profession in the 1970s, utilize Weber's notion of closure and Oppenheimer's proletarianization thesis. They go as far as arguing that Weber actually anticipated Oppenheimer's insights and thus they see no dispute between the Marxian and Weberian types of analysis about modern professions.

As we will see later in relation to the mental health professions, it is now common for sociologists to approach their work eclectically – they draw on more than one theoretical tradition. For some this has become an explicit prescription for analysis. For instance, Turner (1987: 140), when discussing health professions, comments that 'a satisfactory explanation of professionalization as an occupational strategy will come eventually to depend upon both Weberian and Marxian perspectives'.

One important shift in social theory, post-structuralism, now goes beyond eclecticism. One of its main intellectual leaders, Foucault (1980) considers that social analysis entails examining a

> heterogenous ensemble consisting of discourses, institutions, architectural forms, regulatory decisions, laws, administrative measures, scientific statements, philosophical, moral and philanthropic propositions – in short the said and the unsaid.

In particular, Foucault and his followers are concerned to map out discourses associated with particular social periods and places. This notion of discourse includes both forms of knowledge and the practices associated with that knowledge. For this reason, the notion of 'discursive practices' might connote more accurately the focus of the post-structuralists when discussing the professions.

The Foucauldians provide a different way of looking at applied knowledge in professional work. They have no notion of a clear or stable power discrepancy between professionals and clients or between dominant professions and subordinate ones. Power is dispersed; it cannot be simply and easily located in any elite group. While it is certainly bound up with dominant discursive features of a particular time and place, these may change and they may be resisted. For Foucault and his followers, ways in which the person (the body and mind of the individual) is now described or constructed (measured, analysed and codified) are central features of contemporary society. Medicine and professions close to it have had a central role in this regard with their interests in diagnosis, testing, assessment and observation and the treatment, management and surveillance of sick and healthy bodies in society. However, in the post-structuralist account there is a failure to endorse the notion of self-conscious collective activity of professionals, to advance their own interests or to act on behalf of the capitalist state.

As we will see later, the mental health professions have been of particular interest to post-structuralists. This is probably because of the 'psy complex' having a chronic surveillance role in relation to mental patients and because it has been associated with two types of discourse. The first of these emphasized segregation and acting on the body (physical treatments) and the second emphasized the construction of the self via a set of psychological accounts (counselling and psychotherapy). The attack on the body and the construction of the self represent two key ways of understanding the activities of mental health professionals.

A final point in this section relates to how we understand health professions compared to others. As Starr (2009) has noted, the peculiar organizational context they operate within and the particular expectations the public have of them, about an emotive topic (health and illness), create particular pressures upon them. They are endeavouring to maintain a dominant authoritative position in relation to patients and colleagues, in a peculiarly emotive and politicized context. Health and illness bring with them substantial intellectual contention about research and clinical priorities and political contention about professional authority.

The above four general sociological frameworks have been the most influential in understanding the professions. As we will see below, in relation to mental health work, other sociological approaches have also been influential. These include symbolic interactionism, the sociology of knowledge, the sociology of deviance and feminist sociology. Before we discuss these let us look at the relationships that mental health workers have with other key social actors.

Mental health professionals and other social actors

A number of professional groups contribute to mental health work. The most obvious collection – psychiatrists, clinical psychologists, social workers, psychiatric nurses, occupational therapists, art therapists, counsellors and psychotherapists – is employed with the explicit assumption that mental health work is their main role. For this reason, they, or their practice and knowledge, are sometimes referred to as 'the psy complex' by post-structuralists (Ingleby 1983). One way of approaching the sociology of the mental health professions is in terms of seeking out examples within the above sociological frameworks which apply to mental health specialists. However, it would be misleading to give the impression that this core group in the mental health industry provides the only professional input in terms of contact with people entering the patient role or in terms of the negotiation of what constitutes a mental health problem. A variety of other personnel are also implicated, including GPs, the clergy, the police and social services care or case managers.

De Swaan (1990) makes the point that members of the public are encouraged through personal contact with professionals and their clients, and through the media, to frame their personal difficulties in professional terms. He calls this process 'proto-professionalization'. For De Swaan, what start as personal troubles or discomforts about a person's relationship with others can be framed as problems amenable to specialist help, even before contact with professionals occurs.

While De Swaan focuses on the voluntary presentation to professions by those seeing themselves as suffering these difficulties, as we noted in Chapter 6, Coulter (1973) points out that members of the public also look to professions to rescue them from discomfort or threat caused by
others whom they deem to have a mental health problem. Thus, the public are centrally involved
in inserting mental health problems into the domain of professional activity in two senses. Sometimes they label themselves in advance as having a problem amenable to specialist help. At other
times they look to professionals to help them cope with the distress, threat or anxiety which results
from the conduct of others.

Thus, consideration of non-specialist professionals and lay people is important to understand
how specialists obtain and retain their mandate of authority about mental health. We can think in
terms of four groups of social actors who interact with one another to define the field of mental
health problems:

1   the State (represented by politicians, civil servants and managers);
2   mental health specialists;
3   professionals who are implicated in mental health work some of the time (GPs, the police,
    the clergy) but who do not claim a specialist role;
4   that section of the general population that is already convinced of the need to frame their
    own distress or other people's troublesome conduct in professional terms – lay people
    who have been 'proto-professionalized'.

The increasing recognition of the coalescence of lay and professional perspectives and involvement in mental health, evident in the work of De Swaan, highlights a parallel process of the changing knowledge base and territory of mental health professional work. There has been a blurring of
boundaries between mental and physical health work and models of health and illness. Disciplines
across medicine and nursing have embraced the notion of 'holism'. Portmanteau models such as
the 'bio-psycho-social' model are gaining increasing popularity, particularly as a paradigm which
challenges the reductionist and bio-medical emphases of traditional health professionals (Dowrick
et al. 1996; Pilgrim 2002a).

'Emotional labour' has also become a focus of mental health specialist and generalist health
workers alike as well as forming a focus of the analysis of work of non-professionals undertaking 'people work' (e.g. air hostesses) (Hochschild 1983). The terrain of professional health work,
particularly mental health work, has also changed. More work now takes place in the more 'open
systems' of primary and community care. Institutionalized ways of responding and relating to
patients inside organizations have given way to community-focused work. The need to obtain
entry to patients' houses in order to carry out work has reduced the gap between professionals
and patients – in so far as access becomes the object of negotiation between two parties, whereas
in institutionalized settings it has frequently been taken for granted.

'Fringe work', which refers to a series of activities that professionals are not expected to do
or 'supposed' to engage with (de la Cuesta 1993), assumes a higher profile when professionals
work increasingly in the community. The growing recognition of the mental health component of a
wider range of health problems among different population groups and presented in primary care
is evident in the rise in numbers of primary care counsellors employed to deal specifically with
referrals from GPs and other primary care professionals.

Sociology and the mental health professions

Let us now return to the models described earlier within the sociology of the professions. The
neo-Durkheimian approach is rarely visible in the contemporary sociological discourse about

professional life, although it can still be found in the writings of mental health professionals when they are generating a 'public relations' view of their own work. Examples of this can be found in relation to psychiatry (Clare 1976) and clinical psychology (Marzillier and Hall 1987).

Below, we start by acknowledging that many studies have drawn upon more than one theoretical framework. We then look at some purer sociological frameworks before addressing the influence of theoretical models from the study of deviancy, professional knowledge and patriarchy. The latter are important in addition to the work of the sociology of the professions because they come at the question of professional practice from a starting point other than the specialists themselves.

In regard to the other groups we have just noted (non-specialists and lay people), deviancy theorists are interested in the negotiation of deviant roles, like that of becoming a psychiatric patient. While professionals are central to this, they are not the only group of social actors implicated. Likewise, sociological investigations of the transmission of knowledge start with an interest in knowledge but then look to how professionals are a vehicle for its reproduction, possession and modification. Feminists start from a wider interest in the male domination of women in society and then look to particular sites of this domination, like professional practice.

Eclecticism and post-structuralism

Many of the attempts to understand mental health professionals have drawn upon more than one theoretical base. For instance, the extensive work of Andrew Scull on the development of psychiatry during and since the nineteenth century draws heavily upon Marxist ideas. Scull (1979) explains the rise and maintenance of psychiatry in terms of its functional value for economic order and efficiency under capitalism. The segregation of the mad and the delegation by the State of powers to doctors to keep madness under control are central to Scull's thesis. His emphasis is on the role of psychiatrists as agents of social control employed by the State to contain the threat of one section of a poor underclass – the mad. However, when explaining the finer dynamics of how doctors purged lay administrators from the asylums and sought upward social mobility for themselves, he uses a Weberian notion of 'closure'.

Similarly, a work which builds heavily on the work of Scull is Baruch and Treacher's (1978) analysis of the functioning of psychiatry in Britain, which emphasizes the professional dominance of psychiatrists. In the Marxian tradition, they highlight the economic factors which both precipitate mental distress and are consequent upon a person entering the role of psychiatric patient. However, they also draw liberally for the latter purposes on the work of Parsons, albeit with critical reservations. They also refer positively to the post-Marxian social critic Illich, as well as to Scull, in their 'medicalization' thesis about the transformation of madness into mental illness by doctors.

Indeed, while Baruch and Treacher, like Scull, could be labelled as 'Marxist functionalists', they begin their book with a long quote from Illich's *Medical Nemesis* (1974). (The ideological position of Illich is contested. His antiprofessionalism has given comfort to critics of both right and left, and his alternatives to current forms of social organization contain a mixture of libertarian and authoritarian elements.)

The medicalization of madness thesis and the emphasis on psychiatrists as agents of social control is by no means limited to neo-Marxians. Right-wing libertarian critics from within psychiatry have constructed social histories of their profession with these emphases as well. The best example of this is the work of Szasz (1971), who argues that psychiatrists are for the modern State what witch-finders were for the Church in mediaeval times. The work of Szasz also echoes some of the analysis of Foucault, which is described later.

In another analysis of twentieth-century psychiatry, Ramon (1985) looks at services and the professions of psychiatry, psychiatric nursing and psychology. She dubs these for her purposes the 'psy complex', echoing a post-structuralist term but at the same time firmly endorsing the political economy approach to welfare professionals given by the Marxist Gough (1979) we noted earlier (Ramon 1985: 21).

Turning to the analysis of a different profession – clinical psychology – eclecticism is evident again. Pilgrim and Treacher (1992) describe the historical development of the profession and its recent functioning. The profession in Britain has gone through four phases: psychometrics (1950s), behaviour therapy (1960s), therapeutic eclecticism (1970s) and managerialism (1980s). When theorizing the meaning of their description, Pilgrim and Treacher endorse the partial advantages of post-structuralist, neo-Weberian and neo-Marxian models for their data analysis. Psychologists have been mainly concerned with voluntary relationships (see discussion of post-structuralism later). They have tried to usurp the role of a dominant profession (psychiatry) to some extent and they have sought, via a campaign of registration, to attain a State-endorsed monopoly over psychological practice. Psychologists have demonstrably served the social administrative requirements of the capitalist State by seeking to regulate the behaviour of children and people with mental health problems and learning difficulties.

In addition, Pilgrim and Treacher draw attention to questions of gender and race in understanding some of the features of the profession being white and male dominated (see later). These examples of eclecticism reflect that the earlier advice of Turner (1987) about the need to integrate Weberian and Marxian frameworks has been anticipated by a number of sociologists.

Foucault's (1961; 1965) early writings on mental health began quite close to the Marxian emphasis on social control. However, he diverged from Scull's analysis on two counts even at this stage. First, he puts the beginnings of segregation at an earlier point, the 'great confinement' of the mid-seventeenth to mid-eighteenth century. Scull (1977, 1979) argues that most of the mad were still roaming free in society at the beginning of the nineteenth century and it was not until the mid-nineteenth century that the State asylum system was well established to segregate madness. Second, Foucault emphasized the moral, not the economic, order. While Scull argued that psychiatry functioned to aid and abet economic efficiency, Foucault argued that psychiatry existed primarily to deal with those who offended bourgeois morality and rationality. For Foucault, segregative psychiatry was not concerned with either medical cure or economic efficiency *per se* but with moral regulation.

Miller (1986) notes that Foucault's work is essentially a 'prehistory' of psychiatry. It is then extended by Castel (1983) into the period when the profession became more firmly established in the nineteenth century. The moral regulation theme continues about the role of the alienist or psychiatrist. Madness now had to be dealt with within the rules of the emerging bourgeois 'contractual' society. During this period the psychiatric profession did not go unchallenged but it retained its central role in relation to the asylum.

The third phase of interest to post-structuralists has been the changes in psychiatry during the twentieth century (Armstrong 1980; Miller and Rose 1988). Here, four interweaving themes can be identified:

- psychiatry as a professional enterprise is no longer restricted only to the asylum;
- its practices are no longer only associated with coercive social control;
- large bands of the population have been induced into an individualized state of psychological mindedness about their existence, via the media and education; and
- following from the last two points, voluntary relationships involving lengthy conversations about the self are now sought out by the public and deployed by professionals (versions of counselling and psychotherapy) (Rose 1990).

The move beyond the asylum can be linked roughly to changes in practices during the First World War when the problem of shellshock required a new response to mental distress (Stone 1985). Psychotherapy began in earnest at this point: outpatient clinics were set up after the war and centres of excellence, like the Tavistock Clinic, which celebrated the legitimacy of psychoanalysis, were established. Psychoanalysis had been attacked or ignored by psychiatrists before 1914. After the war, the Tavistock Clinic became associated with a wider cultural emphasis on the individual and the family: for instance, by promoting explanations of delinquency and mental distress, which were purported to arise from poor mothering.

Of central importance in this account is the rejection of the coercive social control emphasis of Scull and the 'anti-psychiatrists'. For instance, Miller and Rose argue that the psy complex has increasingly emphasized a voluntary relationship which is sought out and appreciated by clients: 'We argue that it is more fruitful to consider the ways that regulatory systems have sought to promote subjectivity than to document ways in which they have crushed it' (Miller and Rose 1988: 174). De Swaan's notion of 'proto-professionalization', mentioned earlier, also operates with a similar assumption about a cultural consensus between professionals and lay people that their everyday troubles can be solved by conversations (counselling and psychotherapy) which focus on, celebrate and construct the 'self'.

However, the post-structuralist account still emphasizes the role of professionals in 'regulating' the everyday lives of their clients (Donzelot 1979). Thus, differences of opinion between sociologists about the regulatory role of professionals seem to hinge on differences of emphasis. The post-structuralists (and Parsons (1951) in his discussion of the sick role) emphasize a process of consensual decision-making, some of it implicit or unconscious, wherein the client either comes to agree with, or already accepts, professional definitions of the nature of their problem. Social regulation occurs by agreement and with actual (or perceived) benefits to the client. By contrast, the Marxian tradition emphasizes the enforced imposition of a view on the client by professionals acting as agents of the state. The first of these suggests that the power to regulate emotional life and norms of conduct is diffuse or dispersed. Power cannot be located 'inside' any one particular group of social actors. Rather, it is understood as a relationship or discourse shared by several parties. The second account clearly locates power in the hands of professionals who dominate their clients at the behest of their state employers.

Maybe both types of account are credible. Patients do seek out help in voluntary relationships. In addition, sometimes, professionals impose themselves on patients – they lock them up and give them treatments they do not consent to freely. Because post-structuralist writers about mental health have tended to focus on twentieth-century developments, their emphasis has tended to be on the disciplinary, rather than repressive, power of psychiatric experts. This has led to a skewed post-structuralist interest, with Foucault's early concern with repressive power being replaced by an emphasis on psychological interventions which are 'anxiously sought and gratefully received' (Pilgrim and Rogers 1994). This shift emphasizes the role of the secularized confessional in modern society in Foucault's later writings:

> The confession has spread its effects far and wide. It plays a part in justice, medicine, education, family relationships, in love relations, in the most ordinary affairs of everyday life and in the most solemn rites: one confesses one's crimes, one's sins, one's thoughts and desires, one's illnesses and troubles; one goes about telling with the greatest precision whatever is most difficult to tell.
>
> (Foucault 1981: 59)

This role of the confessional is discussed in more detail in relation to mental health work by Rose (1990). He suggests a number of points in this regard:

1   Psychotherapeutic assumptions can be found to operate now in general medicine, education, advertising, and journalism and business management. They are not limited to the work of mental health experts.

2   A countervailing discourse has also emerged from some social critics about a 'modern obsession with the self' and a 'tyranny of intimacy in which narcissism is mobilized in social relations'.

3   Modern psychotherapeutic rituals mimic and displace the older emphasis on religious or spiritual pilgrimages. The growth of Protestantism with its emphasis on individual guilt and responsibility marked a bridge between mediaeval religion and the modern culture of the self and individualism. Alongside this emerged the 'civilizing process' (Elias 1978) in which self not State control became important; the growth in importance of etiquette and manners. Thus, a repressive State form of control was increasingly superseded by self-control.

4   New versions of the confession such as counselling and the psychological therapies became means by which identities were inscribed upon their subjects. Mental health work produces 'the subjectification of work', 'the psychologization of the mundane', 'a thera-peutics of finitude' and a 'neuroticization of social intercourse'. What Rose points to in these phrases is the way in which work, common life transitions, disappointment, death and our intimate relationships are now framed within mental health discourses.

5   Following Foucault, Rose offers a triple aspect on psychological treatments. First there are moral codes in the language and ethical principles of therapy. These imply some notion of 'the good life' and are thus implicitly or explicitly normative. Second, there are ethical scenarios which are the sites or contexts in which the moral codes operate – social work practice, the courts, the private consulting room and so on. Third there are techniques of the self, which are developed to codify the exploration, definition and con-frontation of the self in therapy (Foucault 1988). These techniques are not a unitary body of knowledge but a wide range of models which produce narratives of the self – hetero-geneity of approach characterizes the psychological treatments.

6   These features of mental health work are not guided by the hidden hand of capital (cf. the neo-Marxian view of the professions) nor by the conscious collective self-interest pursued by professionals according to the neo-Weberians (see later). Instead, the main orientation of modern mental health work is one of reconciling or aligning the needs of individuals with the social, political or organizational goals which form the social context of therapists and their clients.

Having outlined the post-structuralist perspective of mental health work, we now turn to the appli-cation of an older sociological approach.

The neo-Weberian approach

This has already been mentioned in relation to clinical psychologists seeking a monopoly on psy-chological practice and on their boundary dispute with psychiatry (Pilgrim and Treacher 1992). It was also an important aspect of the study of a psychiatric unit by Baruch and Treacher (1978), in terms of the strategies which consultant psychiatrists used to maintain their dominant position in the mental health team working with inpatients.

In another study of psychiatrists, their relationship with the police has been analysed in terms of professional dominance. The transactions that occurred between the two occupational groups when people deemed to be mentally disordered in public were taken for psychiatric assessment by police officers (under section 136 of the Mental Health Act 1983) were studied. The same study also found that psychiatrists operated a number of strategies to exert control over how the patient was dealt with. The technical knowledge of the profession was a focus for psychiatrists' dominance over police officers. Even though police officers identified mental disorder with the same technical efficiency as psychiatrists, the latter insisted on depicting the police as lacking in the credentials to understand or manage the client group. The police were not in fact interested in encroaching on the territory of psychiatric practice. Nonetheless, psychiatrists acted to ward off a form of encroach-ment on their professional power that they perceived to be coming from police officers.

Sociologists who try to understand specific groups of professions usually find it necessary to appreciate how practitioners perceive their own role and that of others. The next wider sociological tradition to be discussed highlights this.

Symbolic interactionism

This approach can be found in Goffman's (1961) classic study of asylum life and of how the patient role is imposed on admitted psychiatric patients. What matters in this 'microsociology' are the meanings which are negotiated by various social actors involved in a drama or ritual. Goffman talks of 'degradation rituals', when the patient's identity is removed as they enter the psychiatric patient role (see later); this type of approach was extended by Braginsky *et al.* (1973).

The symbolic interactionists can also be found in studies of how psychiatrists and other mental health workers see and justify their role. Goldie (1977) interviewed psychiatrists in order to understand the meanings they attached to their knowledge base and their perceived superior status compared with non-medical staff. He also observed and took accounts from other members of mental health care teams about how they understood their particular expertise and powers. From this data he built up a picture of how psychiatrists maintain their mandate of authority in the field of mental health and how subordinate professions both challenge and maintain that mandate.

More recently, another study has examined the different mental models held by different members of mental health teams within this negotiated order (Colombo *et al.* 2003). While a pragmatic imperative exists to make a service work and to complete daily tasks, it is clear that these contain strains and compromises about implicit models which permeate the intentions and actions of staff. For example, psychiatrists still overwhelmingly operate a diagnostic treatment approach to mental illness. They work alongside others who do not share this view but prefer an alternative model (psychotherapeutic or social).

In another study of a psychiatric team using participant observation and interviews, Emerson and Pollner (1975) investigated the ways in which professionals classified their work with different types of patients. In particular, the investigators were interested in looking at how less acceptable work, such as the compulsory detention of patients in emergency duties, was conceived by workers. They found that this 'dirty work' or 'shit work' was accounted for by workers who preferred the morally superior role of being benign therapists.

The dirty work conception derives from earlier work by Hughes (1971), who sees it as an aspect of all professional activity entailing a practitioner being obliged to 'play a role of which he thinks he ought to be a little ashamed morally'. For Emerson and Pollner, the dirty work of acute psychiatry is that of social control – involuntary admission to hospital. In order to distance themselves from this explicit and morally dubious role, practitioners will point out that it is not really typical of their duties, that it is forced on them by circumstances or that they use the opportunity to help the patient as best they can.

The symbolic interactionist approach has been given new relevance, given that mental health service reformers are seeking to take account of the role of lay people in quality improvement programmes (Milne *et al.* 2004). (We return to the importance of 'users and carers' in the final chapter.)

The influence of the sociology of deviance

It is not surprising that some investigations of mental health work have started with the social negotiation of psychiatric patienthood, rather than looking at a particular profession. Coulter (1973) studied how social crises in the domestic arena became reframed as psychiatric illnesses. A similar approach can be found in the work of Scott (1973), who tried to map out the powers available to professionals, prospective patients and significant others to establish or maintain the deviant role of mental patient. Scott talked of the 'treatment barrier' to describe the loss of agency occurring once the identified patient was labelled as ill. This process of placing illness inside an individual obscures the roles and responsibilities of all the parties in the transaction and is consequently an impediment to change.

Goffman's work has already been mentioned, but it is important to note that his study of hospital life supplied us with important concepts related to the negotiation of deviance: 'the betrayal funnel' and the 'degradation ritual'. The former refers to the conspiratorial relationship which necessarily develops between relatives of identified patients who have been forcibly admitted to hospital and the receiving professionals. Goffman called this conspiracy 'the circuit of agents that participate fatefully in the passage from civilian to patient status'. The 'degradation ritual' refers to the removal by professionals of a person's everyday identity and a stripping away of their usual sense of self. They are labelled with a diagnosis and normal signals of their individuality (such as their own clothes) are removed.

This emphasis on the involvement of professionals in negotiating a deviant role can be found in Bean's (1980) study of psychiatrists, social workers and GPs who compulsorily detain patients. In this study, Bean was testing the validity of claims arising from Lemert's (1974) work on group interaction, an extension of labelling theory about the treatment of one set of rule-breakers (criminals) and checking how this model applied to another group of rule-breakers (those diagnosed as being mentally ill). The principles of this model of deviancy are concerned with rules, their enforcement by parties (i.e. professionals) with designated powers, and how rule enforcement may or may not lead to an outcome which is intended. Bean's interest in testing the limits of this theory in the field of mental health work involved his observing the conduct and statements of professionals (the 'rule enforcers') in their work when admitting patients to hospital compulsorily.

The influence of the sociology of knowledge

Some sociologists have tried to understand the workings of particular professions in terms of the knowledge base they employ. Within the neo-Weberian tradition this sociology of knowledge approach is evident in the work of Freidson (1970) when examining the general character of modern professional life. In relation to mental health workers, Sheppard (1990) compared psychiatric nurses with social workers within such a framework. He took the lead from Atkinson (1983), who advocates the need to examine 'the relationship between education, practice and the organization of occupational groups'. The rationale here is that a close look at that relationship will reveal how the assumptions about the knowledge will shape professional practice and illuminate how practitioners defend the legitimacy of their particular role. Following from this, empirical studies of professionals should attend to the meanings that practitioners attach to their work (in line with symbolic interactionism discussed above).

Sheppard (1990) suggested that social workers and community psychiatric nurses (CPNs) might in some respects overlap in the type of work they do with clients, but a closer look at the knowledge base of each profession also points to differences. Social workers are influenced, albeit inconsistently, by social science. In contrast, CPNs are preoccupied more by a focus on mental illness – how to account for it and how to respond to it. This means that practitioners accept psychiatric (i.e. medical) models of explanation and treatment or they react against them (i.e. take on board 'anti-psychiatry' arguments). Their background is not within social science but is tied instead to a medical body of knowledge. Also, because of their role in relation to mental health law (social workers approved for this purpose are required to detain patients compulsorily), social workers may be more concerned with legal definitions of work rather than the nature of distress and its treatment.

The influence of feminist sociology

Feminist sociology has emphasized the subordinated role of women in three senses when discussing the caring professions (Gamarnikow 1978; Hearn 1982; Crompton 1987):

1   women are more likely to be subordinated as clients;
2   women on average occupy lower-status positions within professions;
3   those occupational groups which are numerically dominated by women (like nursing) are more likely to be subordinate to male-dominated professions (like medicine).

However, because of the history of male asylum attendants being used to physically control lunatics in the nineteenth century, psychiatric nursing has been more male dominated (and working class) than general nursing (Carpenter 1980).

Pilgrim and Treacher (1992) found that female clinical psychologists were less likely to occupy managerial and professional leadership positions than men. Moreover, they found that conservative male elements in the profession also lamented the greater proportion of women to men on the explicit grounds that this implies an inferior status and induces a decline in salary levels (Humphrey and Haward 1981; Crawford 1989). Feminism has also stimulated new forms of therapeutic practice which are tailored to women's needs (Eichenbaum and Orbach 1982).

Legislative arrangements, service redesign and the social practice of diagnosis

We deal in a general sense with legislation in Chapter 10 but there are specific implications of legal arrangements relevant to discussing the role of mental health professionals. In the current British context, four can be noted.

First, after 2007, with the introduction of a new Mental Health Act in England the role of the Approved Social Worker was replaced by a more inclusive one of Approved Mental Health Practitioner. Likewise the role of Responsible Medical Officer under previous legislation was superseded by that of Responsible Clinician. These wider roles involve other senior mental health workers joining social workers and psychiatrists in sharing statutory powers of compulsory detention and treatment.

Second, after many years of controversy about compulsory powers being exerted outside of hospital, the 2007 Act does now include Community Treatment Orders (CTDs). These were established by government despite extensive disquiet from the mental health professions in the run up to the Act. Community Treatment Orders have been deployed at a moderate rate by professionials (about 4000 a year since their introduction). However, they have failed to reduce the number of psychiatric admissions for people with psychosis and so can be considered to have failed to do what they originally intended (Burns *et al.*).

Third, the range of separate regulatory arrangements for the clinical psychologists, occupational therapists and art therapists have now been displaced by a single body (the Health Professions Council, which at the time of writing is also responsible for 11 other health professions) under new legislation in 2001. The registration of nurses and doctors remains as before. However, these alterations in the bureaucratic organization of state regulation of professions leave intact control over specific practices, which cut across occupational groups working in mental health (such as psychotherapy). As Price (2002) notes, there is an important logical and political difference between the State regulating specific practices and it regulating professional groupings that award titles and maintain a professional register. The more the activities of a profession are specified (rather than its practitioners' credentials being simply formally held on a register) the more its legitimacy can be undermined (Hayes 1998).

Fourth, with major re-organizations to key institutions, problems of who provides what sort of input have arisen; fragmentation had led to problems about which organization did what. Thus devolution and localism have been tempered with the need for the State to step in at times to issue top-down guidance from government about legal matters and professional behaviour. The Harris report (Department of Health 2013) stipulated that every organization in the NHS should undertake a process of due diligence with responsibility to ensure a clear and 'secure' location of responsibilities across the system. It should also have the capability and capacity to carry out its functions and there should be a process of continuing audit and annual governance statements, confirming arrangements for the discharge of their current statutory function irregularities and legal compliance (Department of Health 2013).

At the start of this chapter, we noted that critical accounts of professions displaced credulous ones in sociology but that lay people still retain a positive concept of professionalism. However, this lay view is now being undermined by major scandals about respectable professions. Examples of this in Britain have included the detection of the mass murderer GP Harold Shipman, the removal of body parts of dead babies at Alder Hey hospital without parental consent and a recurring pattern of sexual misconduct among mental health professionals (Allsop 2002; Pilgrim 2002b). This sort of very publicly debated evidence about the professional abuse of power has increased the confidence of politicians in introducing specific rather than general forms of legal regulation.

Another point to note is in relation to quasi-legal constraints on professional autonomy. These refer to formal government policies and structures, which hedge around 'clinical freedom'. For example, after 1997 the government introduced clinical governance arrangements in the NHS which were designed to ensure service improvements. The implementation of this policy necessitated the bureaucratic subordination of professional power to managerial power. Another example was the setting up of the National Institute for Health and Care Excellence (NICE) and the Commission for Health Improvement to provide guidance on good practice and to monitor service standards.

Sociological ambivalence and the deployment of diagnosis in mental health work

For mental health professionals diagnosis as a social practice can be understood as a heuristic device. The latter produces a standardized diagnostic story, with the aim of bringing an individual's experiences of distress and their dysfunctional conduct into view for the purposes of management by mental health workers within their daily practices and routines. However, at the same time the use of codified knowledge, such as diagnosis, is an enduring problem for professions in terms of maintaining professional autonomy. The use of psychiatric classification has been said to create a 'sociological ambivalence' for psychiatrists, which arises from the tension between the desire for autonomy in practice and the professional goal of legitimacy within the system of mental health professions on the other. A space for autonomous practice is carved from what is termed 'workarounds' that in fact undermine the use of diagnostic classification. Workarounds include the use of alternative diagnostic typologies, 'gaming' the numbers on official paperwork and negotiating diagnoses with patients.

All this highlights the limitations of the bio-medical approach to diagnosis and treatment. In the search for autonomy through the creation of opportunities for patient input and resistance to fixed diagnoses doubt may be raised for psychiatrists about the role and use of the bio-medical models and classifications of mental illness such as the DSM (Whooley 2010). The 'workaround' by negotiation with patients about diagnosis is likely to fit better with patient accounts which oscillate in and out of the medicalized discourse of major categories of mental illness, such as 'depression' (Kokanovic et al. 2013). The DSM has also been seen as a platform for inter-professional rivalry and competition in relation to legitimate knowledge. It has been argued that its origin lies in a series of conflicts among psychiatrists, psychoanalysts and clinical psychologists (Strand 2011). These arguments about epistemological authority in service contexts, which are bound up with 'tribal' interests, recall the explanatory importance of professional dominance, from the Weberian tradition. Moreover, there have also been some signs of de-professionalization or 'proletarianization' in the mental health workforce, which we consider now.

The blurring of lay and professional work

The debates about specific, versus general, State regulation are occurring at a time when the UK government is also redesigning health and social care services. This is having substantial consequences for occupational roles under current and envisaged service changes. In the field of mental health, psychology graduates have been introduced to support low capacity in primary mental health care. The increasing integration of health and social care has generated new models of mental health support workers. New forms of service, such as crisis resolution, assertive outreach, early intervention (for psychosis) services and treatment centres for those with a diagnosis of personality disorder are merging. They are generating new roles, blurring the distinctions between the existing mental health professions and a new division of labour between lay people and professionals. In mental health, as well as elsewhere, professional labour involved in the management of illness is increasingly bureaucratic in form. It reflects the 'new public management' model intent upon controlling costs, producing evidence-based and protocol-driven care and minimizing individual and systemic risks.

These comprehensive changes being made to health care (e.g. use of monitoring systems) and new routinized ways of working with Fordist, or 'Post-Fordist', notions of task-centredness reduce work tasks to simplistic components. If successful, as intended, then these tasks are downwardly delegated to other workers but also to patients. Key complex assessments and management decisions are retained higher up the clinical and managerial ladders but much previously in that domain is delegated 'below' (in terms of seniority and levels of training). To an extent this delegation has given rise to an army of primary care mental health workers delivering short-term therapy in primary care (Harkness et al. 2005).

'Self-management' as a set of skills learned by the patient provides a continuum with this professionally delegated work. A set of particular tasks addressing specific elements of what is seen as the core set of patient work, for example communicating with the doctor and action planning, are packaged together in a formulaic way. As professional care becomes more protocol-based, so too does the 'work' of patients; the latter is underpinned by new configurations and distributions of types of knowledge. These were previously clearly demarcated and possessed as formal professional knowledge. For example, self-help programmes are now seen as filling a gap between the supply of trained cognitive-behavioural therapists to treat depression and demand for care in the community. In this example, self-help interventions require less input from a therapist and so are judged to be cost-effective (Khan et al. 2007).

Tacit knowledge, which has gained recognition as an important source of knowledge that informs clinical judgement, also makes a contribution to spontaneous self-help and to formalized responses adopted by the State (Rogers et al. 2009). Modern systems of quality assessment and feedback have highlighted the marginality of the effectiveness of professional input into therapy and treatment and the greater relevance of family, friends, peers and faith as sources of hope and support (Alexander et al. 2009). In the mental health field this traditional ambivalence about professional input makes it an area where the amount of lay input into mental health work is likely to grow as new consumer-based or run services grow in popularity and are able to show levels of retention and support. These could challenge professional services (Schutt and Rogers 2009).

However, in the case of risk management (rather than risk assessment) professional authority is likely to remain important, especially in relation to the risk of harm to self or others. If this proves to be correct then specialist mental health workers may be pushed, even more than in the past, into a coercive social control role where third-party interests are privileged over the expressed needs of identified patients.

The survival of psychiatry?

In the light of the consumerist emphasis just noted alongside the psycho-social orientation of recovery-orientated service philosophies, typical now at the turn of the twenty-first century, the authority of bio-medical psychiatry is under particular challenge. Elsewhere, we have examined whether or not psychiatry is struggling with a particular legitimation crisis (Pilgrim and Rogers 2009). Since the 1980s, in the wake of deinstitutionalization and a new shared service commitment to recovery the profession has been under particular threat. This threat was noted in the *British Journal of Psychiatry* by Craddock *et al.* (2008):

> This creeping devaluation of medicine disadvantages patients and is very damaging to both the standing and the understanding of psychiatry in the minds of the public, fellow professionals and the medical students who will be responsible for the specialty's future. On the 200th birthday of psychiatry, it is fitting to reconsider the specialty's core values and renew efforts to use psychiatric skills for the maximum benefit of patients.
>
> (Craddock *et al.* 2008: 6)

This complaint from a group of conservative British psychiatrists reflected a new context in which other professionals could claim a mandate for authority which did not require medical training. Moreover, user involvement and user criticism (see Chapter 12) have undermined the reputation of the very sort of medical authority the authors were demanding in their special pleading. Ironically, psychiatry's best chance of survival may well reside in concessions to such criticisms and power-sharing with other disciplines, rather than in attempts to re-establish old medical authority.

This question about the survival of psychiatry as a profession has been particularly evident since the contention provoked by the launch in 2013 of DSM-5, noted above and in Chapter 1. British psychiatrists at times have noted that ICD, not DSM, is their official system of classification. However, the arguments we have rehearsed in this chapter suggest that from a variety of directions (including at times dissent from *within* the profession) the political and scientific problems of diagnosis, in principle, are likely to ensure that psychiatry remains precarious as a medical specialty for the foreseeable future.

Discussion

This chapter ends by drawing attention to the twin problems of uncertainty when discussing the mental health professions. The first problem is about the professions themselves. What are they up to? Are they concerned with ameliorating distress or with controlling deviant behaviour (or both)? To what degree are they effective in either of these roles? This question is addressed when we discuss treatment in Chapter 8. In whose interests do they work – themselves, their clients, the general public, the State, patriarchy? What role does power play in their operations? Are they impartial benign practitioners or partisan oppressive enforcers of social conformity, deriving their role from wider inequalities of power (based on race, class and gender)? Do they crush individuality or celebrate and construct it? Any critical student of the mental health professions or critical practitioner within their ranks is drawn to these types of questions in one form or another.

The second problem relates to the lack of consensus on the part of sociologists when attempting to provide answers to these questions. Answers are provided but sometimes they concur with the work of others and sometimes they do not. The mental health professions represent a contested area of sociological inquiry, which is rendered less contentious by eclecticism but remains contested nonetheless. Post-structuralism is only an acceptable resolution for those accepting the epistemological current of post-modernism. Although many are part of that current, not all sociologists are post-modernists.

Both sides to this uncertainty characterize the discourse about mental health work at present. Two questions in particular will continue to tantalize social scientists for the foreseeable future. First, how do mental health professions with such a weak, controversial, contradictory and poorly credible body of knowledge (see Chapters 1 and 8) continue to maintain a mandate to regulate the lives of those they deem to be mentally unfit? Second, with the apparent mixture of coercive and non-coercive power operating in mental health work, how might the tensions and contradictions of the professions be understood?

The post-structuralists seem to come nearest to providing answers to these questions but they leave a number of loose ends. They notoriously ignore gender relationships (Rose 1990). They also understate the continuing role of coercive social control enjoyed by professionals and suffered by service users. Also, traditional epidemiological research seems to suggest that predictable inequalities in mental health derive from real differences between social groups, which are independent of a professional discourse or set of interventions. Arguably, professionals diagnose and respond to these differences, they do not simply create them in cahoots with other social actors. How then do we resolve questions about whether apparent differences in mental health between social groups are real outcomes of social inequality or constructed by-products of psychiatric discourse?

The work of mental health professionals is important to sociologists not only because of the character of their operations, strategies or practices. Professionals might also be deemed to account for the very existence of 'the mentally ill' in modern society on the one hand, or they might represent a set of occupations which respond to real socially determined forms of personal distress and social deviance defined by lay people on the other. Thus leaving aside traditional Weberian concerns about professional dominance, mental health work also raises Foucauldian ones about disciplinary knowledge and the reality or otherwise of mental illness.

This chapter has explored a variety of sociological approaches to mental health work. The diversity reflects wider unresolved disputes within the field of the sociology of the professions. In turn, these disputes are connected to divisions within social theory, with post-structuralism representing the most recent participant in debates about how health professionals are to be understood in society. As we note in the latter part of the chapter, sociological currents outside work on the professions have also been influential in some investigations of mental health work. The sociological perspective taken determines the reader's sympathy for, or criticism of, mental health workers.

Questions

1 Compare and contrast two perspectives from the sociology of the professions and apply them to mental health work.
2 'Mental health professionals and their patients are trapped in the same discourse' – discuss.
3 Are mental health workers agents of the State?
4 Whose interests are served by the work of psychiatric professionals?
5 What advantages are offered by sociological eclecticism when understanding the mental health professions?
6 Discuss the role of non-specialists in mental health work.

For discussion

Would you trust a mental health professional to help you if you were distressed? Consider this question by rehearsing what would encourage you to seek help and what would make you cautious.

8 The treatment of people with mental health problems

Chapter overview

Psychiatric treatment implicates the nature and resolution of personal troubles, which are concerned with an individual's character, biography and the immediacy of their milieu and everyday social life. However, it also implicates public issues; the way in which institutions and broader social interests and power have influenced the production and consumption of medication and therapies and in turn the discourses about them. This connection between private troubles and public issues was put forward by Wright Mills (1959) as an important focus for our attempts at exercising a 'sociological imagination'. This chapter will examine the ways in which the treatment of people with mental health problems might be understood sociologically. In particular the two connotations of 'treatment' will be explored – one related to technical aspects of therapy, the other to do with the way in which people are treated as part of a moral order. The chapter will cover the following topics:

- therapeutics
- a brief social history of psychiatric treatment;
- criticisms of psychiatric treatment; resistance and de-medicalization;
- the moral sense of 'treatment';
- the social distribution of treatment;
- the impact of evidence-based practice on treatment;
- alternative and complementary therapies.

Therapeutics

The term 'treatment', when used to refer to therapeutic procedures and technologies, assumes a view of people being ill and reflects a commonly shared 'therapeutic discourse'. Terms such as 'talking treatments' or 'drug treatments' or 'electroconvulsive treatment' (ECT) (in North America called 'electroshock treatment') are common within that discourse. Here we examine these procedures and technologies within a broader notion of 'treatment' of how people with mental health problems are treated in a broader moral and political sense. This first section will summarize the social history of psychiatric treatment before examining some recent criticisms of that legacy.

A brief social history of psychiatric treatment

Sedgwick (1982) noted that two broad responses to emotional problems can be traced to antiquity. On the one hand, attempts have been made to tamper with the bodies of people with emotional afflictions, for example douching them in water or drilling holes in their skulls to allow evil spirits to escape. On the other hand, in ancient times good counsel was also purported to be of help. Thus, there are certain stable trans-historical themes, one somatic (today's biological psychiatry) and the other conversational (today's 'psychological therapies' or 'talking treatments').

In the twentieth century, Western psychiatry developed an eclectic mixture of these interventions. Those now entering the role of psychiatric patient will be prescribed physical interventions (drugs or ECT) or some version of psychological treatment, or a combination of the two, with the former typically predominating. In the late nineteenth century this was not the case. Psychiatrists at that time had a narrow interest in lunatics in their asylums. These were assumed to have disordered brains and were therefore treated accordingly. Physical treatments were very limited and crude. By the 1930s, psychotic inpatients were being treated with only a few crude physical interventions such as paraldehyde, chloral hydrate, laxatives and cold baths (Bean 1980).

There was little or no interest in psychological treatments or in non-psychotic disorders until the First World War created a crisis of legitimacy for the dominant bio-determinist model of psychiatry. The latter assumed that lunacy, alongside other forms of deviance such as criminality and idiocy, was a result of a 'tainted' gene pool. This hereditarian emphasis was associated with the emergence of the pseudo-scientific discipline of eugenics during the late nineteenth century (Pilgrim 2008a). Eugenicists were convinced that racial improvement necessitated the resistance to external contamination by an alien racial stock and to the internal contamination by the tainted genes of the lower classes. The latter threat was amplified by their purported greater fertility.

With the First World War, 'England's finest blood' began to break down with 'shellshock'. Later this psychological disability was called 'battle neurosis' and then 'post-traumatic stress disorder'. The officers and gentlemen and their lower-class volunteer subordinates could not be construed as being genetically inferior. Consequently, the tainted gene model of psychiatry virtually constituted a form of treason. To add to the problem for the hereditarian position, officers were breaking down at a higher rate than lower ranks. This crisis of legitimacy for the hereditarian model created a space for other approaches to mental disorder, especially psychoanalysis and its derivatives. Versions of psychotherapy were the stock-in-trade of the 'shellshock doctors' of the time and in the treatment centres like the Tavistock Clinic, set up after the war to treat compensation cases of the new disorder. A fuller version of this shift from biological to psychological approaches in treatment can be found in Stone (1985).

Thus, by the end of the war, psychiatry began to become more eclectic, although a pattern was already discernible of neurosis being treated psychologically and madness being treated with physical means. The latter began to predominate again in the inter-war years, boosted in confidence by the appearance of insulin coma therapy in 1934, prefrontal leucotomy in 1935 and ECT in 1938.

Mainstream psychiatry after the Second World War marginalized the aetiological role of psychological factors and talking treatments. The main textbooks of that period, which were to dominate post-war psychiatric training, reasserted the Victorian bio-determinism of the profession's founders (Mayer-Gross *et al.* 1954). Once major tranquillizers were introduced in the mid-1950s, psychiatrists could begin to make the claim, which is often repeated today, that these drugs opened the doors of the hospitals and paved the way for community care. This claim, though common, is unfounded. Inpatient numbers were already dropping before the introduction of major tranquillizers, and the reasons for deinstitutionalization are multiple.

It is generally conceded by most commentators on twentieth-century psychiatry that it developed eclecticism (Ramon 1985) but the bias towards physical treatments remained strong. Despite the incorporation of social and psychological aetiological factors into modern psychiatry, it has tended to reject the centrality of their relevance compared with purported biological causes (Royal College of Psychiatrists 1973), and this has been reflected in the predominance of biological treatments. However, while there is still legitimization of the disease model and the authoritative power of medicine in the diagnosis and treatment of people with personal and social problems, this has been modified with the growing popularity of psychological, social and mixed models of psychopathology (e.g. bio-psycho-social) and its management.

By the 1970s, this revision of the medical model by Clare (1976) was described as a 'portmanteau model' by Baruch and Treacher (1978) to indicate that the disease formulation now takes more on board without being undermined. However, by the 1990s such a portmanteau or 'bio-psycho-social model' found itself once again in competition with and from biological psychiatry (Guze 1989; Pilgrim 2002a).

In the USA, there have been two major presidential campaigns about neuroscience and mental disorder that have legitimized bio-reductionism. The first was the declaration from George Bush Snr. that the 1990s would be the 'Decade of the Brain'. The second was the announcement from Barak Obama that $100 million would be invested in the BRAIN neuroscience initiative. We noted in Chapter 1 that 2013 was also the year when DSM-5 was announced, marking over thirty years of neo-Kraepelinian dominance in the APA, which reflected that ideology of 'hoped-for-biological-reductionism'. However, in the light of criticisms of this approach, a number of British psychiatrists in recent years have argued for a case for a return to eclecticism, with a bias towards social aetiology (Priebe *et al.* 2013). At the same time their colleagues have lined up in multi-authored petitions in the psychiatric literature to complain that their profession has been undermined by a psychosocial emphasis and its diversionary impact on psychiatry as a proper bio-medical specialty (Craddock *et al.* 2008). We considered this point at the end of Chapter 7.

The constraints on eclecticism of psychiatry over most of this period are illuminated by trends in the content of mainstream psychiatric journals during the twentieth century. While there was a broadening in the scope of psychiatric interest to include mental disorders – such as neurosis and substance misuse, and personality disorder – there was an enduring interest in biological treatments of mental illness with relatively little coverage of the alternatives, such as psychoanalysis or social psychiatry. Thus there seems to be a lack of evidence to support the notions that explanatory paradigms used by psychiatry changed much over the course of a century (Moncrieff and Crawford 2001).

As well as psychiatry now offering a mixed therapeutic approach, other mental health professionals vary in the types of treatment they offer. Psychiatric nurses might provide client-centred counselling following the humanistic psychologist Carl Rogers or psychoanalytically oriented 'psychodynamic' psychotherapy, either individually or in groups. Some nurses are trained as specialists in CBT. A similar eclectic mix can be found in the approach of clinical psychologists to treatment (Cheshire and Pilgrim 2004).

A critical appraisal of psychiatric treatment

Throughout medicine, therapeutic preferences are evident. Certain treatments may predominate, but they coexist with lesser-used alternatives. They also wax and wane in popularity with clinicians. They have also been subjected to wider social and cultural influences. The media and 'public opinion' have been influential in changing the regulatory frameworks and provision of drugs. Mental health work is no different in this sense. However, it has been controversial for particular reasons, which go beyond the pattern of fads and fashions typical of wider curative medicine:

1   There is still a broad and unresolved tension between somatic and conversational modes of treatment. The overwhelming dominance of the first of these, especially in response to madness, has led to disaffection among service users and the growing popularity of non-drug based treatments. The latter are increasingly adopted by the state in the form of short-term talking interventions (e.g. CBT).

2   All therapeutic approaches have been attacked for their iatrogenic effects. Iatrogenic effects are those caused by the treatment itself; the term 'side effects' is a common version of this notion when talking about drug therapy. It is more accurate to speak of 'unwanted effects' or 'adverse effects', rather than 'side effects'.

3   Each approach has received critical scrutiny for its ineffectiveness in ameliorating distress.

Why have physical treatments tended to predominate?

From those on the receiving end, the fact that psychiatric treatments are indeed biased more towards drugs and ECT is indeed a problem. Not only do patients (understandably) expect their subjective sense of well-being to improve as a result of psychiatric treatment, they have higher expectations of the helpfulness of psychological and combined treatments than physical interventions alone (Noble *et al.* 2001). In most mental health services physical treatments have predominated as the only form of treatment offered or imposed. However, this picture has changed with the state-sponsored use of talking therapies, particularly CBT, in service responses. Bio-medical professional preferences at the expense of user choice have effectively been affected by the introduction of treatments in primary care settings. This shift in 'place' is discussed more towards the end of this chapter.

Six mutually reinforcing contributory factors can be put forward to suggest why a bio-medical bias in treatment has existed in modern mental health interventions provided in health service settings.

1   The medicalization of psychological abnormality in the nineteenth century entailed a biological emphasis. For doctors to ensure their jurisdiction over madness they had to assert or prove that it arises from some sort of physical pathology. Accordingly, the use of physical treatments is consistent with a bio-deterministic aetiological theory. If such a position is not persuasive, then arguably mental illness is actually a sort of social, educational or existential, not physical, problem. As an indication of this, psychoanalysis, the prototype of the modern talking treatments, became divided in its early years about whether analysts needed to be physicians.

2   During the 1960s, when large mental hospitals came under attack from a variety of sources, an opportunity was created for psychiatrists to shift their site of operation into mainstream medicine. Their preferred service delivery model was that of the DGH psychiatric unit. Baruch and Treacher (1978) point out that this allowed psychiatrists to make a bid to rejoin mainstream medicine and thereby compensate for the low status traditionally enjoyed by their medical specialty. Whether this has actually led to an improvement of their status within medicine is uncertain. However, aligning itself with general medicine was made more credible by the content of its interventions being like other medical procedures. In the USA Kleinman (1986) also noted that medication use and the professional image of psychiatry as a poor relation trying to improve its medical reputation were intertwined.

3   Physical treatments are legitimized and encouraged by the profit motive. Drugs are a well-known source of profits for their producers. In addition to the profits accruing from the sale of psychotropic medication, these companies also sell drugs to offset the side effects of major tranquillizers (e.g. induced Parkinson's disease). Drug companies promote their products through expensive advertising campaigns and sponsored events. These are orientated to professionals, but direct marketing to potential consumers is also increasing.

4   Although millions in each international currency are spent yearly on psychotropic drugs, they are still arguably cheaper to deliver than labour-intensive talking treatments. For instance, minor tranquillizers are a cheap and quick way of disposing of emotional problems in the surgery. Likewise, a reliance on major tranquillizers to dampen down the agitation of psychotic patients, older people and those with learning difficulties has been a cheap alternative to crisis intervention, intensive family support and psychological programmes.

5   If psychiatry exists, among other things, to control disruptive and unintelligible conduct, then physical treatments are highly suited to this purpose because they can be imposed in the absence of co-operation. Medication, psychosurgery and ECT can, in certain circumstances, be imposed on people against their will, whereas it is very difficult to conduct talking treatments with resistant subjects. Indeed, most psychotherapists argue that consent is a necessary precondition for any form of their treatment and that this condition of free choice is clearly compromised by a client being captive (Pilgrim 1988).

6   Although discoveries about the behavioural impact of psychotropic drugs have often been a result of accident rather than design, once the effects are demonstrated, and they are patented and marketed by drug companies, they provide a spurious illusion that bio-determinism has been proven (bringing us back to point 1 above). The drive for pharmaceutical companies to produce both innovative and 'me too' compounds for profit has entailed their stimulation of biological psychiatric research both directly via research funding and indirectly. In the latter regard, Healy (1997) noted that even the patient who is drug 'treatment' resistant becomes a curious conundrum for neuropsychiatric researchers to solve using expensive medical technology to scan (live) and slice (dead) brains. The very use of that expensive technology then confirms the legitimacy of biological reductionism within psychiatry.

Minor tranquillizers

Benzodiazepines are a class of psychoactive drugs, which have been used at various times for treating depression, anxiety, insomnia, agitation, seizures, muscle spasms and alcohol withdrawal, and as a type of premedication for minor surgical procedures. The effects associated with these drugs include the induction of sleep (hypnotic), the reduction of anxiety (anxiolytic) and muscle relaxation (Olkkola and Ahonen 2008). In recent years there has been a significant reduction in the use of benzodiazepine drugs largely as a result of the sustained criticism they have received (see below). A question has arisen about what should replace them as a strategy for managing anxiety-based mental health problems. Nonetheless, despite criticisms, they are still prescribed albeit ambivalently by doctors, and they remain a quick and relatively cheap response to some psycho-social problems in primary care settings.

The benzodiazepines have mainly been discredited for their addictive qualities. They are only effective in symptom control for around 10 days, with 58–77 per cent of recipients reporting sedation effects of the drugs (drowsiness, lethargy and memory disturbances). Thirty per cent of those taking these drugs for more than a few weeks will develop withdrawal symptoms, including panic attacks, insomnia, tremor, palpitations, sweating and muscle tension (Tyrer 1987). In a small percentage (under 5 per cent) more severe problems, including epileptic seizures and paranoid reactions, might occur. During the 1980s, the scale of iatrogenic addiction prompted a popular protest movement which led to litigation against the drug companies supplying minor tranquillizers (Lacey 1991). When they are used in older patients, minor tranquillizers can also lead to mental confusion and falls, necessitating emergency medical treatment.

Sociologists have illuminated the role and impact of wider social influences, institutions and processes on the use and acceptability of minor tranquillizers. Bury and Gabe (1990) demonstrated the role of the media in legitimizing the social problem status of minor tranquillizers. The same authors presented an analysis of events surrounding the suspension of the licence, by the British Licensing Authority in 1991, for the widely used sleeping tablet Halcion (triazolam) (Gabe and Bury 1996). They identified four elements within these events: the claims-making activities of medical experts, legal challenges, the role of the media and the response of the State. Together these have made a contribution to minor tranquillizers becoming a public and governmental issue rather than a purely clinical matter.

In relation to the same controversy about Halcion, micro-sociological factors within organizations such as the Licensing Authority have been offered as an alternative to the account by Gabe and Bury (Abraham and Sheppard 1998). These micro-factors include professional interests and the internal organizational arrangements and processes within institutions for reviewing and presenting data. Abraham and Sheppard suggest that these are more important than broader extra-organizational social influences in determining whether or not a drug remains widely available or is withdrawn from use (cf. Gabe and Bury 1996). It may well be that both accounts are applicable – it seems likely that social processes at both micro and macro levels are likely to sway the extent to which drugs are viewed as acceptable by authorizing bodies, the medical profession, the public and the State.

Despite criticisms of the drugs they are still prescribed, although in primary care this is restricted to short-term use for phobias and they are no longer used as a widespread quick and cheap response to complex psycho-social presenting problems. The impact of campaigns against the drugs and criticisms about poor cost-effectiveness from services commissioners have impacted on GPs' prescribing and so they are no longer habitually prescribed. A recent study suggested a sensitivity to previous criticisms and a much more restricted view of the GP's role. This includes greater awareness of risks and addiction (Rogers *et al.* 2007).

Antipsychotics

The first generation of antipsychotics, which with the advent of a 'second generation' have come to be known as typical antipsychotics, were first introduced in the 1950s. The second generation, known as 'atypical antipsychotics' were developed and introduced into clinical practice in the 1970s, and since the 1990s have been increasingly used in routine practice. Both 'typical' and 'atypical' medication block receptors in the brain's dopamine pathways. Negative effects are common and include weight gain, white and red blood cell disorders (e.g. agranulocytosis), tardive dyskinesia and tardive akathisia (movement and feeling disorders), and neuroleptic induced psychoses. The iatrogenic problems of Parkinsonism (trembling), akathisia (inner restlessness) and tardive dyskinesia are a group of disabling and disfiguring movement disorders, including pronounced facial tics, tongue flicking and jerking limbs. Estimates of their prevalence in those prescribed major tranquillizers vary from 0.5 per cent to 50 per cent with a mean of 20 per cent (Brown and Funk 1986). The probability of the iatrogenic effect occurring increases the longer the drug is prescribed, the larger the dose and the more other drugs are given in a 'cocktail' (technically called 'polypharmacy') (Hemmenki 1977; Warner 1985). When larger doses are given ('megadosing') fatalities are also risked, warranting the invention of a new diagnosis for iatrogenic death from phenothiazines – the 'neuroleptic malignant syndrome' (Kellam 1987).

Given the serious negative effects associated with neuroleptics, until recently the perceived degree of complacency about their use on the part of professionals has attracted sociological interest. Brown and Funk (1986) traced how the evidence about tardive dyskinesia was available to psychiatrists in the late 1960s. And yet, throughout the 1970s and 1980s major tranquillizer prescription rates were undiminished (they actually *increased* in frequency and in dose levels). Active and passive forms of professional resistance to the recognition of tardive dyskinesia as an iatrogenic epidemic were evident in this period. Some clinicians acknowledged its existence but challenged data on its claimed prevalence or argued that the therapeutic benefits outweighed the iatrogenic risks. Others simply failed to change their prescribing habits without comment.

Brown and Funk claim that two theories (professional dominance and labelling) have some merit in accounting for this professional resistance to change. Both acknowledge the importance of the powerless social position of patients. The labelling theory account suggests that the powerless position and low social status of psychiatric patients renders them both unimportant and invisible. Consequently, their treating psychiatrists do not take their complaints about 'side effects', or their concerns about the debilitating effects of the drugs, seriously. Instead, doctors tend to be concerned only with the effectiveness of the drugs in symptom reduction (assessed by them, not the patients themselves).

The professional dominance theory focuses on the relationship between the status of psychiatry as a medical specialty and the role of physical treatment (see earlier). Brown and Funk endorse a similar picture, with psychiatry tying itself to physical medicine and its attendant biological trappings. Given this preoccupation with collective professional status, unfortunate consequences of biological treatment (like tardive dyskinesia) are ignored, denied or rationalized by clinicians. According to this theory, the needs of patients are ignored in favour of the political needs of their treating psychiatrists. A study of psychiatrists and recipient views of major tranquillizers (Finn *et al*. 1990) showed that both groups concur on the risks and 'bothersomeness' of side effects. However, 'psychiatrists saw side-effects as significantly less bothersome than symptoms when considering costs to society' (Finn *et al*. 1990: 843). It is, perhaps, not surprising that patients who experience the side effects of antipsychotics are often reluctant to comply with the regimen. In its depot form this type of medication results in an even more disempowered perception of the treatment process (Kilian *et al*. 2003). What is, perhaps, more surprising is that given the range and severity of side effects, non-adherence rates for major tranquillizers are the same as for other types of non-psychiatric medication.

The problems associated with traditional major tranquillizers (the phenothiazine group of drugs) purportedly applied less to the second generation of drugs. When introduced the claim was that these 'atypicals' were more efficient at symptom reduction and less liable to create movement disorders in patients. However, there is the risk of life-threatening blood disorders with some versions of the new antipsychotics. A range of new problems and adverse effects have become apparent as they have been used on a more routine basis, Indeed, some psychiatrists comparing the use of old and new antipsychotics are now querying these purported advantages of the newer drugs. They argue that the older drugs in low doses are as good as the new ones (Lewis and Leiberman 2008).

> Within psychiatry a sharper focus and use of 'evidence-based' practice has resulted in a more reflexive view about the traditional use of antipsychotics suggesting a greater alignment with both user views and the critique previously made by sociologists such as Brown and Funk. This new view emanates from recognition of the results of clinical trials, which failed to show a superior outcome when the new atypical drugs were compared with the older generation drugs.
>
> (Tyrer 2008)

Others have gone as far as to suggest the possibilities of non-prescribing, as suggested by Morrison *et al*. (2012: 83):

> Given that mental health services appear to have overestimated the strength of the evidence base for antipsychotic medication, while underestimating the seriousness of the adverse effects, it seems sensible to re-evaluate the risk–benefit ratio of such drugs. This risk–benefit profile may be a factor in the high rates of non-adherence and discontinuation of medication found in patients with psychosis; thus, some decisions to refuse or discontinue antipsychotic medication may represent a rational informed choice rather than an irrational decision due to lack of insight or symptoms such as suspiciousness. Given accurate and honest assessment of both risks and benefits, it should be possible to prescribe antipsychotics in a more thoughtful and collaborative way, and these considerations should involve explicit discussion of the possibility of not prescribing at all.

The sociological significance of the prescribing of and compliance with antipsychotics extends beyond the issue of the adverse effects and practices of the profession of psychiatry.

Psychiatric patients' 'non-compliance' with medication has emerged as a significant social problem. Images of deinstitutionalization, often promoted via the media, have become synonymous with the occurrence of socially unacceptable behaviour by ex-psychiatric patients living in the community. Within this oft-publicized scenario, medication has been depicted as an unambiguously valid means of managing and controlling people who are viewed as a potential threat to the social order. Compliance with these drugs has come to be seen as an indicator of the success or failure of 'care in the community'. In this sense, the need for patient compliance derives not only from public pressures about managing psychiatric patients appropriately but it is also a central tenet in the management of mental health problems more generally.

The closure of mental hospitals was predicated on the assumed effectiveness of major tranquillizers. The introduction during the late 1960s of depot medication can be seen as an early attempt to devise a strategy for the more efficient control of patients' behaviour in the community. (It involves patients being injected with long-acting drugs in their home or at a clinic.) Depot medication was uniquely marketed as a means of ensuring the receipt of medication, which did not rely on the patients' daily consent to treatment on their reliability in self-administering daily pills.

The effectiveness of antipsychotics has been assumed by professionals, politicians and relatives' groups who emphasize the importance of treatment compliance for discharged patients. This has extended to legal proposals to enforce medication compliance in community-based patients in Britain – a policy already implemented in some parts of the USA (Dennis and Monahan 1996). However, the effectiveness and acceptability of major tranquillizers have been strongly challenged. For example, Cohen (1997) notes that:

- only one in three medicated patients fails to relapse;
- chronic use of the drugs leads to a reduction in social functioning;
- to date, few researchers have attended to user views of being medicated.

The reviewer concludes that 'the overall usefulness [of neuroleptics] in the treatment of schizophrenia . . . is far from established' (Cohen 1997: 195). In relation to their iatrogenic effects Cohen concludes that the 'neuroleptics' near-sacred reputation as 'antipsychotics' is equalled only by their record as one of the most behaviourally toxic classes of psychotropic drugs' (1997: 201).

Extending the point about assumed utility of the drugs, major tranquillizers have been viewed as the principal means of preventing 'the revolving-door patient' phenomenon. They are a central plank of 'outreach' care, case management, the care programme approach, supervised discharge and the management of those with 'a severe and enduring mental illness'. However, the centrality of medication to mental health policy has been problematic. The iatrogenic effects of medication have also become a focus of critical scrutiny and this has received greater publicity than at the time when Brown and Funk were discussing the topic in the 1980s.

The negative effects of major tranquillizers have been the focus of criticism from campaigning and mental health user organizations. Policy-makers are now faced with balancing the need to maintain medication adherence, with the risks of iatrogenesis (Rogers and Pilgrim 1996). This dilemma has become increasingly difficult for policy-makers to manage in a cultural context of high sensitivity to risk, the emergence of a consumerist philosophy within the health service, and the growing acceptance of the legitimacy of lay perceptions and assessment of medicine within modern health care systems.

The receipt of major tranquillizers occurs in a context of the wider meaning and symbolic significance that 'schizophrenia' has for patients in their everyday lives and of a policy context which stresses the need to survey and control the behaviour of people living in the community. For this reason, self-regulatory action in this group of patients has been found to be less evident, and the threat and application of external social control is greater than in relation to other groups of patients taking medication for chronic conditions (Rogers et al. 1998).

People taking antipsychotic medication do not see – as mental health professionals do – side effects and symptoms as separate issues. Instead, they describe drugs as 'good' or 'terrible', an indication of the total impact of their treatment and the impact that it has on well-being. The latter is defined by service users as normality of function, feelings and their appearance to the outside world (Carrick *et al.* 2004).

Antidepressants

Antidepressants, and most notably the newer types (selective serotonin re-uptake inhibitors or SSRIs) are now widely prescribed drugs globally. Annual sales of these drugs run into billions of pounds (Greenberg *et al.* 2003) and yet despite increasing rates of prescribing and the intro-duction of new variants ('me too' drugs), recent systematic reviews suggest that their effective-ness is limited. For example, Kirsch *et al.* (2008) point to 'modest benefits over placebo treatment, and when unpublished trial data are included, the benefit falls below accepted criteria for clinical significance'.

Antidepressants have been associated with a number of disabling effects, including tiredness, dry mouth, impotence and loss of libido, blurred vision, constipation, weight gain and palpitations. The tricyclic version of this type of drug was implicated in around 10 per cent of deaths from self-poisoning in Britain in the early 1980s. Tricyclics have now been superseded by SSRIs, which are less toxic. In older people a decline in suicide has been directly attributable to prescribing this type of antidepressant (Gunnell *et al.* 2003). However, as these drugs have gradually superseded the tricyclics, new issues have emerged which suggest that the newer antidepressant drugs carry serious risks that may outweigh any benefits. This is particularly the case when prescribing these drugs in the treatment of depression in childhood and adolescence, and warnings have been issued regarding the increased risk of suicide-related behaviour (Whittington *et al.* 2004).

The prescription of antidepressants for a range of psycho-social problems and their asso-ciated distress (reduced diagnostically and monolithically to 'clinical depression' (Pilgrim and Bentall 1999; Dowrick 2004)) is shaped by a number of factors. These include patient and profes-sional characteristics, the interaction between them, the type of treatment setting and form of health care system. Sleath and Shih (2003) found in the USA that insurance status is influential in determining which type of antidepressant is prescribed. Patients belonging to a health manage-ment organization that had capitated visits were four times more likely to receive older rather than newer antidepressants.

As with the newer 'antipsychotics' discussed above, the regular use of newer antidepressants has met with accusations of another false dawn, as new iatrogenic problems are identified and initial hopes of curative power are queried. For example, reviews of studies of antidepressants ver-sus psychological therapies in randomized controlled trials (RCTs) suggest that both are clinically effective in the short term, separately and combined, but no treatment is good at preventing long-term relapse in those who have had a depressive episode in their lives (Fisher and Greenberg 1997).

Initially it was claimed that the SSRIs were not dependency forming. This has now proved to be a false claim. Moreover, and more dramatically, they have been linked to claims of raised risk of both homicidal and suicidal behaviour (Healy 1997). The drugs have also played a role in extending the medicalization of a range of ordinary experiences of distress. For example, Metzl and Angell (2004) examined an increasing range of female experiences which have been medical-ized by their treatment with the newer antidepressants. These include 'pre-menopausal dysphoric disorder (PMDD)', 'post-partum depression' and 'peri-menopausal depression'. Moreover, catego-ries of depressive illness have expanded to incorporate what were previously considered normal life events such as motherhood, menstruation and childbirth.

These points about antidepressants indicate that medications have complex life cycles, with diverse actors, social systems and institutions influencing who they are prescribed to and how they are used. Cohen *et al.* (2001) point to the way in which a medication life cycle evolves and mutates with social and technological change. The drug companies, the medical profession and patients themselves contribute to these changes in prescribed drug use, a relationship explored in depth by Herzberg (2009) in his historical analysis of *Happy Pills in America*. The typical cycle of legitimacy is that a new drug is launched with grand claims in their marketing that they are safe and effective. They are prescribed extensively until their disadvantages (such as addictiveness, limited effectiveness and adverse effects) start to be reported by patients and in the medical literature. Eventually the pharmaceutical industry develops a new 'generation' of drugs that is marketed to replace the old now discredited ones. At this point the problems of the old (once new) drugs are conceded as a form of marketing leverage to sell new products and the cycle repeats.

The scientific theories and the public understanding of science knowledge and theories about antidepressant medication build a complex and ambiguous picture about the social acceptance of antidepressants and lay response to their value in modern society. Pharmacogenomics have increasingly promoted a view of tailoring to individual needs through, for example, the exploration of the role of possible genetic variation in how antidepressants are metabolized by individuals. This implies a more sophisticated means of increasing the tolerance and effectiveness of antidepressants. While there has been considerable marketing and endorsement of genome-based therapies for depression (including medication), lay experience of the use of antidepressant medication contradicts this view of progress. Discussions of the clinical acceptability of genome-based therapies for depression cannot be divorced from some of the wider issues regarding depression and antidepressants. Public perceptions about the benefits and progress of pharmogenetics in the development of antidepressants, which are associated at times with a genetic test for depression (Rose and Barr 2008), sit alongside doubts about and experience of the use of antidepressant medication, ambivalence about a medical model, resistance to dependence on medication and a preference for autonomy and self-direction in managing adversity. A sense of positive selfhood and identity in dealing with adversity (Edge and Rogers 2005) and positive cultural connotations with depression particularly in young people (Biddle *et al.* 2007) increase the likelihood of rejection and ambivalence.

This uncertainty may result in a negative impact on the acceptability of the antidepressants (Barr and Rose 2008). However, any such loss of confidence needs to be put into the context of evidence about their routine use. When the SSRIs emerged in the early 1990s Peter Kramer in his well-known *Listening to Prozac* was an advocate of that wide market for these drugs (Kramer 1993). However, their critics considered that the scale of psychotropic drug consumption in the USA was not warranted, given the recorded evidence about poor efficacy and clinical iatrogenesis (Breggin 1994).

By 2000 in the USA around 25 million patient visits were made for 'depression' per year, with 69 per cent of these visits resulting in prescriptions for SSRIs. By 2004, an estimated 1 in 10 American women were taking an SSRI. By 2007 antidepressants were the most prescribed among all classes of drugs, with a total of 227.3 million prescriptions in the USA alone. In the UK since 2008, in some economically depressed areas, prescriptions of antidepressants have been increasing. At the time of writing, some of those localities have one in six of the population in receipt of antidepressants.

The expanded ambitions of the drug companies and their constraints

The criticisms about the way in which psychotropic drugs have been used for the major categories of mental health problems have led to the commercial interests – notably the drug companies – promoting their drugs in new places for new conditions and 'non' conditions. The activities of drug companies previously hidden from public and scholarly scrutiny have been made more transparent as a result of a combination of investigative journalism and a systematic approach to evidenced-based medicine. With regard to the latter, the results of systematically reviewing both the evidence and methods used to produce evidence have cast doubt upon the rhetoric of drug-company marketing campaigns.

For example Ioannidis (2008) refers to 'a seemingly evidence-based myth on antidepressant effectiveness' in exploring the claims for effectiveness by drug companies. He found that these had been based on a series of small RCTs, which included outcomes that did not appear to be relevant and 'improper interpretation of statistical significant, manipulated study design, biased selection of study populations, short follow up, and selective and distorted reporting of results'. Short-term benefits were found to be small, and the balance between negative and positive impacts on health were not considered in the longer term.

Promoting the use of drugs to include a much larger population is another way in which commercial interests have acted to promote drugs. Reflecting the weak treatment specificity in biomedical psychiatry, psychotropic drugs are rarely matched and tailored to particular diagnosed conditions. For example, all the types of drug discussed above are used across diagnostic boundaries. While this is one aspect of why psychiatric diagnoses have weak validity, the benefit to the drug companies is that they can market psychotropic agents as offering benefits to a very wide range of conditions. For example, olanzapine, an atypical antipsychotic developed to treat 'schizophrenia', is also used to treat bi-polar disorder and dementia and has recently been aggressively marketed in primary care for this 'blunderbuss' utility and to encourage GPs to spot symptoms linked to these categories. An analysis of documents released by Lilly, the manufacturer of the drug, found that the targets for use had been extended to include those in primary care, who were demonstrating mild and arguably normal 'non-symptoms'. The marketing of olanzapine has, according to Spielmans (2009), depicted bi-polar disorder as a common, rather than unusual, illness.

The drug companies are now facing a number of challenges about their products. Few 'blockbuster' drugs are now apparent, and research and development costs are extensive. Patents expire and it is expensive to develop new drugs that are demonstrably safe and effective. Apart from the newer antidepressants developed in the late 1980s, little genuine research advance has been made by the medical–pharmaceutical alliance since the 'pharmacological revolution' of the 1950s, leaving the drug companies to develop secondary marketing strategies to re-cycle older drugs. Healy (2004) notes how the diagnosis of 'panic disorder' after 9/11 became a marketing opportunity to prescribe existing antidepressants for this condition.

Psychological therapies

As far as the psychological therapies are concerned, it is not self-evident that they are benign, simply because they are physically non-invasive and generally preferred by service users. Two types of iatrogenic problems arise in psychotherapy. The first is the so-called 'deterioration effect' – where symptoms get worse during the normal course of therapy (Bergin 1971). The second set of problems is to do with the personal abuse suffered at the hands of unethical practitioners who exploit the power discrepancy existing, under conditions of privacy, to gain emotional or sexual gratification from their clients (Jehu 1995; Pilgrim and Guinan 1999).

By the mid-1990s over half of the malpractice suits taken out by people with mental health problems about their treatment at the hands of psychiatrists and clinical psychologists in the USA involved the distress created by sexual abuse by therapists (Schoener and Lupker 1996). Such has been the crisis of confidence thrown up by evidence of these iatrogenic effects of psychotherapy that some previously committed therapists have recommended the abandonment of therapy in favour of some type of self-help or have issued strong warnings to patients about the risks, as well as of the potential benefits, of psychotherapy (Masson 1988b; Smail 1996; Pilgrim 1997a).

Nonetheless, users of inpatient services still ask for talking treatments, complaining that these are on offer less frequently from psychiatric services than physical treatments. Exclusion from such treatment seems to reflect a tendency to treat neurotic patients more readily in this way.

There is mixed empirical evidence on this issue. On the one hand, psychotic patients seem to be more prone to deterioration effects than less disturbed patients (Bergin and Lambert 1978). On the other hand, there are claims of significant positive effects of psychotherapy with psychotic patients (allowing the latter also to avoid the problems associated with major tranquillizers) (Karon and VandenBos 1981).

Just as medication use and the professionalization of psychiatry are interconnected (see earlier) professional questions also surround the differential use of psychological treatments. During the early professionalization of clinical psychology, its bid for therapeutic legitimacy centred on the behavioural treatment of neurosis. Psychologists tended to leave the treatment of madness to biological psychiatrists (Eysenck 1975). However, since the early 1990s psychologists have taken an increasing interest in the treatment of psychosis (Bentall 2003). As a consequence, the costs and benefits of physical and psychological treatments now need to be considered for all groups of patients as the unstable division of labour between psychiatrists and clinical psychologists has shifted.

Despite the user disaffection about bio-medical treatments in psychiatry and an expressed preference for talking treatments, given the risks of the latter, this does not imply that they are more cost-effective than drugs and ECT. Indeed, it could be argued that in some ways drug regimes are more open to public accountability than are the talking treatments. For example, provided that clinicians co-operate with them, drug protocols can make prescribing practices amenable to audit (by managers or even service users). By contrast, the effective elements of talking treatments largely relate to 'non-specific' effects of the therapist or therapist–client interaction. Good outcomes in psychotherapy are not linked to particular models but to these benign, supportive or inspirational practitioner variables, or the synergies for change created by some client–practitioner interactions but not others (Lambert and Bergin 1983). It is much more difficult to audit such inter-subjective factors than it is to set down guidelines about good drug-prescribing practice. Also drug-prescriptions are public and impersonal, whereas psychotherapy is private and personal. The latter features seem to be linked to user preferences (to have their idiosyncratic experiences taken seriously). However, these are the very reasons why talking treatments are liable to create deterioration effects because incompetent or abusive practitioners are shielded from public view.

Talking treatments, as their name indicates, rely on talk as a resource for personal change. In doing so, they professionalize ordinary human processes: the production and co-production of human narratives. Psychological therapies professionalize narrative work and then generate expert metanarratives. The latter then inform the preferred model of the practitioners through illustrative and justificatory case studies. Psychotherapeutic expertise implicitly or explicitly privileges these preferred metanarratives, with competition existing between professionals about which one is superior.

Thus, this professionalization of narratives could be criticized for undermining the legitimacy and effectiveness of ordinary relationships, which when working well contain elements of clarification, reflection and social support. Indeed, the 'non-specific' effects indicated earlier from psychotherapy outcome research suggest that the main elements of change are common to any helpful conversation between human beings such as rapport, empathy, trust and support (Barker and Pistrang 2002; McQueen and Henwood 2002).

Forms of lay and professional talk are on a continuum with shared characteristics. The professionalization of talk may obscure this continuum when privileging therapeutic narratives. One way of viewing psychological therapies is that they provide the opportunity for helpful conversations which, for contingent reasons, are missing from a client's personal and social context.

Why is there a problem of legitimacy about the effectiveness of psychiatric treatment?

In addition to criticisms about the role of psychotropic drugs in sedating disruptive individuals, drug treatments have been criticized for being ineffective at symptom control. Mention has already been made of the short-term value of minor tranquillizers. Public knowledge about debates of the effectiveness of major tranquillizers is less evident. The psychiatric literature indeed suggests that they are effective at reducing the probability of relapse (Hirsch 1986). However, the extent of this impact is quite modest according to one oft-quoted study. Crow *et al.* (1986) reported that 58 per cent of patients receiving the drugs were deemed to relapse within 2 years, compared to 78 per cent of a control group receiving a placebo. Indeed, there was only a 12 per cent difference between the two groups, according to the original data. (The latter were corrected statistically but without explanation prior to publication.) Subsequent research provides further doubts about efficacy and acceptability. One study found that patients discontinued their assigned treatment with either old or new antipsychotics owing to inefficacy or intolerable side effects or for other reasons (Liberman *et al.* 2005).

We have already mentioned that there is mixed evidence about the effectiveness of psychotherapy. Behavioural critics of verbal psychotherapy have maintained that spontaneous remission from symptoms accounts for positive change in two-thirds of neurotic patients (Eysenck 1952; Rachman 1971). These doubts, plus those mentioned earlier from internal critics about deterioration effects, have certainly rendered psychotherapy problematic. Indeed, the overall estimate of psychotherapy is that it is only of marginal (though positive) utility because the gains it achieves are offset by deterioration effects and spontaneous remission (Bergin and Lambert 1978).

As for behavioural psychotherapy, this has been subjected to two types of criticism. The first relates to the limited value of behavioural work for the gamut of mental health problems referred to psychiatric services (Yates 1970). The second criticism is that it slavishly adheres to, rather than challenges, cultural norms. An example of this was the role taken up by behaviour therapists in seeking to convert homosexual men into heterosexuals by using electroshock (electroconvulsive) aversion therapy (see Chapter 3).

Thus, the legitimacy of psychiatric treatments is undermined by different but inter-related dissatisfactions. First, there is the problem of effectiveness *per se* (i.e. no form of treatment can genuinely claim startling improvement rates, let alone 'cure'). The increasing use of evidenced-based research now provides a cumulative case that the efficacy of *any* psychiatric drug has been exaggerated and that the results of psycho-social treatments and placebos have been in comparison under-played. And even when the latter are properly considered, although they may be more acceptable to their recipients, they are not effective for all people; they too are not cure-alls. This draws our attention to a fundamental problem with the discourse of 'treatment' (whether it is biological or psychological): is the language of 'treatment' conceptually adequate for how madness and misery should be responded to in society? Can those responses be considered adequately by framing them narrowly as medical treatments?

Second, given this poor showing in symptom reduction, the iatrogenic effects of treatment become particularly salient. 'Side effects' might be tolerated if significant therapeutic benefits were also experienced by patients but with high iatrogenic effect rates and low symptom reduction rates, treatments become highly problematic (Breggin 1993).

Third, the use of treatments to ensure conformity (e.g. aversion therapy for sexual deviations in the past) and quell disruptiveness (e.g. antipsychotics, still today) has highlighted, and stimulated opposition to, the normative and coercive role of psychiatric interventions.

Fourth, currently there is a variable gap between the evidence for effective interventions in clinical trials and these treatments being used effectively in actual services (see later discussion on evidence-based practice).

The moral sense of 'treatment'

In everyday parlance 'treatment' has moral as well as medical connotations. Certain medical specialties have been exposed to particular critical attention as far as this non-medical notion of treatment is concerned. One of these is gynaecology and the other is psychiatry. This might imply that certain aspects of the person need to be treated with particular sensitivity by medicine.

The final essay in Goffman's (1961) critique of the mental hospital, *Asylums*, is subtitled 'Some notes on the vicissitudes of the tinkering trades'. He analyses the mental hospital, and the medical model of treatment, as if it were a service industry directed towards the repair of damaged parts of society (psychiatric patients). If we accept Goffman's metaphor of psychiatry as a repair industry then we can examine how its 'customers' are treated.

To begin, the scope of psychiatry needs to be restated. At one end of a spectrum of psychiatric service provision is a picture of enforced detention and imposed treatments. In Britain we have the maximum security special hospitals, regional secure units and inpatients detained under 'mental health law' in open hospitals or psychiatric units. At the other end of the spectrum are outpatients who attend voluntarily to see a therapist of their choosing in a variety of state-provided and private therapeutic facilities. In between are patients who hover around a centre-ground of services, which contains a mixture of both voluntary and coercive practices. Depending on their conduct, they may drift or be propelled suddenly towards one or other end of the spectrum.

What separates the two ends of the spectrum is essentially the question of free choice. If the mental health industry does indeed provide a service to its patients then we would expect it to manifest certain characteristics. Service industries provide options and opportunities for customers in pursuit of a product of their preference. Rotten products which customers found noxious or aversive would quickly disappear from the range of offers made by the industry. A person experiencing some form of self-defined psychological problem or distress would have the resources (financial and cognitive) and the options to freely choose a form of amelioration. How does the mental health industry fare over this issue of free choice? We will explore this question by addressing two more which are raised. Who is psychiatry's client? And what is the extent of informed consent given to patients?

Who is psychiatry's client?

One of the ambiguities surrounding psychiatric work is whether or not the identified patient is the actual client of the service. Clearly, some party other than the patient is being served under those sections of the Mental Health Act which empower professionals to remove a person's liberty and/or impose treatment interventions against the patient's will. Coulter's work (described in Chapter 1) on decision-making about madness in the lay area traces such a process. Professionals are summoned in order to resolve a distressing drama to those around the patient. Similarly, when members of the public contact the police about a person acting bizarrely in the street it is clear that the client of the police-psychiatrist 'disposal' is not the patient, although quite who psychiatry is serving in this instance is ambiguous. Is it the distressed and perplexed member of public making the first police contact, is it the police themselves, or is it both?

Clearly, if a person is detained without trial, and they are interfered with without consent, then it is difficult to conceptualize them as 'customers' or 'clients' of psychiatry. Instead, the terminology favoured by disaffected psychiatric service users would seem to be more appropriate, of 'recipients' or 'survivors' (see Chapter 12). On the other hand, if a person chooses freely to make contact with a mental health worker, to seek help with a personal difficulty, in this instance they would seem to have a genuine 'client' status. However, even with this voluntary contact there is still a sense in which the client does not enjoy the same rights and privileges as other types of customers accessing a service industry.

The question of informed choice

This can be examined with reference to five criteria set out by Bean (1986). Bean suggests that to understand whether or not genuinely informed consent takes place in psychiatric services, we must ask the following questions:

1   Are the patients aware of themselves – are they competent at making judgements on their own behalf?
2   Do those who are assumed to be aware of themselves (relatives and professionals) use that awareness to act morally?
3   Do professionals supply comprehensive and comprehensible information to patients?
4   Are patients subjected to pressure or coercion when they are in receipt of psychiatric treatment?
5   Is consent to specifiable actions offered by professionals to patients?

Answers to these questions, suggested below, point towards psychiatric practice being problematic on all five counts.

Insight

Professionals may over-ride the need to seek consent from patients about treatment if they believe that the patient is lacking in insight into their condition. However, three problems with the notion of insight can be noted:

1   Insight tends to be defined in a circular way. That is, insight means that a patient agrees with their psychiatrist. Sanity and madness are socially agreed notions and where agreement breaks down in a psychiatric encounter between doctor and patient, then the more powerful party has their view upheld. Consequently, the patient may lose their right to refuse treatment.
2   Even if we take it to be non-problematic, on the first count, then mental illness is conceded by professionals often to be episodic in nature. Given this, how do psychiatrists know for sure when a person is aware and when they are not aware?
3   Given that professionals concede that psychotic patients who lack insight may be competent in certain regards (for instance the paranoid patient who can wash, dress and make money on the stock market) how can psychiatrists specify what insight actually means in terms of cognitive and social competence? Clearly, a patient may be aware of some things when they reflect on themselves but not of others; this is probably true of everybody. None of us can be aware of everything relevant to our existence all of the time. None of us can know our own minds for certain. (Indeed, if we are exposed to the tenet of psychoanalysis we are all encouraged to believe that the bulk of our mind is unconscious.) And yet, despite our ubiquitous failure to be fully self-aware, we get by most of the time in most of our lives.

Beck-Sander (1998) deconstructed psychiatric literature referring to insight and found it to have weak construct validity. She found that the concept was used by professionals to indicate four separate patient features:

1   Treatment compliance – when this is a defining feature of insight, then it is assumed that to resist treatment is necessarily irrational. This is a dubious assumption given the iatrogenic effects of psychiatric treatments discussed earlier. Indeed, if all patients were fully informed of these effects, treatment compliance would probably decrease generally.
2   Psychological mindedness – this can be found in the psychiatric literature as another proxy indicator of insight. It refers to insight as a reified defence operating inside patients which purportedly protects them from the pain of their illness. Thus, those with more insight are deemed to be more distressed, whereas those lacking insight are cut off from the pain of the purported disease process they are experiencing.

3   Prognosis is also used at times by psychiatrists as a circular indicator of insight – those with more insight are deemed to have shorter periods of relapse into psychosis and the inverse is deemed to be true for those with less insight. This professional reasoning is post hoc and tautological. Moreover, given that prognosis is determined by a number of external as well as patient characteristics, such as socio-economic opportunity and societal discrimination, then how can we ever know whether insight is a defining single feature when prognosis is good or bad for a particular patient?

4   Pathophysiology – this is offered at times by some psychiatrists as a correlate of insight. That is, purported neuropsychological dysfunction in psychosis is offered as an explanation for why psychotic patients lack insight into their condition. This is, of course, a possibility, much as cerebral bleeding accounts for the brain damage which affects the short-term memory and orientation in time and space of some dementing patients. The problem with this argument is that, by definition, the functional psychoses are not organic conditions, at least they are not demonstrably so at present. They are defined by symptoms alone because biological markers (true signs) are absent, despite substantial bio-medical and neuropsychological research into the psychoses.

Thus, the whole question of competence or self-awareness is problematic. Despite this, professionals have powers to treat patients without their consent and they do so using the notion of 'lack of insight', as if it were non-problematic. Moreover, this purported lack of competence on the part of psychiatric patients is the very rationale for why negotiation about consent is either deemed to be unnecessary or futile. Despite this, there is no evidence that psychiatric patients are actually less able than medical patients to understand what is told to them. Soskis (1978) found that, in fact, psychiatric patients knew more about the adverse effects ('side effects') of drugs they were receiving than did medical patients (showing that if they are told they understand). However, the psychiatric patients were less likely than the medical patients to be told *why* they were receiving the medication. This indicates that psychiatrists are less willing than physicians to discuss diagnosis and rationale for treatment with their patients.

The morality of others

The discussion above showed that, collectively, psychiatrists have not acted morally in relation to the needs and vulnerabilities of patients. Major tranquillizers are one of the main groups of treatments imposed on resistant recipients. Practitioners have also acted immorally in the case of the abuse of patients by psychotherapists. Thus, psychiatric therapists are prone to fail Bean's second criterion.

Comprehensive and comprehensible information

This question is the one most commonly addressed by disaffected users of services. Whether the disaffection is caused by drugs, ECT or psychotherapy, the recurrent complaint is that patients are not supplied with enough information about the advantages and disadvantages of the treatment offered or imposed. The minor tranquillizer campaign led to litigation against the drug companies and the prescribing doctors, which focused on both iatrogenic effects and the withholding of information at the time of prescription about these effects. The same has been true of litigation about major tranquillizers in the USA (Brown and Funk 1986). Rogers and colleagues (1993) found that 60 per cent of a sample who had received major tranquillizers reported not being informed of their purpose, and that 70 per cent of this group were unhappy about the amount of information they had been given. Similar findings have been reported in studies in the USA (Soskis 1978; Lidz *et al.* 1984). These complaints would indicate that psychiatry is found to be lacking according to Bean's third criterion.

Coercion

Despite legal safeguards under mental health legislation, detained patients may be injected forcibly with drugs or given ECT or psychosurgery against their will. They can also be forced into isolation ('seclusion') without consent. One of the questions raised is whether informal patients are genuinely in the patient role voluntarily when some do not feel that they are genuinely voluntarily admitted. In the past when admission to hospital for a mental health problem was more readily resorted to, about a fifth of voluntarily admitted patients reported some degree of coercion – this appeared to be the same in the USA as it was in the UK, suggesting that Bean's fourth criterion was failed by psychiatry. Recently a more significant role has been given over to treatment and management in outpatient contexts and only a small minority of inpatients is admitted on a truly voluntary basis.

Two hypotheses have emerged about the role of coercion in relation to treatment in this new more community-orientated context. The first suggests that the use of coercion might aid engagement with treatment through making a contribution to reducing symptoms, which over time can lead to a reduction in stigma. The second suggests the reverse: coercion acts to *increase* stigma because of associated feelings of low self-esteem and a compromise in the person's quality of life. Empirical testing of these hypotheses (Link *et al.* 2008) found that that costs and benefits of coercion are mixed. On the one hand the treatment of symptoms was found to lead to improvements in social functioning and assignment to compulsory outpatient treatment was associated with better functioning and improvements in quality of life. On the other hand, self-reported coercion increased felt stigma (perceived devaluation and discrimination) and it eroded quality of life and lowered self-esteem.

Consent to specifiable actions

Real informed consent cannot be consent to anything and everything. Instead, it must be consent to a specific action or circumscribed set of actions. If it were consent to anything then this would give arbitrary powers to professionals. Indeed, in secure psychiatric provision, in particular, it is commonplace for patients to be subject to the regime of what Goffman called a 'total institution': all activities and interventions are determined by the regime of the hospital. When this is the case, patients have little or no moment-to-moment powers of decision-making. In effect, they abandon their right to agree or disagree to specifiable actions on admission or it is taken away from them.

Even in less coercive surroundings, if professionals do not give a full account, in advance, of what is to happen when a treatment is carried out, then they are not giving patients the right to agree to specifiable actions. For example, biological psychiatrists may be paternalistic about withholding information on major tranquillizers (in case it may worry the patient). Psychoanalysts may evade questions about their technique as part of their technique (to provide a blank screen for the patient's projections). Thus, for different reasons, both physical and psychological therapists may evade specifying their intended actions in relation to the patient they treat.

Having now discussed both the problems of identifying psychiatry's client and informed consent, let us return to Goffman's criteria of a good repair service industry. In essence he argues that such a service would have the following features (with our queries about the gap between principle and practice in brackets):

1   The workshop of the industry would be benign and would prevent a deterioration in the condition that required repair. (Mental health services are clearly not always benign. Coercion is ever present and treatments can be damaging.)
2   Transporting the part in need of repair to the workshop would not introduce new forms of damage. (Entering services is stigmatizing and can be distressing.)

3   The damaged part is not linked inextricably to its possessor. That is, the owner can be separated from their damaged part for a defined period of time until it is repaired. (The damaged part and its possessor are one and the same. Mental illness is about a flawed or deviant self. This is why a psychiatric diagnosis has such profound implications, as a patient's credibility as a social actor or citizen is questioned, possibly for life.)

4   Those providing the service and those using it enter into the repair contract voluntarily and with mutual respect. (Mental health law exists to enforce the relationship between service providers and service recipients.)

The social distribution of treatment

One of the paradoxes of psychiatric treatment is that it inverts the 'inverse care law'. The latter, which generally holds true for people with physical health problems, refers to the phenomenon of those in the greatest need, as a result of their socially created illness, having the poorest access to the health care system. The opposite is true of mental health care systems, which are numerically dominated by a poor patient group. In the light of the stigma attached to mental health services and the role of psychiatry some of the time, in the coercive control of socially disruptive behaviour, then it is little surprising that some social groups are more vulnerable to service receipt than others:

1   Black and ethnic minority populations receive greater inpatient attention and physical treatments than white populations in Britain and the USA.

2   Inpatients are usually poor. They are often unemployed and unemployable.

3   Women are in receipt of more psychiatric treatment than men, although a caution here is that more men are treated coercively than women.

When we examine the research on receipt of voluntary outpatient attendance in mental health services, then a different picture emerges:

1   The utilization of long-term psychotherapy is inversely related to age (over 65), race (black) and years of schooling (Olson and Pincus 1994b).

2   In the USA black and Hispanic women utilize outpatient facilities less than white women (Padgett et al. 1994).

3   Black war veterans in the USA receive less intensive treatment for post-traumatic stress problems than white veterans.

4   Black people drop out of outpatient family therapy earlier on average than whites (Kazdin et al. 1995). This finding needs to be seen in the context of the failure to incorporate cross-cultural counselling into mainstream services.

The impact of evidence-based practice on treatment

During the 1990s research knowledge and evidence emerged as potential means of controlling and improving the development and quality of health care services. The extent of its formal academic impact in the field of mental health is shown by the appearance in 1997 of a dedicated journal, *Evidence-Based Mental Health*.

The rising popularity of 'evidence-based practice' (EBP) was linked to the imperatives of health policy-makers to control service costs. It was overlain by a discourse of concern to assess the health benefits and risks of technology and treatments (Faulkner 1997). These concerns can be seen as rhetorical devices, which include the purported strengths of multi-disciplinarity and benefits to users of cost-effective treatments. It is common now for all parties to accept, in principle, evidence as a basis for clinically effective and cost-effective interventions. The RCT remains the 'gold standard' of EBP, while evidence-based or lay knowledge and qualitative methods are afforded a lesser place. In the area of mental health there are particular problems in applying the experimental conditions of the RCT to services:

> In RCTs, treatment fidelity is ensured, contaminating variables such as dropouts are eliminated and specific symptom reduction outcomes are investigated. In contrast in actual services, treatment fidelity cannot be assumed, people drop in and out of service contact and their presenting problems are often complex and not limited to specific symptoms . . .
>
> (Pilgrim 1997b: 569)

However, there have been specific aspects of treatments which have been evaluated along standardized criteria and guidelines in actual services. There is evidence too that the rhetorical devices of quality and evidence can be harnessed to empower mental health users to challenge mainstream psychiatric practices. Notwithstanding the relatively weak position of mental health quality standards, compared to physical ones, the trend towards EBM is increasing in the mental health arena. While this is very much a nascent and marginal trend, the insertion of criteria of quality into mental health services is likely to influence what comes to be acceptable knowledge about mental health service development. Two examples are given here of how a user perspective on treatment effectiveness can challenge professional definitions of EBP.

Disputed evidence about ECT

The use of ECT, controversial since its inception, illustrates the challenge of addressing patients' perspectives in the evaluation of health care technology. Despite widespread professional acceptance of ECT, service-user groups have often opposed its use. This illustrates how differing conceptions of evidence can affect the evaluation of technology. It also provides an example of the value of a more complex definition of the significant outcomes of treatment and the way in which they can shape health policy (Heitman 1996). Professional definitions of good outcomes and those offered by treatment recipients may not always coincide. While some users' groups focus on ECT as an irredeemable barbarity perpetrated by professionals, some individual patients endorse it as a life saver, while others harbour life-long resentment about its use in their care (Rogers *et al.* 1993).

Official professional accounts of ECT (Royal College of Psychiatrists 1995) have given no hint of this mixed consumer perspective on the treatment and insist that it is safe and effective, even for children. With such discrepant views about outcomes between psychiatrists and their patients about ECT, services became a contested site for competing interest groups both in terms of their viewpoints and the evidence invoked to support them.

A literature-review-based study designed to ascertain patients' views of the benefits of ECT (Rose *et al.* 2003) suggested that at least one-third of patients reported persistent memory loss. This 'meta-analysis' of patient perspectives suggested that the conventional wisdom from the Royal College of Psychiatrists that over 80 per cent of patients are satisfied with ECT and that memory loss is not clinically important is misleading.

Alternative and complementary therapies

The emphasis on control and responsibility is evident in the use of 'alternatives' to mainstream therapies on offer in mental health services. Giddens (1992) talks of the notion of 'lay re-skilling' where technical knowledge is reacquired or re-appropriated by lay people and routinely applied in the course of their day-to-day activities. 'Lay re-skilling' can be framed as a trend towards the demedicalization of society with a return to notions of 'natural' rather than technical forms of healing, non-compliance with medical treatment and the growth of complementary therapies. Complementary and alternative therapies have grown in popularity in recent years both for physical and mental health problems partly as a result of dissatisfaction with conventional medicine. The popularity in mental health of trying alternative therapies in the form of food, diet or herbal medicine is likely to have been accentuated by the lack of autonomy and choice inherent in some of the more conventional mental health treatment. Thus, while some alternative therapies do sometimes get incorporated into mainstream services (mindfulness, for example) complementary therapies in mental health can be defined as those approaches found to be therapeutic which are not usually or routinely provided or accessible to individuals from mainstream services (in the UK this would be the NHS). The growing recognition of the use and appreciation of alternatives to conventional treatments is evident in the way in which professional bodies now include information about these different approaches to mental health while acknowledging caveats about the 'lack of evidence'. (See, for example, the Royal College of Psychiatrists' web page on well-being www.rcpsych.ac.uk/healthadvice/treatmentswellbeing/complementarytherapy/cams1references.aspx.) The use of some drugs such as cannabis represents something of a paradox as being seen as both a cause and alternative form of management. Cannabis use is most prominently seen within the psychiatric literature as being associated with detrimental effects on and risks to mental health (e.g. the onset of psychosis). This has led to calls for the curtailment of its use for recreational purposes (Patton *et al.* 2002). However, cannabis is a popular alternative therapeutic approach to managing mental health among users. Users have identified cannabis as valuable as a form of self-medication for the relief of symptoms and the side effects of traditional anti-psychotic medication. The benefits of using marijuana are illustrated by this account from a mental health professional working in a community counsellor centre in the USA:

> Typically, the people I worked with at the counseling center felt a fondness for marijuana that they did not feel for prescribed psychiatric medications. Zyprexa and Lamictal were difficult facts of life, but pot was a friend. Many said they found cannabis relieved their anxiety and depression, made it possible for them to leave the house and face the world. Judging by my own experience and that of many of my colleagues, as well as a host of online message boards, marijuana is one of the most popular and widely-used unprescribed treatments for mental health problems, ranging from anxiety and depression to attention-deficit and bipolar disorders.
>
> http://crosscut.com/2012/12/27/health-medicine/112098/
> marijuana-and-counseling-where-do-we-go-here

This intuitive alternative use by services users has links to some scientific evidence that an element of cannabis (Cannabidiol) is effective. Other areas where there is strong commitment by users or potential users of services include the power of spirituality and prayer as a means of overcoming mental health problems. The clandestine use of alternatives such as spirituality arises from a fear that they will not be recognized as legitimate by conventional services. This means that alternative spiritual approaches to coping and help-seeking that are valued by users are not used as part of a holistic approach to managing mental health problems (Edge 2013).

Discussion

Some sociologists have argued that we now live in a therapeutic society in which therapeutic ideas are not confined to clinical and hospital settings but permeate most areas of everyday life. 'Governmentality' in contemporary societies is achieved by the self-regulation of our conduct and feelings, and the internalization of psychological knowledge (Rose 1990; De Swaan 1990).

This sociological emphasis has increasing salience for understanding cultural trends and the popularity of psychological ideas and therapies, and for the promotion within official policy-making of therapeutic interventions designed to promote individual responsibility and control through population-based training programmes (such as the Expert Patient Programme in Britain or Chronic Disease Management Programme in the USA). These public health policies are designed to encourage individuals to take control and responsibility for their illness and their lives. They emphasize self-assessment, self-monitoring of risk and self-efficacy in managing health and illness in everyday life.

The sociological exploration of psychiatric treatment has tended, itself, to be divided between the poles of the spectrum of service delivery mentioned earlier. On the one hand, it has been concerned with critically exposing treatment as mystified coercive social control. On the other hand, it has become preoccupied with those psychological interventions which are 'anxiously sought and gratefully received'. Sociology is a mirror to the divided territory of psychiatry and, arguably, it contributes to that division.

Psychiatric treatment remains in a precarious state of legitimacy. This uncertainty is then amplified by the doubts about the effectiveness of both physical and psychological therapeutic approaches and the complaints that have accumulated about the iatrogenic effects of these treatments. The contradictory picture of psychiatry, mixing as it does both coercion and voluntarism, and an eclectic range of treatments from leucotomy to psychoanalysis, also increases the gap between expectation and reality. If patients entering the psychiatric system expect lengthy explorations of their biography and actually get a cursory interview, followed by a prescription for anti-depressants, then the chances of disappointment are great. Likewise, if people look to psychiatry as a source of comfort during times of personal confusion and distress and actually encounter an impersonal controlling regime, with professionals who serve third parties rather than the patients they are supposedly treating, then disaffection is, again, likely.

The uncertainty surrounding the legitimacy of psychiatric treatment is amplified by the structural inequalities in access to the range of its interventions. In other words, as we have explored elsewhere in the book, not all social groups are represented evenly throughout the spectrum of psychiatry. Some receive harsher treatment than others. Black people are less likely to receive psychotherapy and more likely to receive medication and ECT. They are also more likely to be treated coercively than white people. Richer clients can afford to pick and choose between therapists in private practice, whereas poorer clients have to take what is given by state-employed professionals in their particular locality. Those diagnosed as being psychotic are less likely to receive psychological treatments than those who are diagnosed as being neurotic. Men are over-represented at the 'harsh' end of services.

If entering the psychiatric system ipso facto entailed being treated well, then those groups which are over-represented (like black people) would view themselves as being in receipt of preferential treatment. The fact that over-representation is instead a source of concern and anger to these groups reflects the suspicion with which psychiatry is viewed (as being an oppressive part of the extended state apparatus of control). Sociological investigations of how psychiatric patients are treated (in both senses of the word) may need to take on board this complexity and these contradictions. Up until now, two main 'camps' of sociology might be seen to have been warring about how to describe and understand psychiatric treatment. The humanistic bias of symbolic interactionism, exemplified in the work of Goffman, contributed to the notion of 'anti-psychiatry' and focused on the degradation of the individual and their loss of citizenship. The anti-humanistic bias of the post-structuralists conceives only of discourses which patients and therapists contribute to (or are trapped in). According to this view, individuals are produced, rather than destroyed, by psychiatry.

The psychological technologies, like the psychotherapies, are indeed now deeply implicated in modern secular society, contributing to the regulation of a moral order and promoting the contemporary importance of the 'self'. Arguably, the same is true of an approach which emphasizes the promotion of positive mental health. The problem for the post-structuralist position is that the old humanistic, anti-psychiatric arguments about the coercive power of the State are still highly pertinent to those groups which continue to be its particular target. It is not surprising that such groups remain hostile to psychiatry, rather than receiving it gratefully when contributing to 'productive power'. Sociology cannot ignore either the productive technologies of the self or the destructive potential of coercive psychiatry. Both have to be considered together.

In this chapter we have covered a wide range of considerations about psychiatric treatment. This has included reviewing the literature on specific forms of treatment and the social forces which shape its production and maintenance. Sociologists have contributed to a critical discourse about treatment along with the 'anti-psychiatrists' and disaffected service users. At other times, sociologists have suggested that psychiatry is part of a wider set of processes of governmentality. Overall, sociological scrutiny (exemplified in the work of Goffman) has tended to expose the logical contradictions of treatment. At the same time, the influence of Foucault has focused more on productive power rather than the coercive role of psychiatry in society.

For the foreseeable future, sociologists are likely to retain an interest in both of these aspects of professional mental health work. However, the notion of social exclusion and the need to reverse the effects of the role of being a psychiatric patient through social and economic opportunities suggest a broadening focus to the traditional notion of treatment. This may mean that mental health workers and psychiatrists in particular will be placed in the increasingly ironic position of ameliorating the distress caused by the labelling, treatment and management created by their own professional actions.

Questions

1 To what extent are treatments used to manage private troubles, and public social and structural issues?
2 Does psychiatry produce or crush subjectivity?
3 How can non-compliance with psychiatric treatment be understood?
4 Why does the 'inverse care law' not apply in psychiatric services?
5 What problems are associated with the concept of insight?
6 To what extent does Goffman's work on large mental hospital life still apply today?
7 Discuss the rationale for evidence-based mental health care and barriers to its success.

For discussion

Consider whether you would be prepared to volunteer for psychiatric treatment if you became psychologically distressed. What would be the pros and cons to consider in this decision?

9 Prisons, criminal justice and mental health

Chapter overview

Since the disappearance of asylums as part of the mental health institutional landscape there have been a growing number of inmates classified as suffering from a mental disorder and more of a focus on prisons constituting a mental health system of major significance. It is well documented that the prevalence of mental health problems is higher among prisoners than in the general population (Bradley 2009). Post-institutionalization arrangements have acted to underscore the fact that prisons are effectively asylums of last resort for some people. This is demonstrated, for example, by a direct link being established between an increase in the private-for-profit share of inpatient psychiatric beds and a higher number of prison inmates (Yoon 2011). In dealing with mental health problems as part of their routines, prisons are deserving of sociological attention because they give rise to a particular tension between care and surveillance/punishment. They are also sites for understanding society's complex of moral sentiments about mental health, crime and punishment, which we return to in our conclusion to this chapter. Prison care is often viewed as not merely anti-therapeutic but *actively detrimental* to mental health. Factors such as overcrowding, separation from family and friends, boredom and loss of autonomy have all been implicated in this regard (Nurse *et al.* 2003).

Reforms to prison provision in recent times reflect moral and humanitarian values of the need to prevent and ameliorate suffering among prisoners, while accommodating demands for increased social control and retribution coming from socio-political forces in the general population and articulated by politicians. This picture presents certain complex challenges for those working and living in prison settings. Professional work will be guided, more than in other settings, by a constellation of coexisting logics, derived from broader society about punishment on the one hand and therapeutic and rehabilitative expectations on the other. A system that prioritizes the logistics of punishment can sit uneasily with the need for enhanced and intensive therapeutic approaches, in response to the diverse psychological needs of inmates.

This chapter covers the following topics:

- mentally disordered offenders and the criminal justice system;
- the prison as a dedicated mental health place and space;
- patients as prisoners or prisoners as patients?;
- treatment in prison: medication, therapeutic communities and other approaches.

Mentally disordered offenders and the criminal justice system

Secure mental health services are concerned with the management of those who are 'doubly deviant'; they have committed a criminal act *and* they are deemed to be mentally abnormal. When that dual status is negotiated varies sequentially from case to case. For example, it might be decided at the point of trial or it might emerge after the prisoner is incarcerated.

Forensic psychiatry and psychology deal with the management of lawbreakers and others who come before the courts (and in exceptional cases take violent patients from open psychiatric settings). Thus, their area of jurisdiction is principally in relation to referrals from the criminal justice system and those patients who are detained in hospitals, subject to restriction orders. This introduces substantial ambiguity into the role and functions of these services and professionals employed by them. Is their primary loyalty to the courts, the general public or the patients they detain and treat? Are they concerned with risk assessment and risk management or with enabling mental health gain? These tensions permeate work in secure settings with offender patients.

The view of control discussed at the start of this chapter locates power in the hands of State organizations and agencies and their professional employees (psychiatric staff and lawyers). Foucault provides an alternative view of the emergent relationship between psychiatry and the law. Psychiatry's involvement with penal law in the eighteenth and nineteenth centuries came about with the shift from a criminology that focused on the offence and penalty, to one concerned with the criminal. This shift meant that the focus changed from *what must be punished and how, to who must be punished*:

> It is not enough for the accused to say . . . 'I am the author of the crimes before you, period. Judge since you must, condemn if you will.' Much more is expected of him. Beyond admission, there must be confession, self-examination, explanation of oneself, revelations of what one is.
>
> (Foucault 1978: 2)

For Foucault, psychiatry took its place in the legal machinery through the concept of 'homicidal mania' (a killing that took place in a domestic setting in the absence of any apparent motive) in the latter half of the eighteenth century. From this moment, crime and insanity became conflated. He illustrates this type of crime/insanity with reference to notorious cases: a mother who kills her child; a man who breaks into a house, kills an elderly woman and departs without stealing and fails to hide himself; a son who kills his mother with whom he has always got on well. Psychiatry justified its involvement in order to make the unintelligibility of this type of crime intelligible by offering its preferred medical explanations.

Foucault links forensic psychiatry to a type of public hygiene, where the focus is on the 'societal body' and social danger rather than the 'individual soul'. Homicidal mania represents insanity in its most harmful form – minimum warning, maximum consequences – which only a specialist eye can detect. According to Foucault, forensic psychiatry's claim to violent monomania did not include a desire to take over criminality and was not a form of psychiatric imperialism. Rather, there was the more limited ambition of justifying its function, namely the control of danger emanating from the human condition.

In its current manifestation, forensic 'mental health work' carried out now by doctors, psychologists, nurses and occupational therapists remains contentious in this regard and Foucault's observations remain highly pertinent. Two points of contention stand out. One, already noted, relates to ambiguity about the primary client (is it the patient or is it a third party?). The other relates to the open-ended nature of psychiatric detention, compared to imprisonment with its defined sentences. The fact that mentally disordered offenders are not given a clearly defined date for discharge, whereas a prisoner does have a latest release date, defined at the point of sentencing, disadvantages patients compared to prisoners. They are left in a state of existential limbo, in which it is not obvious how they can warrant their eventual release and when, if ever, that day will arrive (Pilgrim 2007b). In contrast to this confusing predicament, the prisoner simply 'serves their time' and can prepare themselves for their eventual release. However, it is also clear that prisoners have poor access to mental health care. For example, therapeutic needs of prisoners (such as the need to take prescribed medication) are routinely subordinated to an ideology of retribution and penal control (Bowen *et al.* 2009). Thus there are unique features of prison as a mental health place.

The prison as a dedicated mental health place and space

The extent to which prison as a place is associated with the generation of, and a repository for, mental health problems is highly significant. Fazel and Danesh (2002) found that those in prison are ten times more likely to have anti-social personality disorders than the normal general population, and in relation to depression and psychosis had several times the rate in the general population.

Prisons operate as unique places in terms of both fashioning and exacerbating mental health problems. In *Discipline and Punish*, Foucault (1975) highlighted the primacy of the penal management of its inmates through a triadic regime of surveillance, the organization of spatial activity, and forms of classification designed (literally) to 're-form' the inmates.

Goffman (1961) conceptualized both mental hospitals and prisons as total institution – in other words, places of residence cut off from wider society and governed by de-humanizing systems of administration and routines. The 'encompassing tendencies' of total institutions for Goffman invariably lead to an inmate's sense of self being eroded by processes that impact on individuality, in order that the goals of the institution can dominate. Becoming a prisoner involves a process of drawing in the labelling power of being institutionally committed. The prisoner internalizes the dominant framing of their own criminal nature, and he (typically it is a man) comes to accept the technologies used to identify them, such as the court system of conviction, and to manage them after release.

Prisons as places of correction, rather than therapy, are governed by the architecture of a unique type of total institution. It is one in which the presence of health care, and personal access to it, is of secondary importance to other organizational rationales and so has to be continually negotiated. For this reason, policies and practices surrounding mental health that are politically determined by custodial, rather than health, priorities can create difficult and delayed routes into care.

The architectural and regulatory construction of prison treats the prisoner as a depersonalized unit where their loss of agency is normalized. The prisoner's movement through the geographical space of the prison is regulated at all times by custody policies, routines, economies and spur-of-the-moment decision-making. The latter arbitrariness removes personal control from the individual prisoner. These policies and practices, primarily determined by custodial priorities, can create significant delays and distortions of access. The notion of 'anti-place' has been applied to describe the lack of empathy for inmates by those charged with their care, who primarily have to act as custodians (Stoller 2003).

As suggested above, compared to the general population, people in prison experience poorer mental and physical health and many have adopted, or are exposed to, lifestyles that put them at risk of mental ill-health. Evidence of the detrimental aspects to the prison environment has been a focus of concern to social campaigners and policy-makers in liberal welfare democracies, where therapeutic optimism and values stand alongside, and in tension with, the urge not just to provide punishment as an organizational disposal but to impose punishment as a psychological process during incarceration, as well as ensure temporary risk reduction to wider society.

While prison environments are often not seen as conducive to mental health, paradoxically at times the penal system has been viewed as holding out new possibilities for its improvement. Prisoners are a transient population but time spent in prison has been viewed as a potential 'window of opportunity' to promote health and prevent disease, in a high-risk section of the population. This aspiration of promoting the mental health of prisoners has become a claimed core activity and focus for the prison service in the UK and USA.

In the UK, this shift is embodied in institutional and organizational reform, with responsibility for prison health care provision in England shifting from the Home Office dealing with penal matters to the NHS. With this shift, prisons have come to be seen as aspirational 'therapeutic landscapes' with attempts to offer prisoners the same standard of mental health care as in the rest of society. This is indicated in the attribution of new responsibilities for penal establishments, to carry out the assessment of health needs and develop local health improvement plans, commensurate with mainstream health policy. As Reed and Lyne (2000) put it:

A period in prison should present an opportunity to detect, diagnose and treat mental illness in a population often hard to engage with NHS services. This could bring major benefits not only to patients but to the wider community by ensuring continuity of care and reducing the risk of re-offending on release.

The policy objective behind these changes has been predicated on the notion of equivalence in the range and quality of services available to prisoners, and the integration and normalization with NHS services. An emphasis has been placed on the impact of the early stages of custody. Measures which have been implemented have included: increasing the availability of day care facilities to provide therapeutic settings, in which members of community mental health teams (CMHTs) can run appropriate interventions; the expansion of wing-based in-reach services; the engagement of community-based health professionals to assist in promoting continuity of care on entry to prison and post-release; and the promotion of the prisoners skills in self-care.

Within this broader context of attempts to make changes, in prisons the structural barriers to reform may remain entrenched. There is an inherent tension between security needs and health improvement schemes, because the over-riding priority for enforcing security puts constraints on attempts to enable individuals to improve their health. Contextual factors relevant are the built environment and prison regime, the demographic characteristics of prisoners and the health behaviours accompanying them into prison. The notion that prisons can be supportive and healthy environments is at odds with the view that a therapeutic approach to mental health is undermined by an ethos that disempowers and deprives, through processes devoted to discipline and control. The tension between medicalized and punitive solutions for those with a mental health problem are reflected in the criminalization versus psychiatrization debate now discussed.

Patients as prisoners or prisoners as patients?

During the 1960s and 1970s in the USSR, the Communist Party categorized and dealt with ideological deviance by diagnosing and institutionalizing so-called 'counter-revolutionaries' with mental illness. Citizens could be deemed psychotic, simply on account of their political views. Dissenters, who were often seen as both a burden and a threat to the system, could be easily discredited and detained. To accommodate to this extreme form of psychiatrization, Soviet definitions of mental disease were expanded to include political disobedience. This crude form of psychiatrization amounted to little more than political abuse and repression.

However, while the extremes of criminalization versus psychiatrization are not always as stark as the Soviet example, we noted earlier that there is an inevitable ambiguity when the State detains people who are deemed to be mentally disordered. The competing logics of care and punishment discussed above still recur and are ubiquitous. The navigation and construction of statuses in the criminal justice system are blurred. Fernandez and Lézé (2011) suggest that prisoners are selected and converted into 'patients' as a result of earning attention by their honesty, sincerity and role compliance. In other words, the non-disordered offender is treated with caution and suspicion because of their knowingly resistive, deceitful and manipulative ways, whereas those warranting patient-hood do not present in this manner to staff but are accepted as being less self-serving. Treatment thereafter is orientated to the therapeutic and moral expectations of responsibility, recognition of guilt and self-esteem.

However, this separation in the prison population does not mean that those with mental health problems are less criminalized at the outset. Those with mental health problems are *more* likely to be criminalized than those who have not been considered to have a mental health problem. For similar offences those with a label of mental illness have a greater chance of being arrested than non-mentally-disordered people (Teplin 1984). However, the criminalization versus psychiatrization paths are evident in discussing the dilemmas of the apparently psychopathic or psychotic patient who acts dangerously. These patient groups emerged in the UK with institutions like Broadmoor and subsequent asylums for the 'criminally insane'. (As another indication of the blurring of different forms of the State apparatus of coercive control, the Prison Officers' Association (POA) in the UK was established at Broadmoor after it was built in 1863. Broadmoor was and is still not a prison but the POA remains there and in other high-security hospitals.)

By definition, the mentally disordered offender qualifies for entry into both the criminal justice and mental health systems. This raises particular dilemmas and questions, which arise out of the conceptual merging of two types of deviance: criminality and mental disorder. Explicitly stated, should individuals be dealt with in the system designed to deal with the criminal aspects of their behaviour (i.e. in prison) or should they be treated for their mental disorder in hospital?

The arguments for psychiatrization are made on the grounds that hospitalization of mentally disordered offenders is less stigmatizing and hospital treatment benefits patients more than do prisons. Prisons, the argument goes, are unable to provide the environment or range of treatments that a health care regime can (Abramson 1972). A policy initiative stemming from this reasoning was the diversion of mentally disordered offenders from custody projects which were informed by the prevailing ethos of community care in the 1980s.

However, others (Monahan 1973; Fennell 1991) see psychiatrization as resting on dubious logical and empirical grounds. They point out that mental hospitals are far from stigma free. Arguably, in Britain the association of the high-security hospitals, like Ashworth and Broadmoor, with notorious serial killers and gangsters means that they are far more stigmatizing than prisons. For example, when poor care has been exposed in these places, staff defending their traditional role have been keen to emphasize the notoriety of their residents (Pilgrim 2007b). This both confirms stigmatization of these patients and offers a basis to rationalize their mistreatment by staff accused of wrongdoing (see later).

Even though many official bodies overseeing mental health care in prison settings argue for more transfers to medical settings (e.g. Mental Health Act Commission 2008), there remain substantial doubts over whether medical treatment regimens are superior, as was noted earlier. Those labelled as 'personality disordered' make up a significant proportion of those in high-security hospitals, yet there is little evidence to suggest that there is an effective treatment for antisocial behaviour in every case.

There is evidence that the 'recidivism' rate is lower for those coming out of hospital; in other words, discharged forensic patients are less likely to re-offend than mentally disordered offenders discharged from prison (Fennell 1991). But this may be attributed to the conservative discharge policies of hospitals, noted earlier, which are driven as much by 'security' considerations, as it is to changes in the mental state of patients. 'Psychopaths' in high-security hospitals receive longer periods of detention, on average, than their counterparts in mainstream prison provision, as judged by equivalent index offences (Peay 1989). Logically this leads then to false positive biases being possible in hospitals (patients continue to be detained in case they are dangerous, when actually they would not go on to re-offend). By contrast, prisons are more likely to have a false negative bias: prisoners are released at the end of their defined sentence and might and often do re-offend. For example, re-offending in sex offenders is a case in point here.

There are two main arguments underlying a criminalization position. The first relates to a moral and philosophical argument that *both* those who are designated mentally ill *and* those who are not should be treated as humanely as possible. That is, poor and 'brutalizing' conditions should not exist *in either* the prison or the mental health systems (Monahan 1973). Reforming the prison system has also been argued for on pragmatic grounds. Fennell (1991) suggests that there will always be situations which do not permit the rapid transfer of mentally disordered offenders out of the prison system.

Prisoners may not meet the legal criteria for transfer or transfer cannot be arranged quickly enough. Additionally, transfer may not always be the fairest option for prisoners. Sentences are often suspended for prisoners who spend time in hospital and recommenced if a person is transferred back to prison. (That is, there is no remission for the period that they have been treated as patients, and so their detention is actually extended beyond their sentence.) Moreover, increased diversion into psychiatric facilities is unrealistic, given the burden on existing facilities and the failure to rapidly develop more regional secure facilities.

Fennell argued for a proper legal framework for psychiatric treatment in prisons to be established as a means of improving the standard of care that is currently provided. One policy option, which tried to bridge the gap in the UK between these two positions, was proposed by the Tumin Report (Woolfe and Tumin 1990). This suggested that adequately staffed psychiatric intensive care wards from the NHS be provided inside prisons.

Finally, we can note here that a focus on the challenges of humane mental health provision in the prison services would not disappear if suddenly all mentally abnormal offenders were dealt with under mental health law in hospital settings instead. For example, the high security hospitals in England (Broadmoor, Ashworth and Rampton) have experienced recurrent scandals related to patient abuse, which has sometimes been linked to iatrogenic deaths (Boynton 1980; NHS Hospital Advisory Service 1988; SHSA 1990, 1993; Blom-Cooper et al. 1992).

Moreover, as we noted earlier, prisoners know their time of release, whereas patients in secure psychiatric provision do not. Being detained indefinitely can be considered as a human rights violation, and even a claim of torture can be claimed (Levin 1986). For example, the indefinite detention of asylum seekers and terrorist suspects has been discussed by ethicists in terms of *both* human rights violations *and* its negative impact on mental health (Silove et al. 2007; Freckleton and Keyzer 2010). With these considerations in mind, a patient detained indefinitely in secure psychiatric conditions is being subjected inherently to the same risks.

The convergence of an actuarial approach to risk

The debates about the comparative merits of criminalization and psychiatrization are mainly in relation to different ways of controlling and containing offender patients. Alongside these arguments about which institutional structures (penal or health care?) should take precedence is evidence of a convergence of organizational philosophy. There has been a shift in both mental health and criminal justice facilities towards an actuarial policy (Armstrong 2002; Gray et al. 2004). The latter refers to the emphasis on risk calculation as the main procedural guide to professional action in both systems.

While the penal system traditionally aimed to rehabilitate offenders, and the psychiatric system aimed to treat patients, in recent years both aspirations have been displaced by an emphasis on risk assessment and minimization. Treatment and rehabilitation in different ways are orientated towards the reform of the deviant individual. Treatment ideologies, prior to the emergence of 'actuarialism' had, to some extent, influenced rehabilitation interventions for some prisoners. For example, prisons have contained therapeutic communities as part of their rehabilitative strategy. By contrast, actuarial management is more about using observational and psychometric methods to efficiently deal with the social threat of groups of deviant people, *wherever they are contained.*

Both actuarial and treatment approaches are examples of how mental health assessments and interventions have permeated the criminal justice system. For example, in prisons we find concerns about prisoners at risk of self-harm and suicide, which might require the input of complex psycho-social interventions. These require risk assessments at the outset. Similarly, we find the link of risk assessment to the warranting of treatment provision in relation to abused and bereaved women, as well as initiatives to improve staff–prisoner relationships and reduce the bullying arising from institutional norms (Marzano *et al.* 2011). In other words, proving risk at the aggregate level can be a rationale for resource requests and with it forms of changes in institutional practice, which can then be audited to ascertain whether interventions have led to risk reduction, as intended. However, the aggregate argument is also one to cast doubt at the individual level. Aggregate data does not help to answer the question, 'will this *particular* patient/prisoner re-offend if discharged/released?'

Treatment in prison: medication, therapeutic communities and other approaches

While the demographic characteristics of prisoners and the health behaviours that they import make an important contribution to health in prisons, the environment, the regime and the organizational culture of the prison are likely to be more important. Medication practices are a key indicator of, and contributor to, the therapeutic prison environment. They have particular relevance in the light of findings that the taking of mood-modifying medication can provide some support and encourage patient engagement. Recent studies suggest that approximately 20 per cent of male and 50 per cent of female prisoners take some form of psychotropic medication, roughly representing a fivefold increase on the general population (Hassan *et al.* 2012). The benefits of prescribing are for staff as well as patients. Psychotropic drugs are prescribed because they help to manage tensions within prisons, easing the work of prison officers and facilitating relationships between prison officers and psychiatrists (Fernandez and Lézé 2011).

Medication management is a predominant form of treatment and support for patients with a mental health problem, reflecting the bio-medical approach to treatment which has predominated in general psychiatry since the 1960s. Medication practices of patients and staff are therefore a key marker of the extent to which the health practices in prison settings equate with those of normalized routines in community and other settings. Psychotropic medication is a psychological prop, a key and valued form of support for people with mental health problems entering custody. Existing regimes of medication and the autonomy to self-medicate established in the community are disrupted and curtailed by the prescribing and medication practices of prison clinical staff and enforced prison routines for the taking of prescribed medication.

Thus the continuity of mental health care (if it is defined by medication routines) can be undermined by the rule changes experienced on entry to prison, exacerbating prisoners' anxiety and sense of helplessness. The disruption to previously experienced routine medication management on entry to prison appears to contribute to poor relationships with prison health staff, disrupts established self-medication practices and discourages patient autonomy and control. Together these can detrimentally affect the mental health of prisoners at a time when they are most vulnerable. Practices such as this inhibit the integration and normalization of mental health management protocols in prison, compared with those operating in the wider community. This may hinder progress towards improving the standard of mental health care available to prisoners suffering from mental disorder.

We noted above that these disruptions are in the context of medication, for now, being the main intervention provided by psychiatry (though with the mainstreaming of CBT as an addition or alternative to norms of practice in psychiatry). Taking the longer view, closed systems such as prisons have been sites of opportunity for non-medicinal approaches to mental health care. We noted in Chapter 6 the rise of the therapeutic community movement. An organizational precondition of therapeutic communities is one of a stable closed system '24/7'. The historical prototype of this could be found in the early asylum system when lay administrators offered 'moral treatment'. By the mid-twentieth century its legacy could be found in the therapeutic communities of military hospitals and then some prison settings.

As far as the latter are concerned the focus on moral responsibility takes on a particular significance, given that prisoners ipso facto have a proven record of immoral or amoral conduct. It is easy to see then why the moral dimension to punishment and rehabilitation coalesces in the regime of a therapeutic community. It is noteworthy that when secure therapeutic communities have emerged, they have been in prison settings and not health care regimes, such as high-security hospitals like Broadmoor, Ashworth and Rampton in England or Carstairs State Hospital in Scotland. The latter have been in many ways less imaginative than prisons in their experiments with incorrigible-offender patients. This may be because the sub group of patients dealt with by therapeutic communities are those with a diagnosis of psychopathy or anti-social personality disorder, as well as those with problems of substance abuse or sexual offending. These are the most challenging group of detainees in the prison system and because the starting premise philosophically of the latter is about the moral responsibility of the offender, then a moral approach to treatment is aligned. By contrast, the bio-medical determinism of psychiatric orthodoxy is not aligned with human agency: patients await 'patiently' for medical treatment to have an impact upon them.

All of these groups could be designated as suffering from forms of mental disorder, under nosologies such as DSM or ICD, but even within that traditional diagnostic medical framework, the role of moral agency becomes central to defining a constituent 'symptom'. For example, is the desire to have sex with children a symptom of a medical disorder or merely an offensive part of the wide and variegated range of human sexual desire? Thus the offender patient of this type raises conceptual challenges for both ethics and epistemology. Despite those challenges, as we have just noted, in practice the moral regime of group exploration and personal feedback in therapeutic communities is explicitly aligned with the essentially *moral aspect* of the offender population targeted.

But an example at the level of social policy about mentally disordered offenders that reflects the link between broader philosophical questions and specific practical outcomes is the Dutch penal policy. In the Netherlands since 1925 they have had an explicit policy of separating punishment from treatment in prisons but with the explicit goal on both fronts to produce new pro-social conduct and thereby reduce prospective risk to the host society (van den Berg and van Marle 1997).

The results of studies of these treatment regimes, in penal not health settings, have yielded ambiguous results, in line indeed with all research on the treatment of 'personality disorder'. For example, in the UK the longest-standing prison therapeutic community has been at HMP Grendon. The first criterion of success measured has been pro-social conduct in prison. Dolan and Coid (1993) found that prisoners with an offending history of violence became less violent there than in other prisons and that the inmates' symptoms of distress also diminished. The second criterion of success relates to data on recidivism, which has been more contested, with some studies showing increases in re-offending (albeit shifting to less violent modes of offence) and others showing a clear decrease (Rice *et al.* 1991; see also Cullen 1994; Marshall 1997).

What the Grendon regime reveals in the context of this chapter is the ambiguity of the competing rationales to remove offenders from society. Apart from their prompt sequestration, which removes them temporarily from the open system in which they might immediately be a risk to others, the prospective role of detention is ambiguous. Is it to reduce re-offending or is it to re-form the prisoner to become a different sort of or psychologically healthier person? Of course the two may coalesce or reinforce one another but they may remain separate processes. For example, the contestation about the rationale of Grendon in relation to its operational philosophy, not its effectiveness, highlights this point. This has revealed a medical-psychoanalytical rationale, about psychotherapeutic insight and reformation of the personality, in conflict with a more techno-centric approach to treatment, which uses cognitive-behavioural approaches to target particular offender behaviours (Cullen, 1997).

The wider shifts in the practices of the mental health workforce are then being mirrored in the psychological therapeutic rationales in prisons. McGuire (2008) notes that since the early days of therapeutic communities dominated by psychoanalytical assumptions other approaches can now be found in prison settings. These include programmes to enhance anger management and self-control, as well as forms of cognitive therapy to improve moral reasoning and increase motivation for change. These are still forms of psychological therapy but they are not based upon the exploratory and insight-focused mode, which was originally associated with therapeutic communities.

The ambiguity just described about the confluence of therapeutic and offence-focused work become evident when mental health professionals and their preferred theory and practice are introduced into penal settings. That inclusion has been warranted by claims that historically health care standards and their governance have been poor in prisons (Birmingham 2002). Once health professionals then become part of that setting then they begin to shape mental health patienthood in new ways.

Fernandez and Lézé (2011) show how professional engagement centres on the moral expectations of prisoners under their care. They show how prisoners are selected and then converted into patients deserving of attention (based on expectations of honesty, sincerity and compliance). Then professional categorization means that patients are divided into three main intervention categories, in which the treatment is both therapeutic and moral, involving expectations of responsibility, recognition of guilt and self-esteem. Similarly, the use of professionalized diagnostic tools, such as the risk assessments noted above, is consistent with a disciplinary regime aimed at 'taming'. This is achieved through mental health professionals posing as being rhetorically progressive, while actually producing their preferred version of governance that regulates rather than supports or empowers offender patients. Central to this shaping rhetoric is the use of a psychological discourse, and labels such as 'borderline personality disorder', together with treatment regimes, such as dialectical behaviour therapy (Pollack and Kendall 2005).

The intersection of mental health professionals with the implicit role of generic work in the criminal justice system can also be noted in concluding this section. For example, prison officers have been found to be able detectors of mental health problems (Birmingham 1999). Outside the prison system itself, the probation service often deal with clients with clear mental health needs. Recent estimates are that 40 per cent of clients are experiencing mental health problems (Brooker *et al.* 2012). This is a cue for the next section about community settings and offenders with mental health problems.

Police officers as street-level bureaucrats

Key workers at the front line of the criminal justice system shaping referrals into prisons (or not) are the police. They operate with a lay conception of mental health problems (this does not imply a lack of sophistication, merely an absence of the discourse of the expert 'psy complex'). They can adopt a rationale born of experience (this practical wisdom was called 'phronesis' in Greek philosophy). The dilemmas of policing mental health at the front line are evident in the blog and social media presence of MentalHealthCop, who describes his work in the following way:

> I'm a serving 24/7 police inspector blogging in a personal capacity. I've had more than my fair share of policing & mental health incidents and **I continue to get them daily** on the frontline of British policing. It was the overwhelming feeling when I joined of *not knowing what on earth I was doing*, that got me asking questions about this stuff. I asked them of other police officers, including supervisors, but it emerged they often knew little of use. I have made it my business to ask psychiatrists, forensic psychiatrists, A&E doctors, paramedics as well as

psychiatric nurses and AMHPs (or ASWs as they were) how we should operate in this area of policing. Anyone who would stand still long enough and talk to me, frankly.

http://mentalhealthcop.wordpress.com/about

The police are at the front line of making decisions about who enters the mental health system, who is diverted to mental health services and who, when circumstances allow, is returned to a domestic setting. In sociological terms the police can be viewed as what Lipsky terms 'street-level bureaucrats' or as 'public service workers who interact directly with citizens in the course of their jobs, and who have substantial discretion in the execution of their work' (Lipsky 1980: 18).

The characteristics which Lipsky considers define street-level bureaucrats include:

- a focus on the need to process workloads expeditiously;
- a substantial amount of autonomy in individual interactions and dealings with clients (in this case members of the public);
- an interest as part of a professional or occupational project in maintaining and maximizing their own autonomy;
- conditions of work that include inadequate resources (both monetary and in terms of personnel and time);
- a context of demand that will always exceed supply;
- ambiguous and multiple objectives;
- difficulties in defining or measuring good performance;
- a requirement that decisions should be taken rapidly;
- clients who are what Lipsky calls 'non-voluntary' (1980: 56).

In the latter regard, these 'clients' have limited (or a non-existent) choice over whether, where or how they present to the service involved.

Lipsky suggests that 'the decisions of street-level bureaucrats, the routines they establish, and the devices they invent to cope with uncertainties and work pressures effectively become the public policies they carry out' (1980: xii). In other words, the pragmatics of an open system, with different and particular constraints and opportunities from one situation to another shape what happens, independently of the abstraction of policies and ideal procedures. In a study of decision-making about psychiatric referrals from the police Rogers (1990) identified this pragmatic process occurring as police officers make decisions about the management of patients they encounter on the street. These are not specified explicitly in the legal terms underpinning the policy but exist in the discretion of the particular contingencies available to help people or simply to deal with an uncertain scenario of personal vulnerability or social threat.

In these conditions of uncertainty police officers try to apply where possible their own version of a routine that works for them in practice. Lipsky pointed to how street-level bureaucrats respond to pressures placed on them by processing people in a routine and stereotypical way. In the Rogers study just noted police officers referred to the need for a routine psychiatric and physical health check, which they called a 'nut and gut', when deliberating on whether to refer a person to hospital or the criminal justice systems. However, as we just noted above there are limits to this police discretion and ability to act autonomously. The latter is constrained by the social context, within which officers become involved in incidents which are constrained by the external influences impinging on police decision-making, such as resources available and immediate competing tasks.

Discussion

This chapter has dealt with a number of ambiguities. First, there is the matter about whether criminality is a version of mental abnormality in principle because it reflects a failure of socialization. This invites the question about whether all criminal deviance could or should be medicalized.

Second, however we might answer that question, it is clear that criminality and mental abnormality often overlap and coexist and, accordingly, it is not clear whether it is easy empirically to separate mentally abnormal offenders from normal offenders. For example, diagnoses such as 'psychopathic disorder' or 'antisocial personality disorder' or 'substance abuse' together would account for the bulk of the male prison population, in the case of the first two because they are defined tautologically mainly by criminal conduct. In the case of substance abuse, criminality is a common source of income generation in terms of the frowned-upon trade in illegal substances and other forms of activity pursued to sustain a habit. The decriminalization of recreational drug use would alter that criminal justice landscape and allow for a clear offer of a policy of voluntary treatment for addicts. Under current legislative arrangements, criminalization inflates the prison population and offers treatment in a coercive, rather than a more auspicious voluntary, setting.

Third, although intuitively we may consider that a psychiatric approach in detention will be more humane, this is not necessarily the case. For example, such an assumption legitimizes the idea that prisons can and should remain brutal for the normal prisoner (which is open to challenge) and that a health disposal will not be brutal (which empirically is not defensible). On the first count, how exactly will a brutal regime encourage pro-social conduct on the release of a prisoner? On the second count, we have noted the many scandals in high-security psychiatric provision, suggesting that it does not protect patients from an oppressive regime.

Fourth, simply being detained and subjected to institutional routines, in either penal or health settings, may be inherently detrimental to mental health, despite the advantage of stability offering a window of opportunity for intervention being available in a closed system. The latter policy shift we address in this chapter seems to be making a virtue out of necessity. Generally coerced relationships are not the best starting point for personal change, a point noted already in relation to the treatment of drug addiction.

Fifth, any putative advantage of a health setting is offset by the personal costs attached to there being no estimated time of discharge in advance. Those detained in prison know in principle when they will be released (within a range of time). Those in a high security hospital do not. The latter is thereby more offensive to a rights-based approach to care than the former, and so which is the more desirable setting for people with mental health problems who have committed a criminal offence? We weighed up that question in the section on psychiatrization and criminalization of mental abnormality.

Overall, we can conclude that the double deviance of being an 'offender patient' or 'mentally abnormal offender' brings with it a double disadvantage of multiple and sometimes competing rationales from the State apparatus of social control. That double deviance also ensures that the mentally abnormal offender will be subjected to a double rejection by society.

Given that the general public are suspicious of both ex-prisoners and former psychiatric patients, then that double role implicates particular considerations about public policy. For example, many in the non-criminal population think that people should be sent to prison not just as a punishment but *to be* punished. A discourse of care and treatment inherently conflicts with such an attitude. Likewise the crimes of sexual and non-sexual violence, which are the typical index offences that invite the criminal justice system to define an offender as 'mentally abnormal', are the very offences which tend to provoke public anger and demands for severe retribution. Those demands, fuelled by the popular press depicting mentally abnormal offenders as animals and monsters (i.e. not human), include expectations of permanent detention (and for some even capital punishment). In the light of these public reactions, few politicians are likely to prioritize the liberalization of the regimes of detention discussed in this chapter or address the human rights questions we note.

Questions

1 To what extent can criminality and mental illness be seen as overlapping categories?
2 To what extent can the management of mental health problems in criminal justice systems be determined by the activities of agents such as the police or prison officers?
3 Is there a justification of arguing for more humane treatment for those with mental health problems over those detained for criminal offences alone?
4 Can total institutions, whether hospital or prisons, ever be therapeutic environments for those with mental health problems?

For discussion

Consider what the merits and disadvantages would be for dealing with mentally disordered offenders if special hospitals were closed down. What would be the implications for inmates of prisons, politicians, policy-makers and health professionals.

10 Mental health and legalism

Chapter overview

This chapter will extend the exploration of the previous one about mental health in secure settings. Its focus though will be on legalism: a governmental approach to the regulation of psychological difference in society. This is humanly constructed and so has been a matter of push and pull, implicating a variety of social groups: politicians, lawyers, the police, clinical staff, social workers, the general public and patients themselves. The law has been used in a double and arguably contradictory way. On the one hand, it has been a way of ensuring social order and is thus directed at controlling the deviant conduct associated with mental abnormality. On the other hand, it has also been used as a break on professional power. The State then *both* delegates powers of control and discretion to what we now call 'mental health professionals' *and* then operates to limit those powers. A further ambiguity has been that the State apparatus of legalism might be viewed as being inherently about third-party interests (those who are sane by common consent) against the interests of patients. Alternatively it might be depicted as a means to protect the rights of the latter, including the right to treatment. In the light of these general comments, this chapter will explore the role of mental health legislation, which is a central feature of the relationship between the State and mental health service activity and professional action and priorities. It will cover the following topics:

- legal versus medical control of madness;
- socio-legal aspects of compulsion;
- the globalization of compulsion and the internationalization of human rights legislation;
- professional interests and legislative reforms;
- dangerousness.

Introduction

Mental disorder represents the main point of contact between psychiatry and the law. The early days of psychiatry in the nineteenth century were heavily influenced by eugenic considerations – it was assumed that a variety of deviant conducts could be explained by a tainted gene pool in the lower social classes. This degeneracy theory, which characterized early biological psychiatry, linked together the mad, the bad and the dim. However, during the First World War and its aftermath such an underlying assumption began to falter. In the forensic field, there emerged a resistance to the old eugenic ideas of degeneracy, which accounted for criminality in terms of an inherited disposition to bad conduct (Forsythe 1990). This was replaced by an increasing interest in environmental or psychological explanations for law-breaking. Since that time, psychiatric experts have played a major role in identifying and explaining criminal conduct. And once there was that shift away from bio-genetic determinism, then this opened up questions, still pertinent today, about *psychological explanations*. Given that the latter contain elements of determinism as well as assumptions about human agency, then case by case the balance allotted to each is always open to consideration and varying perspectives. The norms of the criminal justice system permit this ambiguity. For example, mental illness may be considered as a reason to exculpate criminal action in a context, in which usually intention, and therefore intentionality, is the focus of interest to judges and juries.

Until 2007 in British law the notion of 'mental disorder' included four separate conditions: 'mental illness', 'mental impairment', 'severe mental impairment' and 'psychopathic disorder'. The first of these was not defined; the second and third were references to people with learning difficulties who were additionally deemed to be dangerous; the fourth referred to antisocial individuals who were 'abnormally aggressive' or who manifested 'seriously irresponsible conduct'. The 2007 Mental Act removed these specific categories but retained a more generic definition (Department of Health 2004):

> 'Mental disorder' means an impairment of or a disturbance in the functioning of the mind or brain resulting from any disability or disorder of the mind or brain. . .

Superficially this reads like a coherent English sentence. However, it poses a number of problems for the reader:

- The inter-dependent constituent parts of 'impairment', 'disturbance', 'disability' and 'disorder' are not explained or defined.
- The word 'disorder' is used to mean both the whole and a part, with no clear logical distinction between the two roles in the definition.
- The inclusion of the word 'brain' suggests that any patient suffering from a neurological disease affecting the central nervous system could potentially be framed as being mentally disordered.
- The word 'functioning' is used to connote functional criteria, apparently dealing with the difficulty that most mental health problems are of unknown or contested origins. Confusingly, though, the words 'resulting from' are inserted, implying causal reasoning to the reader. This offer is then immediately retracted. The antecedents suggested are simply a restatement of dysfunction in the mind or brain (the use of the words 'disability' and 'disorder').

The legal framework thus tends to deploy tautological definitions or accepts that mental disorder is what mental health experts say it is. In particular cases tried in court, psychiatric opinion is offered as an expert view on the presence or absence of mental disorder. Because mental illness is not legally defined, judges have sometimes resorted to the lay discourse. In 1974, Judge Lawton said that the words 'mental illness' are 'ordinary words of the English language. They have no particular medical significance. They have no particular legal significance'. Lawton refers to the dictum of Lord Reid in a case where the defendant's mental state was being considered:

> I ask myself what would the ordinary sensible person have said about the patient's condition in this case if he had been informed of his behaviour? In my judgment such a person would have said 'Well the fellow is obviously mentally ill'.
>
> (cited in Jones 1991: 15)

This lay conception of legal insanity has been called 'the-man-must-be mad' test (Hoggett 1990).

In one sense, therefore, the legal framework accepts a psychiatric framework, but when the latter is found lacking then ordinary language definitions are invoked. It also raises the question about whether mental disorder is simply, for legal and lay purposes, incomprehensible conduct. 'Normal' criminal acts are clearly goal directed. 'Mentally disordered' criminal acts are not directed towards obvious personal gain. The boundary between these is not easy to maintain though, especially when making judgments about sex offenders. The latter seek personal gratification even if this is not financial. Under different circumstances, they may or may not be diagnosed as mentally disordered. Sex offenders may end up either in prison or in secure psychiatric units, showing that sexual gratification as a criminal motive confuses those prescribing a judicial response.

Also, some murderers are adjudged in commonsensical terms to be sane, despite the contrary view of expert witnesses. If the legal framework looks to lay people through a jury system to clarify the presence or absence of mental abnormality, then this ambivalence is likely to be reflected in their judgments. Lay people may argue that, on the one hand, a person must be 'sick' to perpetrate heinous acts but, on the other, that the acts warrant severe punishment or even death.

Whatever the logical strengths and weaknesses of the legal framework and the varied outcomes generated by the interaction of legal, psychiatric and lay opinion, it is practically and politically very important for two key reasons. First, it defines the conditions under which mental health professionals can and cannot detain patients and compulsorily treat them, even when they have not broken the criminal law. Second, it makes decisions about those who have broken the criminal law and who provisionally are deemed to be mentally disordered. In criminal law, for a person to be judged guilty, the court must be satisfied that there was malicious intent. Unintended but reckless or negligent acts are lesser crimes than those where 'malice aforethought' or 'mens rea' is evident. For this reason, they tend to lead to less severe sentencing. In the case of British mentally disordered offenders, these judgments about culpability may be modified further in a legal setting, when the defendant's mental state is considered:

- The perpetrator may not be deemed fit to stand trial – they lack a 'fitness to plead'. In these circumstances, they may be sent to a secure hospital without trial, provided that their role in the offence is clear to the court. If their mental disorder is treatable or recovery emerges naturally with time, then they may be recalled at a later date to face trial.
- Whether or not the patient is deemed fit to plead, they may be judged to be 'not guilty by reason of insanity'. When this is the case, then the court, having taken psychiatric advice, decides that the person was sufficiently mentally disordered at the time of the offence that they were unaware that their actions were wrong. The insanity defence is more common in some countries than others. It is rare in Britain, where the next contingency is more likely to operate.
- The defence of 'diminished responsibility' can be invoked, when mentally disordered offenders commit murder, but not in the case of other crimes in current English law. The legal term used in this context is suffering from 'abnormality of mind', which does not map neatly on to diagnostic categories preferred by psychiatrists.
- The most contentious decision is in relation to temporary loss of reason and intention. This might apply to automatism (crimes committed while sleepwalking) and more commonly, but also more controversially, crimes committed while under the influence of drugs or alcohol. Substance abuse is particularly contentious. On the one hand it is deemed to be a mental disorder. On the other hand in some crimes, such as dangerous driving, the intoxicated driver is typically treated much more harshly, by the courts, than the sober one. When this happens, the presence of a mental disorder, where the offender can demonstrate their long-term substance dependence, does not mitigate the action but the reverse occurs.

Having introduced the question of determinism and intentionality in relation to considerations about mentally disordered offenders (which we consider more later) we now turn to the second major consideration about the intersection of the law with mental health work: the tradition in the past 200 years of placing legal limits on clinical discretion.

Legal versus medical control of madness

During the early nineteenth century, in Britain as well as other emerging capitalist economies in Europe and North America, the systematic control of madness began. The system involved the

State setting out laws and prompting, or prescribing, public spending on asylums. The building of county and borough asylums was encouraged by the County Asylums Act of 1808. These suggestions were made mandatory by the Lunacy Act of 1845, which led to a rapid enlargement of the State asylum system. This system came to displace a very varied picture of control. Prior to 1845, lunatics were dispersed in a range of places – small private madhouses, bridewells, poor houses and workhouses. This dispersal was unregulated and cases were not systematically recorded (Donnelly 1983).

The Lunacy Act 1890 prescribed that all admissions to hospitals and treatment would be governed by statute. It also ensured that the control and supervision of inmates would be overseen by government bodies. At first during the twentieth century, such safeguards and powers increasingly involved the legal profession. But later, diagnosis and admission were seen primarily as the concern of the medical profession. Since the Victorian lunacy legislation, in Britain legal reforms in 1930, 1959, 1983 and 2007 have reflected this tension between legal and medical power.

Historically, legalism has been used to counter what have been viewed as the deficits of medical management. Similarly, the assertion of a medical view of mental disorder has been resorted to at times when legalism was considered to have failed. The tension between legalism and medical control permeates the implementation of mental health legislation. This is true of civil compulsory admissions of both non-offender patients and mentally disordered offenders. It is also worth noting here that the current discourse of 'mental health' legislation is essentially a misnomer. Such legislation is not about mental health but about the control of some people who are deemed to be *mentally disordered*. The use of the term 'mental health' in this context of legalism is part of a wider discursive shift in which euphemism is now common (e.g. 'mental health problem', 'mental health services') to disguise or gloss the difficulties with 'mental illness' or 'mental disorder' (Pilgrim 2005a).

It is not only the psychiatric profession that has resisted the intrusion of law into its work. The use of the law in the mental health area has also been criticized by some social scientists. For example, Kathleen Jones (1960), a prominent social policy analyst, argued that there are severe limits to what the law can achieve in mental health services. Jones considered that good practice is likely to be fostered through adequate resource allocation and the development of professional norms and values. She believed that the latter would enhance the appropriate attitudes, skills and treatments needed for the compassionate management of mentally disordered people and inter-professional co-operation. A strict legal framework might inhibit this process. Thus, the use of the law in her view should only be as a last resort.

From a different standpoint, Rose (1986) has argued that legalism is just another form of control that does not ultimately benefit the patient. Instead, he argues that not only does legalism not constrain psychiatric discretion but it also disguises the wider political context of the delivery of mental health services. It thereby depoliticizes the debate over how psychiatry is organized and operates: 'legality is merely one mode of regulation and body of professional expertise amongst others, neither conceptually more rigorous, nor necessarily more effective in bringing power to account' (1986: 209). Rose's criticism centres on the tendency of legal measures to individualize problems.

Legalism has had a chequered history with regard to fostering positive values about mental abnormality. The Lunacy Act 1890, for example, led to wide-scale stigma around madness and 'certification', because it allowed only for the forced admission of people to mental asylums via the courts. The Mental Treatment Act 1930 attempted to rectify this by introducing the possibility of voluntary admission to hospital, which, it is argued, fostered a more sympathetic attitude to emotional deviance.

Bean (1980) found that, under the Mental Health Act 1959, which represented a swing back from a legal to a medical control, there was an absence of adequate checks and control mechanisms. Over-zealous psychiatrists sometimes placed patients in a vulnerable position by permitting them to be deprived of their liberty for considerable periods of time. Bean related this to the nature of 'therapeutic law', with its open-ended clauses and standards, which leads to a tendency towards ad hoc rule enforcement and the playing down of the importance of general rules. In other words, where there is a clash between the views of medicine and legal requirements, medical demands tend to be privileged. At the same time medical paternalism seemingly offers a softening of pure legal measures operating in penal settings, where environmental conditions are typically inferior to hospital settings. Whether this paternalism leads to long-term humane outcomes for mentally disordered offenders remains a moot point (see below).

Since the early 1990s there has been a global trend towards balancing the medical dominance of 'therapeutic law' with a greater legal presence in order to offer greater weight to the individual rights of patients. A recent ethnographic study carried out in Sweden examining such arrangements seems to suggest that nothing much changes when the legal role is formally extended. Psychiatric norms and values still dominate patient–professional interaction and the outcome of assessments.

Even in a legally dominated context, those with mental health problems are treated as patients rather than adverse parties and there is an inbuilt bias to the proceedings; it is assumed from the beginning that they are mentally ill. There is a tendency for their credibility to be viewed as suspect, and expressions of 'sane' behaviour are seen as a temporary effort at self-composure. Where mental health is concerned, an informal atmosphere is often adopted which is atypical of other legal proceedings. This further militates against a view of the patient as a valid legal party (Sjostrom 1997).

The problematic status of personality disorder

Although the overwhelming concern of the State and psychiatry during the nineteenth century was lunacy, 'moral insanity' was also described:

> The moral principles of the mind are strongly perverted or depraved; the power of self government is lost or greatly impaired and the individual is found to be incapable not of talking or reasoning upon any subject proposed to him, but of conducting himself with decency and propriety in the business of life.
>
> (Prichard 1835, quoted in Ramon 1986: 215)

The concern of the State to utilize medical facilities to control bad behaviour (in the absence of formal evidence of psychosis) continued in the twentieth century. Under the Mental Health Act of 1983, the legal definition of psychopathy appeared as: 'a persistent disorder or disability of mind (whether or not including significant impairment of intelligence) which results in abnormally aggressive or seriously irresponsible conduct on the part of the person concerned'. A problem with this legal definition was that it mapped poorly onto preferred professional ones. For example, the use of the term 'psychopathy' in law approximates to those of 'antisocial personality disorder' and 'dissocial personality disorder' codified by the APA (1994) and the WHO (1992) respectively. However, to complicate matters, there is a strong clinical tradition of using the word 'psychopath' to describe people who show overlapping symptoms of three types of personality disorders (antisocial, histrionic and narcissistic) (Cleckley 1941; Hare 1991). Some but not all of those with this clinical profile become criminals. Indeed, the dominant psychological, rather than psychiatric, account of psychopathy suggests that most people fulfilling criteria for the label are successes in politics and business ('snakes in suits') and most of the time they do not fall foul of the criminal law (Babiak and Hare 2007).

The use of the term 'personality disorder' in general, but here in particular in relation to antisocial or criminal acts, highlights again the ambiguity we discussed in the Introduction. These morally offensive patterns of conduct located in their repeated expression by named individuals can be judged as the acts of human agents *and/or* the obvious products of a 'sick mind' (and so not within the personal insight and control of individual human agents).

Moreover, the scenario of judging mentally disordered offenders rather than self-seeking politicians and business leaders seems to be governed less by questions of intentionality (both 'know what they are doing') and more by prevailing social norms and mores. If we *expect* our business leaders to be ruthless and greedy and our politicians to be self-centred and power-obsessed then their actions are normalized. By contrast, violence, sex offending and fraud – which operate more at the personal level of everyday life and so threaten ordinary people very directly, actually or in their anxious imagination – will not be normalized: quite the opposite. For example, in recent times those offending against children ('paedos') have come to represent the most offensive version of being human that is imaginable. Indeed in the current public imagination and media representations they are not human beings at all but have become 'beasts' or 'monsters', a point we noted when looking at mentally disordered offenders in the previous chapter.

At the beginning of the twenty-first century the British government introduced further confusion about this matter. The specific category of 'psychopathic disorder' was dropped and a more generic definition of 'mental disorder' was introduced, which was tautological and applicable to any patient to be detained under legal powers, whether or not they were offenders: '"Mental disorder" means an impairment of or a disturbance in the functioning of the mind or brain resulting from any disability or disorder of the mind or brain, and "mentally disordered" is to be read accordingly' (cited in Pilgrim 2005a: 436).

An additional complication, to be discussed more later, was that the government developed its own preferred and invented *administrative category*, namely that of 'dangerous and severe personality disorder' (DSPD). This was neither medical nor legal in its conceptualization (though it drew partially upon their historical discourses) but was driven by the pragmatic political desire to ensure that high-risk patients were detained and, if possible, treated. The former dominated at the expense of the latter in the definition, providing the State with the opportunity to detain *indefinitely* those deemed to be at high risk to others. Generally these 'patients' are incorrigible sex offenders or ruthless killers, who might be released at some point from prison. Hospitals by contrast can, when required, guarantee true life detention. Thus the one function of mental health care is to offer the State the option of indefinite social control of risky individuals, while circumventing the normal due processes of legal proof.

While early psychiatry was concerned with 'moral insanity', during the twentieth century it began to codify many other types of personality disorder. By 1994 the APA described ten types, in addition to that of antisocial personality disorder (the approximate conceptual legacy of 'moral insanity'). One of these, 'borderline personality disorder', is used commonly to describe female prisoners who are emotionally unstable.

Personality disorder has been controversial for a number of reasons:

- As its aetiology is not known, it is described tautologically by its symptoms and its symptoms are accounted for by the existence of the disorder. (For example, a man is deemed to be 'psychopathic' because he rapes children. His raping of children is then explained by his 'psychopathy'.)
- In the light of the above, it is impossible to disentangle attributions of personal abnormality from social deviance (Blackburn 1988).
- The types of personality disorder described are not coherent and separate but overlap in clinical presentations, undermining the validity of specific diagnoses (Pilgrim 2001).
- Mental health professionals are divided about the 'treatability' of personality disorder. By definition, personality refers in the professional discourse to stable and unchanging personal attributes. If a personality is deemed as abnormal then it cannot (or would not

be expected to) change. Despite this there is some empirical evidence that people with a label of 'psychopathy' offered psychological interventions re-offend less often than those untreated (Skeem *et al.* 2002).

Thus 'psychopathy' or those deemed to have a 'dangerous and severe personality disorder' may not be truly 'treatable', but the overall probability of specific offending behaviours may be reduced in groups of patients with the diagnosis. This implies a further challenge; risk prediction in *particular cases* is difficult. Say only a proportion of mentally disordered offenders, as a group, are an immediate true risk to others at a point in time but the rest are not, the dilemma about discharge then relates to identifying which *individuals* continue to pose a risk and which do not.

Current methods of risk prediction are not capable of making this distinction and so secure services tend towards cautions or conservative 'false positive' risk assessments. That is, an unfairly detained patient (who is not dangerous) arouses no general concern for society (though may create an understandable sense of injustice for the particular patient). By contrast, a dangerous patient released to re-offend creates public outrage and jeopardizes the careers of professional decision-makers. In this context, decision-making bias is readily understood.

The logical and empirical vulnerability of any diagnosis of personality disorder has not deflected either the State or some parts of the psychiatric profession from using 'personality disorder' as a legitimate notion and rationale for social control. Such a continuing political and professional imperative has been divisive though. Mainstream psychiatry showed evidence of wanting to reject 'psychopaths' as patients worthy of their attention, but personality disorder is part of the bread-and-butter work of the specialism of forensic psychiatry. In the Mental Health Act 1983 a treatability clause had to be inserted to prevent open-ended professional decision-making. It stated that if a patient is suffering from psychopathic disorder, treatment must be likely to 'alleviate or prevent a deterioration' of the person's condition. This provided the option for psychiatrists to reject patients they diagnosed as being 'personally disordered' on the logical grounds that they could not be treated.

This treatability clause was removed from the Mental Health Act 2007. Instead now professionals must only be able to demonstrate that they can 'manage' the behavioural manifestations of the disorder. This of course is easily achieved. Simply by detaining such patients in a secure (i.e. *de facto* penal) setting, called a 'mental health facility', this separates perpetrators and their potential victims. Whether this does or does not lead to an improvement in the mental health of the detainee is thus rendered irrelevant.

In the reform of the Mental Health Act 1983, to be superseded by the Act of 2007, the implications of psychiatry's ambivalence towards 'personality disorder' became evident. Not only did the government introduce the DSPD programme and abandon an operational definition of 'treatability' (see below), it also allowed non-psychiatrists to inherit the jurisdiction over detained patients, with the notion of 'Responsible Medical Officer' now being replaced with that of 'Responsible Clinician'. What lay behind this expansion of professional jurisdiction from those, like clinical psychologists, who are not medically qualified was the inability of the government to trust the medical profession to offer a reliable willingness to manage those deemed to be 'personality disordered' patients (Pilgrim 2007b).

Why is psychiatry divided in this way about psychopathy? The answer could lie in the lack of responsiveness to treatment of this group of patients. However, this logic could well apply to other psychiatric diagnoses. For example, the limited success of treating 'schizophrenics' with major tranquillizers has not led to mainstream psychiatry wishing to diminish its contact with this group. A more plausible explanation is connected to changes in segregative control.

Ramon (1986) traces the change in the psychiatric stance towards psychopathy to developments in psychological approaches just after the Second World War. Then, soldier patients showing evidence of psychopathic disorder began to be treated in therapeutic communities. The move away from segregative control in mainstream psychiatry meant that the method to control antisocial behaviour became less feasible. Forensic psychiatry in contrast still had the segregative means to effectively manage such deviance.

Indeed, it seems to be that the precondition of the psychiatric detention of this group is governed by the demands of security and public threat, rather than mental state. As patients who have committed offences, they are likely to be detained for a period at least commensurate with the gravity of their offences (Norris 1984; Peay 1989). This is true also for those who have committed minor offences. An American study, using a large random sample of misdemeanour defendants, found that those with a psychiatric history were 'criminally sanctioned more severely than defendants without psychiatric records, and defendants with relatively extensive psychiatric records were even more severely sanctioned' (Hochstedler-Steury 1991: 358).

At the turn of the twenty-first century, the British State exerted its right to impose an administrative concept of personality disorder in order to cut through or over-ride professional ambivalence (Department of Health/Home Office 1999). This involved the construction of and use of a new category of 'dangerous and severe personality disorder' (DSPD). The impasse over which sector (prison or health service) has responsibility for the management and containment of people with personality disorder was in part been resolved by this State intervention, which included the development and funding of new services.

The solution to the tensions posed by the precarious validity of personality disorder noted above would not have been resolved without the intervention of the State, which refused to rely upon 'medical science' alone. Manning (2002) has shown, through the use of actor network theory (Law 1992) and the analysis of policy networks, the mechanisms behind the effective intervention of the State in this arena. It managed to secure a practical policy outcome, despite the controversies surrounding the description and treatability of personality disorder rehearsed above. The State funded and promoted professional networks and research designed to achieve the outcome it desired. It even named and promoted this sponsored network, as the 'Virtual Institute of Severe Personality Disorder' (VISPED).

Key players within forensic psychiatry and psychology, and others in the academic medical and criminological centres of excellence, were recruited into the policy development. Money was made available to generate both research capability and capacity. Younger people were attracted into the field through PhD, postdoctoral and other research fellowships. 'Pilot' services were funded and evaluated.

The characterization of the new service as a 'pilot', when it actually looked like the final version, acknowledged the difficulties of a thin evidence base. At the same time, it warded off criticism from professionals and engaged them in a policy development, which could build upon what had been started by government initiative. The research capacity and activity was put in place to furnish the technical capability of DSPD diagnosis, assessment and treatment, in the classic manner of the sociology of 'translation'. That is, the network enrolled, co-opted and disarmed the professional interests and stabilized the development and production of new knowledge.

Socio-legal aspects of compulsion

Having extended our discussion from the previous chapter about 'offender patients' or 'mentally disordered offenders' we now turn to the second major aspect of legalism: the lawful coercion of those who are *not* offenders. A key difference in the societal response to people with mental health problems and those with physical health problems is the commonplace use of compulsion. The historical theme, of most societies physically constraining madness, was simply formalized when the legislative arrangements of the nineteenth century we alluded to earlier came into being.

Szasz (1963) has argued that as long as there is legislation authorizing compulsory detention there can be no genuine voluntary admission. The latter status is vulnerable to threats of invoking the former. Bean has used the term 'coactus voluit' ('at his will although coerced') (1986: 5) to describe voluntary admission. In his research into compulsory admissions to hospital Bean found that assessing psychiatrists sometimes gave patients a 'Hobson's choice'. Patients were informed in a non-negotiable way of their impending admission or told that if they did not come into hospital voluntarily they would be compelled to do so (Bean 1980). A substantial minority of patients who are admitted to hospital as voluntary patients regard themselves to be there under coercion (Rogers 1993).

This illusory status of voluntary patients has become less relevant practically in recent years in Britain, in the wake of large hospital closures. A consequence has been that the smaller number of in-patient beds have been reserved overwhelmingly for involuntary cases. In the early 1980s, notionally, only a minority of patients was involuntary and the bulk was voluntary. This balance is now inverted. A second illusion can now be dispelled because of the smaller inpatient infrastructure. While the professional campaign of psychiatrists to move from the old asylums to new DGH units was based on a rhetorical alignment with mainstream curative general medicine (Baruch and Treacher 1978), by the turn of the twenty-first century, these units had been reduced to holding units for risky patients. Many of the latter had multiple social problems and used drugs or alcohol.

By the 1990s, the prospect of these units being true treatment centres, in line with the medical rhetoric and aspirations of the 1970s, had disappeared. They had become 'non-therapeutic', with patients feeling unsafe and often describing a deterioration in their mental health as a result of hospital admission (Sainsbury 1998; MIND 2004). Acute psychiatric units were effectively becoming small madhouses.

The challenge for the State then was no longer been about the lawful control of those admitted to and controlled in hospital (this is taken care of by 'mental health legislation', which defines who can and cannot be lawfully detained without trial and by whom). Instead, the main social administrative challenge began to relate to the bulk of patients living in the community, who previously would have lived and died in the asylum system. When patients episodically developed acute psychotic symptoms they were already in hospital (to be controlled). After the closure of the asylums this was no longer the case. After the policy of deinstitutionalization, the typical socio-legal challenge was about the surveillance and management of community-based patients.

In the US 'involuntary outpatient civil commitment' (IOC) is now widely accepted as a principle in mental health services. Although the use of such powers are still relatively rare, since the early 1980s most States have passed legislation that permits involuntary outpatient intervention on the basis of a need for treatment. Some patients have been placed on IOC indefinitely, and the penalty for non-compliance has varied from no action to automatic readmission, depending on the State involved (Maloy 1992).

Since the early 1990s, CTOs have been advocated at different times in British mental health policy debates which would entail the forced medication by injection with psychotropic drugs of people in their own homes. The Mental Health Act of 2007 has indeed introduced CTOs – a version of this 'long leash' approach to the surveillance and control of non-compliant patients outside of hospital.

Advocates for the introduction of legislation permitting this treatment argued that a small number of patients were prone to 'relapse' and could not be relied on to take medication. This gave rise to a number of philosophical, ethical and practical difficulties. Who would administer the medication? Although psychiatrists would prescribe it, CPNs were reluctant to take on the responsibility for administering drugs, which they viewed as potentially damaging to their relationship with patients. There were also problems related to who would receive compulsory treatment, given the limited effectiveness of major tranquillizers in treating certain patient groups and the strong opposition to the idea on the part of patient advocacy groups.

Although formal attempts by psychiatrists in Britain to negotiate powers of compulsory community treatment failed in the late 1980s, the issue was revisited by politicians in the mid-1990s, when a series of embarrassing incidents occurred in public involving psychiatric patients. As a result, new legislation was introduced to ensure active follow-up in the community with powers to recall non-compliant patients to hospital (the Supervised Discharge Act 1995 modified the 1983 Act). This legal adaptation of the 1983 Act was reinforced by a raft of procedures including a register of 'at risk' patients and the Care Programme Approach. These administrative mechanisms were a governmental attempt to systematize risk management in the community. There has been a steady increase in the use of CTOs. After their introduction their use steadily increased. For example, by 2012 there had been a 120 per cent increase in the use of CTOs over a 4-year period.

On 31 March 2012, 22,267 people were restricted under the Mental Health Act for England and Wales either on hospital sections or CTOs. Of this number, 17,503 people were detained in hospital (an increase of 856, or 5 per cent) and 4,764 people were subject to a CTO (an increase of 473, or 11 per cent). These figures include detentions and CTOs for both NHS and independent sector provider

These reflect powers of the State to legally enforce 'case management', a concept prevalent in mental health policy since the late 1908s in Britain. Huxley (1990), for example, described case management as a system in which care is provided through individually planned combinations of different sources of support. The ideal type of case management began with a collaborative and voluntaristic emphasis. In contrast, once coercion emerges centre stage then different ethical matters must be considered. The term 'aggressive outreach' (used in the USA) as opposed to the British notions of 'Care Programme Approach', 'care management' or 'assertive outreach' suggest tenacity and surveillance on the part of mental health professionals, which goes beyond paternalistic benevolence.

In both types of research positive outcomes include measures of the extent of contact that people with mental health problems have with their worker and a reduction in hospital admission rates. However, existing prototypes of this model in the UK at least have not provided optimistic results. In one RCT, even though participants found assertive community treatment more acceptable and engaged better with it than standard care provided by community mental health teams, no advantage over usual care from community mental health teams in reducing the need for inpatient care and in other clinical outcomes was found (Killaspy *et al.* 2009).

The emergence of inpatient units as crucibles of coercive control (when they originally aspired to be treatment units to generate mental health gain or recovery from acute episodes) poses a major problem now for professional ideology about 'mental health care'. Where legal rules govern admission, discharge and daily decision-making and action in between, in what sense can professions like psychiatry and mental health nursing maintain an ethical stance of caring for patients? Pols (2001) studied this clash of functions and ideologies in the work of mental health nurses in their interactions with inpatients. She found that legal measures to define 'doing good' (the patients' 'right to treatment') and those which were inherited from a non-legal paradigm of professional ethics interfered with one another.

The forced integration of professional paternalism with its preferred voluntary approach and one in which professional action is shaped and expected by legal requirement was highlighted in the Draft Mental Health Bill (Department of Health 2004) preceding the Mental Health Act of 2007. In order to make the Draft accessible to ordinary people, the government produced an 'easy read version' which contained the following the statement:

> It is better if people with a mental disorder can live the life they want with the right help and support but sometimes they have to have treatment which they do not agree to.
>
> (Department of Health 2004: 4)

Once such legal rules were made accessible to all, ordinary people were arguably becoming party to their own oppression. This was part of the rationale in the Bill to shift towards lawful measures of community control, but it continued an older theme in the discourse of professional mental health work. That is, it is presumed that care or treatment, whether given with or without the permission or co-operation of the patient, is still the same care or treatment.

The professional and political assumption here is that the content of care is independent of legal rules. Pols (2001) points out that this is a rhetorical avoidance of actual outcomes in services, where compliance with legal rules inevitably affects patient–staff relationships. It is not merely a matter of patients having treatment 'which they do not agree to'. It is also that any such failure to agree triggers an interaction with staff, which alters the very nature of any treatment received or imposed upon patients.

This point opens up two different interpretations of the link between compulsion and treatment. On one side is the State, most psychiatrists and some sociologists (e.g. Gove 1975) who assume that the impairments of mental disorder include a failure on the part of the patient to request what is needed, due to a lack of insight.

In this view, compulsion ensures that those without insight into their real needs are given access to interventions which are good for them. The law is being used as a vehicle to ensure patients have the treatment they need (one version of 'doing good' in Pols's analysis above). On the other side are those who assume that compulsion is largely driven not by patient needs (actual or assumed, expressed or not expressed) but by the needs of others to maintain social order. This position has been taken in the main by dissident psychiatrists (e.g. Szasz 1963) and by sociologists studying the social control of residual deviance (e.g. Scheff 1966).

Underlying these debates about the ethical status of compulsion in mental health work are two discrepant, and so competing, assumptions. On the one side is the assumption that coercion increases the chances of a patient receiving treatment that will improve their quality of life in the long term (Torrey and Zdannowicz 2001). On the other side there are those who argue that coercion infringes the human right to autonomy and increases stigma, thereby actually aggravating quality of life (Pollack 2004). These competing claims were investigated empirically by Link *et al.* (2008), who tracked outcomes for patients either given CTOs or not by courts in New York. The authors found partial support for both assumptions, one they called the 'coercion to beneficial treatment' perspective, and the other the 'coercion to detrimental stigma' perspective.

The globalization of compulsion and human rights legislation

Variability exists in relation to the extent to which a national or State culture is authoritarian or liberal and this affects the extent to which compulsion is used in its mental health services (Brakel *et al.* 1985; Ramon 1988; Cohen 1989; Dingwall *et al.* 1991). As well as these international variations, there have been signs since the mid-twentieth century of global convergence occurring in relation to mental health law. These include a change from the use of terminology such as 'insane' and 'lunatic', to 'mental illness', reflecting a worldwide trend towards medicalization. Latterly this may also signal globalization. For example, since the beginning of the twenty-first century there has been a gradual convergence of therapeutic law with many countries adopting similar definitions of mental disorder and legal processes. Evidence of this is in the consensus statement issued by the WHO (2001) offering 10 recommendations:

1   provide treatment in primary care;
2   make psychotropic drugs available;
3   give care in the community;
4   educate the public about mental health and mental health problems;

5   involve communities, families and consumers;
6   establish national policies, programmes and legislation;
7   develop human resources (for an adequate mental health service workforce);
8   link with other sectors;
9   monitor community mental health;
10 support more research into biological and psycho-social causes of and treatment for mental health problems.

The list as a whole reflects the interest groups influencing policy in the WHO, and the trends or aspirations for good practice in countries across the globe. For the purpose of this chapter, the third recommendation is important (as the community, not hospitals, will increasingly become a site of compulsion) and so is the sixth.

The WHO suggests then that mental health legislation is a desirable global outcome. It also assumes that such legislation (which defines the conditions of compulsion and safeguards against its misuse by the State and professionals) is an unambiguous sign of progress. Thus the WHO is not signalling the need to abandon legal powers of compulsion, only the need to *standardize* these powers, in the light of 'current knowledge and human rights considerations'. This international position exists despite criticisms of legalism being well rehearsed in developed countries, which have had such legislation for many years (e.g. Campbell and Heginbotham 1991).

An indication that the presumption that legislative powers are inherently beneficent and progressive is problematic emerged prior to the new legislation, established in England in 2007, after many years of controversy. Some of its opponents, in debates in the run up to the new Act, took the opportunity to argue for the abandonment of *any* form of 'Mental Health Act', in favour of a combination of disability legislation and a statute about *dangerousness* (Pilgrim 2007b). Their argument was that is both illogical and discriminatory to legally control the risky behaviour of only one defined social group (psychiatric patients) rather than of *all* citizens, independent of their mental state. While this view did not prevail, the fact that the position was argued at all demonstrates that not all of those involved in deliberating about legislation adopt the political assumption of point 6 on the checklist of progress offered by the WHO above. This contention is noted again below in the discussion of dangerousness. However, it is noted here to emphasize that the very existence of mental health legislation (which is actually not about mental health but about the lawful control of some people who are deemed by others to be mentally disordered) remains contentious.

Professional interests and legislative reforms

In England and Wales, the 1959 Mental Health Act established the medical profession as the key party involved in making applications for compulsory admissions. This was based on the view that mental illnesses require medical treatment. This principle remained unchanged in subsequent mental health legislation in 1983 but, as we noted above about new roles and the ambivalence of the medical profession towards 'personality disorder', by 2007 substantial ambiguity about professional jurisdiction over mental disorder then emerged. As Pilgrim and Ramon (2009) noted, at the turn of this century, revisions in mental health policy were characterized by contemporary arrangements about the following recurring agenda:

- the structures and processes involved in responding to mental health problems;
- the professional jurisdiction for mental health problems;
- the conditions under which mental disorder should be lawfully controlled and the type of control involved;
- links with wider health and welfare policy changes;
- the enhancement of mental health in the population.

The mid-2000s saw new mental health legislation in the form of the Mental Health Act 2007 and The Mental Capacity Act 2005. With regard to the former, while legislation is altered in line with the need to update matters every 25 years or so one of the major drivers to legislate in 2007 was the need to deal with breaches of the European Convention on Human Rights. Another was to provide 'flexibility' in delivery of mental health services through providing for compulsory treatment in the community, for patients deemed to be dangerous. In so doing it has been argued that the government was following a populist agenda created by homicide inquiries into the deaths caused by mental health patients (The National Confidential Inquiry). Government policy followed a line of thinking that homicides would be prevented by broadening the conditions of compulsion to include people with personality disorder and alcohol or drug problems and limiting discretion to discharge from compulsory detention people considered high-risk cases.

The Mental Health Act 2007 altered the definition of mental disorder in the 1983 act to a more inclusive one – 'any disorder or disability of the mind' – and broadened the notion of treatability, requiring only that 'appropriate medical treatment is available' and removing the need to demonstrate that a treatment is likely to alleviate or prevent deterioration of a mental health problem. Notwithstanding these changes, the 2007 act does not appear to have drastically changed matters from the existing legislation and is unlikely to alter the number of patients subject to compulsion in community or hospital settings (Shah 2009) (see Figure 10.1).

Separate legislation introduced in 2005 means that mental capacity is now a core part of UK mental health law (Owen *et al.* 2009). While on the face of things a number of issues changed in the legislation, in this chapter it is the second and third of these points we need to consider. Earlier we noted the shift from the role of the 'Responsible Medical Officer' to that of the 'Responsible Clinician' (open now to non-medical practitioners of a senior grade). Also, there was a replacement of

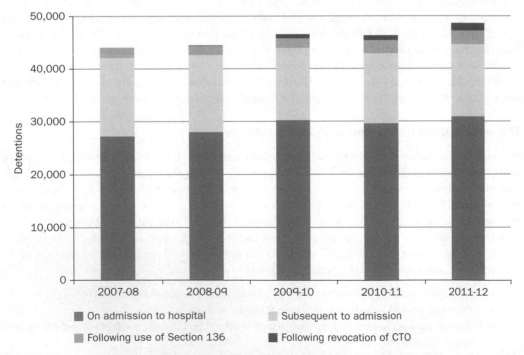

Figure 10.1   Adapted from The Health and Social Care Information Centre showing small increase in numbers of civil compulsory detention & admissions.

the Approved Social Worker (ASW) role with that of the Approved Mental Health Worker (open now to non-social workers).

Bean (1986) noted that the social worker's role in compulsory detention was due to a historical accident. Certainly, as a predominantly female occupation, social work did not have access to the structures and territory that the male medical profession had when capturing jurisdiction over the control and management of mental disorder. This was evident in the position that social workers were ascribed in mental health legislation. Social workers did not see their interests in competing with the knowledge and skills of other mental health professionals by increasing their own expertise in mental health, preferring instead to adopt an industrialization strategy (Oppenheimer 1975).

After 1983 ASWs had the task of co-assessing people in crisis with psychiatrists and GPs, about whether hospitalization was warranted and whether less restrictive alternatives could be identified (Ramon 2006). The ASWs tended to take a psycho-social perspective rather than a medical one and had the right to disagree with psychiatrists and GPs. The change in the 2007 Mental Health Act disappointed ASWs when this designated special role was opened up to others (Rapaport 2006).

There has been further evidence of role diffusion and blurring in the mental health workforce. For example, nurses may now train to become prescribers alongside psychiatrists. This might indicate that nursing is being further medicalized and/or that the restrictive practices of medicine are being eroded and the leadership role of psychiatrists undermined (see Chapter 7). These doctors objected to the implications of the government's programme to re-engineer the mental health workforce, called 'New Ways of Working' (NWW), and its impact on medical authority.

The NWW programme brought together representatives of all mental health disciplines, with a few (carefully selected) users and carers, to shape future services for those working primarily with adults experiencing severe mental health problems. Several conferences and publications came out of this work (Department of Health 2007), highlighting principles of collaborative work with other disciplines, users and carers. Although the programme was formally committed to recovery principles, the discussion focused on organizational efficacy and securing the continuation of professional monopoly. A change in the traditionally medically dominated and fixed hierarchy workforce was also encouraged by accumulating shortages. By 2000 services had unfilled vacancies in psychiatry, nursing, psychology, occupational therapy and social work (SCMH 2000). The shifting emphasis towards community psychiatric nursing, after the closure of the large hospitals, meant that inpatient wards had particular problems with recruitment and retention. They often relied upon temporary ('bank') staff. This trend was amplified by Project 2000 (when nursing became a graduate profession) because student nurses were no longer an extra pair of hands but largely attended placements as learning experiences.

Together these factors created a crisis of recruitment at the turn of the twenty-first century. In response the government set up the Workforce Action Team (WAT), which was charged with developing solutions. Reporting in 2001 it focused on staff recruitment and retention, national occupational standards, a single agreed skill set for the mental health workforce, skill mix solutions, the recruitment of more trained support staff, primary care staff development, tackling the stigma of working in mental health services, and engagement with professional bodies to examine the educational implications of this scoping exercise (Workforce Action Team 2001).

Capacity and compulsion in a post-institutional context

While the notion of 'capacity' has dominated in recent discussions of legalism by the mental health workforce, a counter-trend has been what can be termed 'rights-based legalism'. This refers to the rights of individuals with mental illnesses, predicated, to some extent, on the social model of disability. The latter provides a framework within which pre-existing relationships, attitudes and assumptions that underpin traditional forms of social and legal engagement with people with a diagnosis of mental illness could form the bases of a challenge to augment the notion of 'capacity' in mental health law through a stronger focus on the principle of participation (Weller 2013).

Before we leave the complexities of compulsion and professional interests within it, it is important to note a structural change in context. The above debates about compulsion and social policy progress have been largely one of moral or political principle (the ethics of paternalism versus voluntarism, rights of access versus the right to be left alone, respect for mental capacity and so on). However, many of those debates were triggered during the 1950s and 1960s in a context of wide-scale institutionalization. The liberal and libertarian critiques from sociologists like Erving Goffman and psychiatrists like Thomas Szasz and Ronald Laing reflected that agreed scenario of mass compulsion. This was manifest as well in media representations, such as the film *One Flew Over the Cuckoo's Nest* or the Laingian-inspired film *Family Life*.

However, since the advent of deinstitutionalization in the early1990s, the structure of compulsion has changed but perhaps not as much as one might have anticipated. The principled arguments have not, and so they remain today (as above and the next sections indicate) but the *scale and type of setting* have certainly altered. The restriction on numbers of psychiatric beds may mean now that risky conduct, rather than expressed need, drives admission priorities, but that other means such as CTOs will be used more.

This in not to argue now that critical professionals are unconcerned about the agenda, set by those like Goffman and Szasz in the 1960s. Their current concerns though are about defending State backing and funding for *new* service philosophies that support forms of therapeutic social control, which are voluntaristic, biographically sensitive and user-centred (Romme *et al.* 1992; Calton *et al.* 2007; Thomas and Longden 2013). Thus, while the structure of compulsion in mental health services is now shaped by a post-institutional service context (barring secure provision) and attempts at quick 'throughput' in acute psychiatric wards, the arguments about voluntarism and human rights persist today. This is evident in the perennial debates about risk and dangerousness, to which we now turn.

Dangerousness

This section will first deal with violence to others and then suicide.

Violence and mental disorder

While public attitudes, backed up at times by the views of politicians, err on the side of assuming that mental disorder predicts violence to others, the considered empirical position about this relationship is complex and varies over time. Broadly three phases can be identified:

1   *The negative relationship phase.* Studies of the relationship between mental disorder and violence between 1925 and 1965 suggested that people with mental health problems were actually less violent than the general population (Rabkin 1979).

2   *The small positive relationship phase.* After 1965 this position went into reverse. Link *et al.* (1992) found that after 1965 the median ratio was one of 3:1, with patients being more violent than non-patients. A number of factors could account for this reversal. First, episodic violent acts were historically contained in mental hospitals, when nearly all patients were chronically warehoused, with the range of potential victims being highly restricted in closed settings. This changed as more and more patients were treated in the community. Second, the community settings for patients were often risky environments – poor and socially disorganized with high rates of crime. Third, these environments also contained access to substances which could be abused less readily in hospital settings.

3   *The disaggregated data phase.* During the 1990s a further analysis of the small relationship phase revealed a complicated inter-relationship between clinical factors, personality
factors and contextual factors (Blumenthal and Lavender 2000; Pilgrim and Rogers 2003).
Although a cursory look at the evidence by pressure groups such as MIND suggested that
growing tolerance towards the mentally ill since the Second World War went into reverse
in the 1990s, a more complex picture is painted when an increasing number of studies
which address specific aspects of the relationship between mental state and violence are
taken into consideration. The following summarizes these findings:

- Ambiguous findings have been evident about the link between psychosis alone and
  violence in community settings. Swanson *et al.* (1990) found that psychotic patients
  who did not abuse substances were three times more dangerous than their non-patient
  equivalents over a period of a year. By contrast Steadman *et al.* (1998) found that psychotic patients who did not abuse substances were no more likely to be violent than
  their neighbours. Given that violent acts are quite rare it is also worth noting that even
  in the Swanson *et al.* study, their findings only pointed up estimates of 7 per cent of
  patients who were violent compared to 93 per cent non-violent patients. This is why
  the estimated small aggregate relationship between mental health problems and risk
  of dangerousness refers to a 'trivial contribution'. Interestingly, another British study
  showed that most perpetrators with a history of mental disorder were 'not acutely ill' at
  the time of the offence (Shaw *et al.* 2006).
- Substance abuse predicts violence. People, whatever their mental state, who abuse
  alcohol and some other substances (such as crack cocaine) are significantly prone to
  violence and other risky behaviour, such as dangerous driving. Some drugs do not predict violence though, most notably the opiates (though they do predict other forms of
  criminality to feed the habit). Substance abuse also is the best predictor of violence in
  psychotic patients (Steadman *et al.* 1998).
- The diagnosis of mental disorder which best predicts violence is that of a type of personality disorder (antisocial/dissocial/psychopathic). This is hardly surprising. As we
  noted earlier this diagnosis is typically defined tautologically by persistent violent habits. Broad diagnoses alone of mental disorder (such as personality disorder in general)
  or mental illnesses such as 'schizophrenia' are very poor predictors of violence.
- Ambiguous findings exist about the role of individual symptom and treatment variables. For example, compliance with medication reduces the risk of violence (Swartz
  et al. 1998). Command hallucinations with hostile content predict violent acts
  (Junginger 1995). Taylor (1985) also found that this was the case for hostile delusions.
  However, other studies have not demonstrated a relationship between hallucinations or
  delusions and violence (Teplin *et al.* 1994; Appelbaum *et al.* 1999; 2000). Violent rumi-
  nations seem to predict violence in those who abuse substances (Grisso *et al.* 2000).
  Indeed the consistent theme in the recent literature is that psychopathic disorder and
  substance misuse are strong predictors of violence but psychosis *per se* is not.
- Independent of clinical and personality variables, some times and places shape dangerousness more than others. When patients are discharged into richer areas they are less
  dangerous than in poorer areas (Silver *et al.* 1999). The latter areas of 'concentrated poverty' contain what Hiday (1995) calls 'violence inducing social forces'. In these poor community contexts, patients are more prone to be both the victim and perpetrator of crimes.

Having summarized the phases of empirical investigation about the overall or aggregate link
between mental state and violence a prospective question is suggested: can violence be predicted
in individual cases? A number of criticisms can be raised in relation to the possibility:

1   *The empirical attack.* This is a body of research evidence which suggests that accurate prediction is impossible: 'It now seems beyond dispute that mental health professionals have no expertise in predicting future dangerous behaviour either to self or others. In fact predictions of dangerous behaviour are wrong about 90 per cent of the time' (Ennis and Emery 1978: 28). While health professionals might not be able to predict future acts accurately all of the time, at the individual level there is an increasing evidence base to suggest key points at which individuals may be more likely to commit violent acts to themselves or others which in principle at least could feed into clinical decision-making. For example, tailored support at key points might reduce risk. (Nearly half of post-discharge suicides occur within a month of discharge, with the first week and first day after discharge being particularly high-risk periods (Hunt *et al.* 2009).) Similarly, another study has indicated that in people with a diagnosis of schizophrenia who went onto to commit violent (homicidal) acts, in the month before the offence 32 (56 per cent) had shown a change in the quality, intensity or conviction of emotional response to their delusional beliefs (Meehan *et al.* 2006).

2   *The political attack.* From a libertarian position, Szasz (1963: 46) has argued that prediction violates patients' civil rights:

Drunken drivers are dangerous both to themselves and to others. They injure and kill many more people than, for example, persons with paranoid delusions of persecution. Yet, people labeled 'paranoid' are readily committable, while drunken drivers are not . . . Some types of dangerous behaviour are even rewarded. Racecar drivers, trapeze artists, and astronauts receive admiration and applause . . . Thus, it is not dangerousness in general that is at issue here, but rather the manner in which one is dangerous.

The libertarian critique from Szasz has been echoed by other critics such as Sayce (2000), who argued that singling out mentally disordered individuals for particular scrutiny in relation to dangerousness is discriminatory. This point can be highlighted by the use of a table (Table 10.1) which identifies the contingent judgements and outcomes applying to a variety of social groups. This ongoing contention about types of risk emerged with every mass shooting (which is clouded part of the time by tautological arguments about the mental state of the offender). The attempt by President Obama in 2012 to alter gun control laws in the USA highlights why the *availability* of risky means is a good predictor of risky action, whereas predictions at the individual level are difficult (see earlier point from the empirical attack).

3   Professional dissent. The third source of attack emanates from some mental health professionals. Because predicting dangerousness is tied to social control, some professionals worry that it is incompatible with a caring and therapeutic role. They resent and resist becoming society's police officers for informal rule rather than law infringement. Risk minimization pushes professionals into conservative decision-making to avoid false negatives (predicting the absence of risk when a patient then goes on to be dangerous). This type of decision-making encourages professionals to take a distrusting attitude towards patients in general. The discussion earlier about the way in which legal rules and obligations interfere with professional ethos of care is relevant to this point.

These various examples demonstrate that psychiatric patients are only one of many groups that we might consider when thinking about degrees of dangerousness and socio-legal sanction. The question is whether or not psychiatric patients are offered the same rights as others in the table. For instance, currently in Britain people of known dangerousness (like those in cells 4 and 6) are

Table 10.1 Mental health and dangerousness

	Sick				Well			
	Law breaker		Law abiding		Law breaker		Law abiding	
	Detained	Free	Detained	Free	Detained	Free	Detained	Free
Dangerous	1	2	3	4	5	6	7	8
Non-dangerous	9	10	11	12	13	14	15	16

Cell 1: Mentally disordered offenders.

Cell 2: Mentally disordered offenders prior to detection.

Cell 3: Civil compulsory admissions to psychiatric hospitals.

Cell 4: People who are HIV+ who indulge in unprotected sexual intercourse.

Cell 5: Convicted prisoners.

Cell 6: Drunken/speeding car drivers.

Cell 7: Prisoners of war.

Cell 8: Members of the SAS.

Cell 9: Petty criminal prisoners who are psychologically disturbed.

Cell 10: Petty criminals on probation.

Cell 11: Old people forcibly hospitalized under the 1948 National Assistance Act because they live in insanitary conditions.

Cell 12: People in the community who are depressed.

Cell 13: Prisoners guilty of 'white collar' crimes like fraud.

Cell 14: Unapprehended shoplifters.

Cell 15: Victims of child abuse who are taken into care.

Cell 16: The assumed societal norm.

morally condemned but not legally restrained. By contrast, many psychiatric patients who are no proven threat to others are compulsorily detained under the Mental Health Act.

Suicide and mental disorder

The social control of psychiatric patients, both in hospital and community settings, is not limited to the question of violence to others. Mental health services are also concerned with reducing the incidence of self-harm and self-neglect. Rates of suicide among psychiatric patients are high for a number of reasons. Their labour market disadvantage places them in a demoralized and devalued position. Their primary disability may include profound feelings of anomie, aimlessness, worthlessness, low mood and low self-esteem, as well as angry feelings which can be trapped and turned inwards. The secondary disability created by psychiatric treatment may be both demoralizing (when coping with drug side effects and stigma) and an opportunity to act suicidally (the option to self-poison with prescribed psychiatric drugs).

The differential way in which psychiatric patients are treated when violent or potentially violent is also true of self-harm. In Britain suicide is not illegal. Despite this, suicidal patients, when identified, are treated in a peculiar way – coercion is applied. The question of suicide in psychiatric populations is thus more contradictory in a legal sense than that of violence to others. The latter in any population, general or psychiatric, is judged to be both immoral and illegal. By contrast, suicide is not illegal and its moral status is contested. Another example of the differential rule application to psychiatric patients in relation to suicide is more subtle and implicit.

When psychiatric patients are suicidal, it is often assumed that their intentions are governed singularly by their mental abnormality. However, suicides in non- psychiatric populations are evaluated in a range of ways, which might include a notion of a temporary imbalance of mind, but other motives can be ascribed as well. These include a notion of rational intelligibility, when, for various reasons, it is obvious why a person has little or nothing to live for (e.g. severe pain or physical disability, or traumatic loss of significant others). Similarly, for reasons noted earlier, psychiatric patients might, for very good reasons, feel devalued and disabled. And yet, suicidal intent or action on their part tends only to be interpreted as irrational. Thus, while the post hoc attribution of mental abnormality may be applied to any person committing suicide, there is a greater tendency for this to occur with people who are already psychiatric patients.

Psychiatric diagnosis is a weak predictor of suicide. For example, those with a diagnosis of depression have a 15 per cent lifetime risk of suicide and for those with a diagnosis of schizophrenia it is 10 per cent (Morgan 1994). This means that the overwhelming majority of those with a psychiatric diagnosis do not commit suicide, although more do so than in the general population. When specific personal and social factors are taken into account, rather than diagnosis, then predictive validity increases. These factors include: drug and alcohol abuse, single or separated status, male gender, low social class, unemployment, poverty, previous parasuicide, age (variable according to diagnosis) and recent violence (received or given) (Platt 1984; Jenkins *et al.* 1994).

When suicide is reframed as a social, rather than individual, phenomenon then a range of public policy factors can be identified in relation to primary prevention. For example, in the USA suicide rates are lower in states with tight gun control than those with lax control. An Australian study revealed that 85 per cent of gunshot deaths were linked to distress rather than criminal action (Dudley *et al.* 1996). Suicide increased with motor car use over a period of 20 years (via carbon monoxide self-poisoning) but it decreased when North Sea (non-toxic) gas was introduced in Britain in the 1970s. Given that self-poisoning is a common means of suicide, then lax prescribing of psychiatric drugs by the medical profession is likely to increase suicide rates, as will the widespread availability of some over-the-counter drugs like paracetamol that are toxic in overdose. It is also the case that structural changes have reduced the risk and opportunity of suicide leading to a decrease in incidence, which implies that focus is outwith the individual. The removal of ligature points in hospital wards has resulted in an estimated 40 per cent decline in incidence of suicides in hospital (Gunnell *et al.* 2012). This example suggests the capacity for environmental change to have more traction in bringing down suicide rates, for example, than an over-focus on ameliorating individual distress.

Impact on patients of their risky image

The legal and empirical debate about dangerousness and mental illness and how to assess risk does include considerations of moral and ethical issues. However, notwithstanding the importance of the latter, sociologically there is a much wider agenda than assessing the points at which it may be considered legitimate or illegitimate to use coercive control.

> The conflation of violence with mental illness and its expression in language, its importance as a cultural construct, and its impact on the everyday lives of people with psychiatric diagnoses are also worthy of our attention. There is evidence, for example, that psychiatric patients internalize the stigma of dangerousness in a way which comes to impact negatively on their self-image. This has been illustrated in a study of the meaning and management of neuroleptic medication in its recipients.

> (Rogers *et al.* 1998)

In this chapter we have been mainly concerned with the way in which psychiatric patients have been contained and confined within psychiatric facilities or in the community by the provisions of therapeutic law. The shift towards community settings has nonetheless brought to the fore the issue of the rights of psychiatric patients to be involved in the mainstream of society and to participate in the planning and delivery of the mental health services they receive. British legislation, most notably the NHS and Community Care Act 1990, has encouraged the direct participation of service users in the planning and management of care services. However, legislation which encourages and promotes the notion of consumerism in mental and community services does not, in itself, ensure change.

The meaning and purpose of user involvement and how service users can best be represented and power shared cannot be legislated for, but requires more fundamental changes to take place outside a strict legal framework (Bowl 1996). However, with the rise of the users' movement there has been growing attention placed on the need for a set of positive rights linked to the notion of citizenship. This perspective has stressed the need for equal opportunities about, and rights of access to, employment and housing for all psychiatric patients (Rooke-Matthews and Lindow 1997).

Psychiatric patients are singled out and treated in a separate way by legislation. First, involuntary patients admitted to hospital under civil sections of mental health legislation have no one to act as their advocate to *retain* their freedom at the time of admission. They have only the right to argue for their freedom after their detention. Second, they can be singled out in terms of their *potential* rather than their actual behaviour. Thus, therapeutic law is used for purposes of preventive detention. While criminals have a prescribed period of detention, mental patients do not, in the sense that legal powers allow their periods of detention to be renewed. Criminals lose their liberty as a consequence of a proven transgression of the law. Mental patients can lose their liberty even if there has been no such transgression – to offend public or family rules of decorum is all that is required. And even when a patient has committed an offence, they are not prescribed a defined period of detention if they are sent to a secure psychiatric facility. Earlier we noted the negative implications of this for patients with no estimated time of discharge.

Thus, Szasz is correct to point out that psychiatric patients are indeed treated in a particularly discriminatory way in modern society. Moreover, some people who are not labelled as mentally disordered are manifestly dangerous (like those in cells 4 and 6 of Table 10.1) yet they suffer none of the infringements of liberty imposed on non-offending psychiatric patients. This discrimination against psychiatric patients is not implicit or covert, as is the case in so much of sexual and racial discrimination, but is explicit and legally legitimized.

Although British mental health legislation seemingly exists to protect the rights of patients, it may inadvertently help facilitate this discrimination, rather than alleviating it, since it frequently fails to adequately protect or enhance patients' civil liberties or their quality of life. Instead, the law legitimizes 'the institutionalization of society's unfounded prejudice and fear regarding madness'. The latter phrase is used by Campbell and Heginbotham (1991) when arguing that there is little justification for maintaining a separate legislative framework for those considered to be mentally disordered – a stance as we noted above that was argued by opponents of new English legislation before 2007, even though the objection was unsuccessful. A development in the UK representing recognition by the State of the specific discrimination faced by those with mental health problems is encompassed in the Mental Health Discrimination Act 2013, which removed three legal barriers contributing to stigma. These included the three provisions in the Act:

- repealing section 141 of the Mental Health Act 1983, under which a Member of the House of Commons, Scottish Parliament, Welsh Assembly or Northern Ireland Assembly automatically loses their seat if they are sectioned under the Mental Health Act for more than six months;

- amending the Juries Act 1974 in order to remove the blanket ban on 'mentally disordered persons' undertaking jury service;
- amending the Companies (Model Articles) Regulations 2008 which stipulates that a person might cease to be a director of a public or private company 'by reason of their mental health'.

While on the face of things these components seem relatively small in their remit, the Act represents the removal of discrimination in law towards those with a mental health problem. It represents a shift from the focus on legislating for the effects of mental illness for people participating in society by removing the social and institutional barriers to citizen participation paving the way for accepting full participation in social, political and economic life.

Discussion

The interdependent relationship between the legal and psychiatric systems has been explored in this chapter. As we have reviewed the interplay between legal and medical control, it seems that their conceptual separation, and assumed antagonism, does not always translate neatly into practice. Currently, the two feed off one another or form complementary contributions to the constraint of mental abnormality. In Britain, for instance, both lawyers and doctors sit on Mental Health Review Tribunals. The Mental Health Act Commission, which arose out of legislation (the 1983 Act), contained both doctors and lawyers.

Moreover, although the Commission was a manifestation of legalism, it enshrined the collegial loyalties enjoyed by doctors. For instance, it appointed and paid second-opinion doctors to review the appropriateness of the treatment of detained patients at the hands of other doctors. Disagreements with the 'treating psychiatrist' were uncommon. (Note that the Mental Health Act Commission subsequently became part of a larger organization called the 'Healthcare Commission'.) Thus, arguably, in the field of mental health, lawyers and psychiatrists are bedfellows, not adversaries, and so any sociological reading of 'therapeutic law' must be aware of the reproduction of a particular professionally negotiated discourse. The latter may be limited in focus and divert us from a wider understanding of legalism and psychological deviance.

A wider approach to understanding mental health care and coercion from within the social sciences and health services research is likely to add to analysis provided from within the existing legal framework. A greater focus on social and contextual aspects of violence and mental health suggests a response at a different level (for example, a public health agenda about mental health). Additionally, the adoption of a patient-centred approach to the framing of questions of care and control in coercion research is likely to balance the dominance of disciplinary approaches from within psychiatry and the law. The social construction of violence and mental illness at a sociopolitical level, the wider role played by services and professionals and the risks faced by patients living in the community should arguably be at the centre, rather than at the periphery, of research and analysis on coercion.

Legalism has played an important role in the field of mental health. It has set certain limits on medical power and discretion. It has also codified two separate social processes which are at odds with one another: the rights of patients to exercise choice and the rights of professionals to impose their actions against the wishes of patients. Psychiatric patients have also had special legal provision when they commit criminal offences. The legal rules applied to them have been different from those of other offenders, highlighting the special (arguably discriminatory) way in which people with mental health problems are treated. This special treatment also applies to self-injurious behaviour. Although suicide itself is not illegal, suicidal intent detected in people with mental health problems can trigger peculiar forms of lawful control.

Questions

1 Should dangerous psychiatric patients be treated differently from other dangerous people?
2 Discuss the evidence about mental health status and dangerousness.
3 What contradictions exist in mental health law?
4 In which respects has mental health law in Britain changed since the beginning of the twentieth century?
5 Can consumerism operate while we have coercive mental health law?
6 Should mental health legislation be abandoned?

For discussion

Consider the different ways in which psychiatric patients might be denied informed consent, and examine legal options to improve their lot in this regard.

11　Stigma and recovery

Chapter overview

The notion of stigma, denoting relations of shame and deviations from what is considered 'normal', has a long history within the mental health field. Here, though, we focus mainly on contemporary social processes and concepts to offer some sociological insights into the topic. We discuss the response to stigma through the emergence of a recovery-based social movement and government anti-stigma campaigns. These have entailed a contemporary reconsideration of the source of stigma and the role of professional services in its reduction or amplification. Approaches to these topics have varied from a social psychological emphasis on prejudice to structural critiques, emphasizing a social disability model. That range of understanding is important for students of this complex area of sociological investigation.

　　This chapter considers:

- lay views of psychological differences;
- stereotyping and stigma;
- the backbone of stigma;
- labelling or social reaction theory and its modification;
- the role of the mass media;
- social exclusion;
- recovery.

Lay views of psychological differences and attributions of stigma

In every culture there is some notion of emotional or psychological difference. Not all cultures identify these differences in exactly the same way, nor do they use identical terms. Equally, no culture is indifferent to those who are sad, frightened or unintelligible in their conduct (Horwitz 1983). With or without an expertise in the field of mental abnormality, most people know madness when they see it. Equally, most of us can identify for ourselves when we are sad or anxious. This has become more salient with individualism and resonates with the discussion on self-surveillance which is seen as intrinsic to the psy complex (see discussion in Chapter 1) and with the observation of the increasing tendency to self-label emotions in the context of help-seeking (Thoits 1985).

　　Any of us might be directly involved in invoking a medical diagnosis for a friend, a relative or even a stranger in the street who is acting in a way we find perplexing or distressing. Any of us might reach a point where we decide that our own distress warrants a visit to the doctor or other expert for help. Everyday notions of 'nervousness' suggest that a concept does prefigure a psychiatric label of phobic anxiety or some other version of neurosis. Likewise, if people act in a way others cannot readily understand they run the risk of being dismissed as a 'nutter', a 'loony', 'crazy', 'mad' or even 'mental'. Again, these prefigure notions of psychosis within a professional discourse.

　　Users of mental health services, rejecting the psychiatric notion of 'mental illness', have often opted instead for the term 'mental distress'. A problem with the latter is that it alludes only to the pain of the patient and it gives no notion that they can be distressing, frustrating or frightening to others at times. Indeed, from the lay but non-patient perspective, the latter is often the preoccupying concern. There is considerable overlap between lay and psychiatric notions of mental health and illness. For example, in psychiatric disease categories, such as anorexia nervosa, where there is uncertainty about the cause and a large cultural component to the diagnosis, lay and psychiatric epistemologies have been found to be similar (Lees 1997). And as we note later, psychiatric professionals often simply 'rubber stamp' judgements already made in the lay arena about madness or misery. While this overall trend is apparent there are nuanced differences within lay groups and between lay people and professionals.

For example, in one study African-Caribbean people indicated less stigmatizing and more alternative beliefs towards the symptoms and diagnostic label of 'schizophrenia' compared to white European people. The latter were more likely to follow a Western model of mental illness (Stone and Finlay 2008). Similarly, adolescents who self-label (rather than are labelled by others) report high ratings of self-stigma and depression and a lower sense of mastery (Moses 2009). Variations of lay views seem to be connected to group values and perceived legitimacy of discrimination. For example, high group value and low perceived legitimacy of discrimination predicts positive reactions to stigma (Rusch et al. 2009). There are also differences between lay perspectives and disciplinary and formal knowledge. Notions about antisocial behaviour sometimes appear to be less readily accommodated within the lay discourse of distress and oddity, with mental health professionals more likely to offer pathologizing rather than simple moralistic accounts. This happens when juries are asked to consider the states of mind of mass murderers and sometimes reject expert psychiatric views that people are mentally disordered.

The lay discourse contains a contradiction about mental abnormality and antisocial conduct. As Rosen (1968) points out, in Ancient Rome and Athens madness was defined in pre-psychiatric times by two characteristics: aimless wandering and violence. In Laos, 'crazy' people are called 'baa'. Westermeyer and Kroll (1978) studied villagers' perceptions of the 'baa' people at a time when the country had no mental hospital or mental health professionals. They found that non-'baa' people adjudged their deviant fellows to be violent in 11 per cent of the cases, before their change of character, but, this attribution went up to 54 per cent after 'baa' was identified. It may be that alongside this belief in the inherent link between mental abnormality and violence, those who consider themselves to be sane are suspicious of false claims made to avoid criminal prosecution. The latter of course is logically possible – some criminals do use the insanity defence, favouring florid psychosis (in the case of the 1980s serial killer Peter Sutcliffe, whose sanity remains debated) or in the US context dissociative identity disorder (multiple personality disorder), when seriously heinous crimes are under scrutiny. But whether a person is truly or falsely insane confirms a distinction in principle between two groups of people.

A further example of this point can be given in relation to the 'family colony' which has existed at Ainay-le-Château, France, since 1900. Psychiatric patients are fostered by families in the community instead of being inside an institution. Jodelet (1991) studied the ways in which citizens construed the patients in their midst. She found that the patients were segregated not by walls but by personal constructions – mainly based on fear of contamination by the illness and fear of unpredictable danger. This fear is so great that a taboo has emerged in the colony about patients marrying non-patients. When sexual relationships of this type have developed over the years, which are rare, this has led to the couple being banished from the locality.

As we noted in Chapter 10 the relationship between 'mental illness' and dangerous acts is complex. However, public views tend to exaggerate the extent and link between violence and schizophrenia. This is a cross-cultural phenomenon. In the USA, which has been called a 'psychiatric society' by Castel et al. (1979), the public has mixed views about the association of mental disorder and violence. Research on public opinion undertaken has in the past shown that most people considered that a person diagnosed as 'schizophrenic' is more likely to commit a violent crime than other people (Field Institute 1984). While some have suggested that violent imagery is less pronounced in terms of viewing mentally ill people as more dangerous than others it is still one of the core reasons for social rejection and devaluation (Pescosolido 2013).

Lay people tend to spontaneously view 'mental illness' as being about psychotic or unintelligible behaviour, with violent behaviour seen as reflecting mental illness or disorder. This is why, as we noted earlier, defence lawyers can appeal to lay jurors to consider mental abnormality as an exculpating factor when judging the source of violent acts. However, the commonest diagnosis in psychiatry is actually depression. This particular diagnosis is not the lay stereotype of a mentally ill person. Moreover, depression and the distress linked to stressful personal circumstances now occupy an ambiguous space in the minds of lay people. Terms like 'stress' – as an internal subjective state, not as an external objective pressure – and 'depression' are now part of the vernacular in Western societies. They are seen as an extension of normal existence and are not necessarily seen as mental illness (Pilgrim and Bentall 1999).

What this points to is a recurring theme across disciplinary and lay perspectives. For example, early traditional psychiatric accounts of mental illness focus overwhelmingly on madness (the functional diagnostic categories of 'schizophrenia' and 'manic depression'), and depict anxiety and depression as stress reactions and not true mental illnesses (Fish 1968). This old psychiatric dichotomy has been reinstated in some recent sociological accounts. For example, as we noted in Chapter 1, Horwitz (2002) argues that there are true mental diseases (the psychoses including extreme depression) and there is an extensive range of diagnostic categories, which are merely psychiatric codifications of variations in normal mental states, which vary in quality, prevalence and style of evaluation from culture to culture. This is why one recent criticism of DSM-5 has been not that it offers diagnosis in principle (as DSM has always done) but that it extends pathology to those not warranting it (Wykes and Callard 2010). The latter talk of the 'pool of normality shrinking to a mere puddle', with the publication of DSM-5.

Thus we can see a degree of convergence between lay attributions about mental abnormality, traditional psychiatric accounts and some sociological accounts (see more discussion about this in Chapter 1). This does not imply though that a fixed consensus exists across these three communities of thought. Currently, most Western psychiatrists do see 'anxiety' and 'depression' as being mental illnesses. By contrast, many mental health service users, even those with diagnoses of 'major' or 'severe' mental illness, do not depict their problems in illness terms. Also, many sociologists frame mental illness either as a form of 'residual deviance' or as a cognitive by-product of professional activity (a 'discourse' of the 'psy complex').

Stereotyping and stigma

We have already begun to draw attention to the micro-sociological phenomenon of stereotyping. This refers to the tendency of human beings to attribute fixed and common characteristics to whole social groups. Stereotyping can be thought of as a form of social typing. It is not always negative but it is always narrow and potentially misleading, because it ignores individual variability within social groups and the overlap of characteristics across them. The shift from stereotyping to stigmatization involves an enlargement of prejudicial social typing (an error of reasoning). Two other processes are added to this cognitive error. The first is emotional and entails any combination, depending on the personal target of the stereotype, of anxious avoidance, hostility or pity. A second feature of stigmatization, which goes beyond the cognitive error of stereotyping, is moral. Those stigmatizing others can show caring paternalism or moral outrage and revulsion, depending on the deviance involved. The stigmatized person is thus set apart from their fellows in these additive ways culminating in increased social distance, between the labeller and the labelled. The latter suffers consequent depersonalization, rejection and disempowerment (Jones *et al.* 1984; Braithwaite 1989; Hayward and Bright 1997). According to labelling theory stigmatized people become isolated and demoralized and develop, what Goffman (1963) called a 'spoiled identity' (see Box 11.1).

> ### Box 11.1 Accounts from Erving Goffman and Bruce Link about Stigma
>
> Erving Goffman, in his book *Stigma: Notes on the Management of Spoiled Identity* (1963), describes stigma as a
>
>> special kind of relationship between attribute and stereotype . . . [an] attribute that is deeply discrediting . . . that reduces the bearer . . . from a whole and usual person to a tainted, discounted one . . . We believe that a person with a stigma is not quite human . . . We tend to impute a wide range of imperfections on the basis of the original one . . . We may perceive his [sic] defensive response to his situation as a direct expression of his defect . . .
>>
>> (Goffman 1963: 14–16)
>
> Goffman goes on to point out that stigma is generated in a social situation. It is a reaction by society that spoils a person's identity by a set of imposed norms that are bought to bear on an encounter. According to Goffman these norms
>
>> concern identity or being . . . Failure or success at maintaining such norms have a very direct effect on the psychological integrity of the individual. At the same time, the mere desire to abide by the norm – mere good will – is not enough, for in many cases the individual has no immediate control over his [sic] level of sustaining the norm. It is a question of the individual's condition, not his will; it is a question of conformance not compliance . . .
>>
>> (1963: 52–3)
>
> Bruce Link extends this focus on social psychological aspects of *conformity* to wider social processes about *power* in his conference paper to the American Public Health Association in 2000 *The Stigma Process: Re-Conceiving the Definition of Stigma*:
>
>> We conceptualize stigma as a process. It begins when dominant groups distinguish human differences – whether 'real' or not. It continues if the observed difference is believed to connote unfavorable information about the designated persons. As this occurs, social labeling of the observed difference is achieved. Labeled persons are set apart in a distinct category that separates 'us' from 'them.' The culmination of the stigma process occurs when designated differences lead to various forms of disapproval, rejection, exclusion and discrimination. The stigma process is entirely contingent on access to social, economic and political power that allows the identification of differentness, the construction of stereotypes, the labeling of persons as different and the execution of disapproval and discrimination . . .

The negative stereotypes underlying the stigmatization of people with mental health problems contain three recurring elements about: intelligibility, social competence and credibility, and violence. Although we will now discuss these elements separately, a single personal image may capture or embody all three at once. The strongest negative attributions seem to focus on the spectre of a homicidal madman – a deranged being who explodes violently, erratically and inexplicably (Foucault 1978). However, because stereotypes are characterized by false generalizations and inaccurate claims about social groups, and because the stereotyping associated with mental illness is so powerful, the empirical validity of the main constituent elements described earlier invites particular scrutiny. In Chapter 10 we looked at the evidence about psychiatric patients and dangerousness. Here we will focus on questions of intelligibility, competence and credibility.

The meta rule of Intelligibility

An implicit 'meta-rule', in any social context, is that participants have an obligation, if called upon, to render their speech and conduct intelligible, about any rule transgression or role failure (Goffman 1955; 1971). If rules are followed and role expectations delivered by a person, then this obligation about intelligibility is not demanded of them. Generally, we only want to know why things have gone wrong or why our expectations in a social situation are not being fulfilled. With the peculiar therapeutic exception of psychoanalysis and the peculiar sociological exception of ethnomethodology, which, in different, ways interrogate normality or hold it to account, people are very rarely asked to explain or justify their compliance with role-rule expectations. This would be a tiresome disruption of everyday social interactions and incompatible with the free flow of social activity. However, when and if a rule infraction or role failure occurs, while others may ignore it for a while, at some point they usually expect and demand an explanation or an 'account' (Scott and Lyman 1968). The sane transgressor then will offer this account persuasively (e.g. the apology offered by someone making an honest mistake) or unpersuasively (e.g. the vacuous or dishonest explanation offered by the caught-out criminal) (Tedeschi and Reiss 1981).

This is where the first attribution then arises about madness: sane fellows cannot elicit or recognize an intelligible account or excuse from the transgressor. A person living in a world of their own is not in the social world observing the meta-rule of required mutual intelligibility. The mad person or incipient 'schizophrenic' offers no account to others for their deviant conduct, or offers one that does not make sense. They are said, therefore, to 'lack insight' into their conduct. The term 'lack insight', in this context, refers to the breakdown in an implicit social contract about our obligation to account to others, if required, for our transgressions.

Coulter (1973) points out that the most powerful ascriptions about madness do not come from psychiatrists. The latter only rubber stamp decisions and evaluations already made on common-sense grounds by others. Most typically, this will be the relatives of the patients, but it may come from others, such as strangers in the street. Here for example, Jonathan Miller, the theatre director, gives his account of the implicit social contract of mutual accountability studied by Coulter and its role in defining madness (then codified as mental illness by psychiatry). Miller calls it a 'very complicated constitution of conduct':

> It appears in the family first of all and then of course it appears in public places; there's a vast, very complicated constitution of conduct, which allows us to move with confidence through public spaces, and we can instantly and by a very subtle process recognize someone who is breaking that constitution. They're talking to themselves; they're not moving at the same rate; they're not avoiding other people with the skill that pedestrians do in the street. The speed with which normal users of public places can recognize someone else as not being a normal user of it is where madness appears.

(cited in Rogers *et al.* 1993)

Goffman (1971) analysed the social obligations we have for one another in public places, such as respecting personal space and reciprocating communications. Failed obligations require some form of remedial action, such as an apology or explanation. Miller suggests in his description above that mad people have abandoned, or they are incompetent at, what Goffman (1955) called 'impression management'. The latter refers to the subtle and dynamic range of communications we give out to others to indicate that we are conducting ourselves well and appropriately in a particular social situation.

A sociological rather than psychiatric account defines madness not by an objective decontextualized checklist of peculiar behaviours only recognized by experts. Instead, it takes a step before diagnosis and examines those actions, which are described and evaluated by others in a particular social context. For example, take Miller's point about people talking to themselves in public. He does not mention a public place where this rule does not apply – church, mosques and temples. People may speak to themselves in places of worship with no negative evaluation. He also does not mention a very common street scenario of talking to oneself without inviting an attribution of madness – the use of mobile phones. Hands-free sets now create the uncertain scenario for onlookers about the possibility of the speaker addressing auditory hallucinations.

These give examples of how the ascription of sanity or insanity requires the sort of subtle situation-specific judgements which Miller and Goffman are keen to identify. The praying person and the mobile phone user both act in a context in which others can decode the nature of their speech behaviour. By contrast, praying in the 'wrong place' or speaking out loud with no mobile phone in the hand invites ascriptions of madness. Madness is thus an ordinary social judgement awaiting medical codification. In a society without psychiatrists, the latter would never arrive but the social judgements would remain (Westermeyer and Kroll 1978). In the family, deviance may be noted but ignored (Lemert 1974). This suggests that identifying residual deviance and doing something about it are separate processes.

The point made by Coulter and Miller about a general meta-rule implies a global and transhistorical quality about human interaction. However, the application of this meta-rule can vary over time and place; another reason why judgements about madness need to be qualified by social and cultural relativism. For example, cross-cultural studies show how some peculiar actions, such as those linked to hallucinations, may be valued as mystical powers in one culture but dismissed as symptoms of mental illness in another. This shows that the same deviant action may be positively connoted in one context but negatively in another.

Thus unintelligibility, as a building block of stereotyping and stigma, is only applicable in those social contexts in which it is disvalued. Nonetheless, there is some empirical validity for the stereotype that psychiatric patients are unintelligible. After all, whether we use the term 'madness' or technicalize it as 'schizophrenia' or 'bi-polar disorder', conduct which baffles others is the core basis for the attribution of madness. While these are social judgements made in context (not scientific descriptions) they are still practically justified by the meta-rule about intelligibility.

However, psychotic patients are not invariably unpredictable. Mental health workers and significant others who get to know patients over months and years will describe their predictability (including cues of an imminent period of acute psychosis). Thus single or episodic attributions of unintelligibility do not imply constant unpredictability. The stereotype of the wild and unpredictable lunatic may still exist, but the typical manifestations of mental health problems are more complicated but also more mundane.

The backbone of stigma

The persistence of stigma across eras and countries makes it a culturally enduring phenomenon, maintained as much in degree and kind by social structures and cultural variations as it is by the response of individuals encountering deviant behaviour (Pescosolido *et al.* 2013). A global analysis of the nature of public stigma reveals what has been termed the 'backbone' of stigma.

This universal character of stigma refers to social rejection and personal devaluation in intimate settings. This universality is reflected in a 'core 5' of prejudicial views, which are held by more than two-thirds of a representative sample of people evident in all types of countries.

These items – more in evidence in relation to people diagnosed with schizophrenia – included doubts about those with a history of mental health problems being child-care providers, an enhanced potential for self-directed violence, unpredictability, negative views about the possibility of marrying into one's family or being trusted to teach children. A further consensus about another five items among more than 50 per cent of respondents from the same global sample appears to have potentially serious implications for civic participation and social participation in valued positions within society (e.g. questioning the ability of those with a mental health problems to supervise others in the work place, being difficult to talk to, and assumed potential for violence to others).

The study also revealed some cultural differences (it was a USA/UK comparison). The US sample was more optimistic about the impact of treatment than those responding in the UK. However, the context of greater faith-based ideology in the USA meant that severe mental illness was more likely to be seen as a biological impairment distributed in the population by 'God's Will'. An implication of the continuing biodeterminism in the public imagination about mental disorder is that it does not lead to more compassion or tolerance, but the reverse.

Competence and credibility

To summarize some relevant connecting points made earlier, the first element of stereotyping about mental illness is actually quite persuasive for some patients, some of the time. It is not only reasonable to claim that some people diagnosed as being mentally ill lack intelligibility; this empirical claim has actually been the main sociological rationale for understanding 'major' mental illness, as a form of residual deviance, rather than individual pathology. However, there are also three important caveats here.

First, only some psychiatric patients (those deemed to be psychotic) speak and act in ways that others cannot readily comprehend. Most patients (those who are depressed or anxious) not only obey the meta-rule of mutual intelligibility, they may actually use their distress as part of this obligation.

Second, some psychotic patients are largely intelligible all of the time. For example, there are patients with circumscribed delusions, who only speak and act oddly when these are discussed or prompted.

Third, most psychotic patients are rarely persistently mad. Madness tends to be episodic, with varying time periods of conformity to norms and evidence of a normal commitment to intelligibility in between crazy episodes. Moreover, social niches may exist in which these deviant qualities are functional or are attributed to social value. Here are some examples of these social situations and the value-frame they provide about mental abnormality:

- The first example is in relation to creativity. The latter, like madness, involves transgression. To create something original or to think in an original way requires a suspension of conformity and the production of something which is out of the ordinary. There is some evidence of both forms of transgression overlapping in the same individuals but this is not the same as saying that madness is intrinsically creative. We can neither conclude that all people with a diagnosis of mental illness are creative nor that all creative people are mentally ill. However, the incidence of mental health problems does seem to be higher in creative artists, novelists, poets and musical composers (Chadwick 1997). There is also some evidence that bi-polar disorder has a higher incidence in unusually successful people. This group manifests periods of excessive energy and industriousness and the grandiosity these creative people experience ensures that innovative thought experiments are attempted in practice during manic phases (Jamison 1998).
- A second example of social niches in which mental abnormality enables better performance is in relation to obsessionality. Patients with a diagnosis of obsessive-compulsive disorder are preoccupied with orderliness and rule-following to a point that they even

construct new rules for themselves to comply with (compulsive rituals). If they are not allowed access to this rule-following then they become very distressed. Those with a diagnosis of obsessive-compulsive personality disorder are conformist, hygienic, pedantic and moralistic in their outlook. In the nineteenth century, these types of problems were viewed as a form of insanity, whereas now they are framed by psychiatrists as neurotic or personality problems (Berrios 1985). What psychotic and obsessive-compulsive problems highlight in different ways is that mental health is defined implicitly by a capacity to conform to role-rule relationships. When patients are mad and they act or speak unintelligibly, then they under-conform. By contrast, obsessional patients over-conform. Tasks which require close attention to detail and are repetitive are done exceptionally well by obsessional people. The latter are well suited to any occupation involved in counting money carefully or in slowly checking fine details in a task. Societies which are organized around mechanical rationality would place more of a value in careful rule compliance than those which were more laissez-faire. The obsessive-compulsive personality seems to be an exaggerated version of North American materialistic individualism (a preoccupation with individual work responsibilities defining the person's identity and an emphasis on a person's unique material possessions). In a British context, Marks (1987) notes that the features of an obsessional personality read like a 'list of Victorian virtues'.

- A third example is in relation to spirituality and religious leadership. The close relationship between religion and mental abnormality can be found in psychiatric texts, which, since the mid-nineteenth century have focused on 'religiosity' or have distinguished between healthy and pathological religious commitment (e.g. Donat 1988; Tseng 2003). Between 10 and 15 per cent of people with a diagnosis of schizophrenia are described as having religious delusions (Koenig *et al.* 1998). Also, as an indication of the importance of cultural context, the content of these delusions is closely linked to prevalent religious beliefs in a patient's particular time and place (Wilson 1998). Thus, generally, religious commitment and experience can be a focus of diagnostic interest for psychiatrists. This interest may discredit the patient's right to be taken seriously by others. On the other hand, the charismatic seminal leaders of the main world religions could be diagnosed retrospectively as suffering from some form of psychosis. With the exception of Judaism, the major religions have placed a positive value on poverty, social isolation and even begging. Christ wandered in the desert and knew that he was the son of God (any other person making this claim now would be called 'deluded'). Siddhartha, who became known as the Buddha, abandoned his comfortable aristocratic existence and went into the forest, isolating himself from the world and putting himself in jeopardy. This type of incorrigible social withdrawal has traditionally been associated with madness – the aimless wandering described in antiquity. The prophet Mohammed craved isolation and sought refuge in a cave near Mecca, where he experienced a frequent command hallucination, telling him to cry. These three famous individuals rejected the constraints of daily living and the norms of their host society and acted in a way that would now invite a diagnosis of 'schizophrenia'. However, eventually, their actions yielded not less, but more social credibility. Together, Jesus Christ, the Buddha and the prophet Mohammed are now worshipped by the majority of the world's population – they have what could be called a form of global and transhistorical 'hyper-credibility'. They also reflect and reinforce a tradition, which pre-dates their existence, in Hinduism of a mendicant tradition of holy men, who put themselves outside of society, with no direct means of support. This lifestyle overlaps strongly with that of madness. Holy mendicants, venerated religious leaders and mad patients are separated only by whether their conduct in common is deemed by others to be a product of spiritual choice and duty or of involuntary psychological incompetence.

It may seem, on commonsense grounds, that mental abnormality intrinsically signals social incompetence. However, the above three examples challenge this idea. Much depends on a particular social situation placing a value on, and continuing to support, what the identified patient is expressing.

To summarize the theme of this section, is it fair to stereotype people with mental health problems as being continuously irrational in thought and action and so undeserving of social credibility? The answer is clearly in the negative. People manifesting symptoms of mental illness can be highly goal directed, creative, reliable and even inspirational across many generations. Despite this, the powerful stereotype that they should be denied credibility because of their irrationality leads to stigma and discrimination in most modern societies.

Does labelling matter? The insights of modified labelling theory

We now address a different empirical question. If negative stereotyping is unreasonable but still occurs, does any prejudicial action flowing from it matter? Put differently, what evidence is there that negative social reactions have any detrimental effect on people with mental health problems? When labelling theory was first applied to mental illness (Scheff 1966) it was faced with an empirical critique and consequently lost its popularity within sociology. Studies emerged which did not seem to confirm the detrimental impact of negative social reactions on people with mental health problems (e.g. Crocetti *et al.* 1974; Kirk 1974). These studies were complemented by a strong counterclaim to social reaction theory; that labelling actually gave patients the positive opportunity of access to effective pharmacological and psychological treatments to ameliorate their problems. Gove (1982) suggests that labelling is driven, in the main, not by social contingencies but more by the patient's symptoms. He emphasized that patient behaviour, not the prejudices of others, determines labelling. Primary not secondary deviance is highlighted in this view.

Link and Phelan (1995) revisited the empirical status of labelling theory and drew attention to a number of studies, which, contra the critique of Gove, clearly demonstrate the negative impact of labelling. These studies indicate that disvalued social statuses – such as prostitution, epilepsy, alcoholism, criminality and drug abuse – form a hierarchy of stigma, with mental illness being near to the bottom (Albrecht *et al.* 1982; Skinner *et al.* 1995). Some experimental studies also show that knowledge of a person's psychiatric history predicts social rejection (Link and Cullen 1983; Sibicky and Dovidio 1986). To confirm this, surveys of the general public show that fear of violence and the need to keep a social distance diminish with increasing contact with people with a psychiatric diagnosis (Alexander and Link 2003). Also, some naturalistic studies, even at the time that labelling theory was losing its popularity in sociology, demonstrated that a psychiatric history reduced a person's access to housing and employment (e.g. Farina and Felner 1973).

These types of finding have led Link and his colleagues to offer a 'modified labelling theory', which has empirical support in a series of studies they conducted and are summarized in Link and Phelan (1995). These studies demonstrate two main findings. First, provided that best practice is offered in mental health services, people with mental health problems can derive positive benefits to their quality of life (in a qualified way, thus supporting Gove's claim about the positive impact of labelling). Second, whether or not specialist mental health services have positive or negative effects (a function of their range of quality), independent stigma effects persist from, and are embedded in, social processes in the community.

The theory Link and colleagues developed to account for this second finding, which is supported by their additional experimental investigation of lay views of mental illness, relates not to direct prejudicial action by others but by a shared cultural expectation. The latter is that mental illness will lead to suspicion, loss of credibility and social rejection. All parties, including and especially the person who develops a mental health problem, share this assumption from childhood.

Consequently, the diagnosed person enters, or considers entering, interactions with others operating this assumption. For their part, the non-patient also expects the diagnosed person to be expecting social distance.

This shared field of assumptions then leads to a disruption in confidence to engage in both parties and a self-fulfilling prophecy ensues – the patient keeps their distance and the non-patient expects and lets this occur. Subsequently, this creates social disability and isolation in the patient. Thus, this modified labelling theory is not about the unidirectional impact of the prejudicial actions of one party on another but an interaction that creates social rejection, based upon shared acculturated assumptions.

The modified labelling theory of Link and colleagues is also supported by the work of Thoits (1985), who drew upon studies in the sociology of emotions (Hochschild 1979), which emphasizes shared internal assumptions, rather than social reaction *per se*. Thoits noted that labelling theory was preoccupied with involuntary relationships (as was much of this tradition including that of Goffman (1961)), whereas we know that most consultations for mental health problems occur voluntarily, mainly in primary care services. Thoits's view is that we learn from a young age to self-monitor emotional deviance. For example, we begin to learn when it is appropriate to be happy, angry, sad or fearful. Consequently, we also can identify in ourselves when our emotionally driven actions will be considered inappropriate by others.

Thoits, following Hochschild, describes this as people being aware that they are transgressing 'feeling rules'. For example, the phobic patient knows that their fear is irrational but they also feel as though their actions are not in their control. The depressed adult knows that their low mood and lack of confidence disables them from carrying out normal family and work obligations expected of them, and this knowledge may fuel their depression further.

The implication from the work of Thoits, Link and colleagues that labelling is incorporated into a negative view of self has been challenged by some. For example, Camp *et al.* (2002) studied women with chronic mental health problems and found that such a negative acceptance of stigma is 'neither straightforward nor inevitable'. However, confirming the view of Thoits, the respondents were aware of their symptoms and their social implications. Badesha and Horley (2000) also found that positive and negative views about psychiatric diagnosis varied between patients. Of these different groups, women with a diagnosis of schizophrenia had the most negative view of themselves. By contrast, another study by Wright *et al.* (2000) found a more consistent internalization of negative views from others in psychiatric patients. In the group studied, the stress of chronic social rejection was a key feature in their biographical accounts.

Thus the notion of 'feeling rules' is a useful conceptual adjunct to that of the meta-rule of intelligibility, discussed earlier in relation to madness. Those breaking 'feeling rules' may well be capable of complying with the meta-rule of intelligibility, but they still receive a psychiatric diagnosis; indeed, the latter may be negotiated with their full co-operation, once they have self-labelled their rule breaking or role failure. The diagnosis is a professional codification of the person's own view that they have transgressed a 'feeling rule', just as one of 'schizophrenia' reflects the lay judgement of others that the patient has acted unintelligibly. What all patients then have in common is that they accept that others now will harbour changed expectations about rights of citizenship, personal credibility and social distance.

Once a person has lost their reason or fails to act competently as an adult in situation-specific ways, and others know this, then he or she may well be held in permanent suspicion. For this reason, people with a psychiatric diagnosis are ambivalent about disclosing their problems to others, though once this step is taken some benefits (such as increased self-esteem) as well as costs (such as more prejudicial responses from others) may accrue. These mixed outcomes suggest that any ambivalence from a patient about 'coming out' is reasonably warranted (Corrigan and Mathews

2003). In the section on social exclusion we will extend this discussion of the social consequences of stigmatization and discrimination.

The role of the mass media

Studies of media representations of mental illness have recorded consistent findings about negative images. There has been a recurring emphasis within these media portrayals upon psychosis and its assumed link to violence. This negative image seems to have a transglobal consistency. A focus on violence and madness can be found in the mass media of the USA (Sieff 2003), Canada (Day and Page 1986), Germany (Angermeyer and Schulze 2001), New Zealand (Nairn *et al.* 2001) and Britain (Philo *et al.* 1996; Rose 1998). The style (e.g. dramatic camera work) or mood (e.g. menacing music) in radio and TV accounts of mental illness shape fear in the audience and exaggerate the violent propensity of patients (Wilson *et al.* 1999). Olstead (2002) provides a content analysis of two Canadian newspapers over a 10-year period and their depiction of mental illness and violence. He notes that the journalistic strategy throughout was to depict the 'otherness' of mentally ill people. (We endorse this analytical point in the discussion of race at the end of Chapter 4.)

The link portrayed between mental illness and violence is all the more significant because of the lack of empirical evidence that mental state is a good predictor of dangerousness. Moreover, it is common to find stories and headlines which would not be tolerated about other minority social groups. Even when non-psychotic patients are described, these do not accurately match the symptom profile of patients with the diagnosis. For example, Wahl (2000) examined media depictions of obsessive-compulsive disorder and found that less than one-third concurred with psychiatric descriptions.

Wahl (1995) emphasizes that accuracy of information is relevant because the mass media are the most common source of understanding for the general public about mental illness. It can be noted though that the notion of 'accuracy of information' is problematic, given that psychiatric knowledge is contested. It may be more valid to simply record that media depictions do not always concur with psychiatric ones. Sieff (2003) has noted that the mass media may now be lagging behind the general public. The latter are more likely to have a broader and more subtle view about types of mental health problem than the mass media they encounter.

Less attention has been given by the newsprint media to depression than other diagnoses, but a content analysis of the Australian press in 1 year (2000) (Rowe *et al.* 2003) revealed three discourses (the bio-medical, the psycho-social and the administrative/managerial). A consistent message was the need for protection of these patients (rather than the protection of others) and depression as individual pathology. Apart from violence, the other negative image found in the mass media is that of pathetic dependency or silliness (Corrigan 1998). Patients may be depicted as being naïvely cheerful, childlike and quirky, leading to their social incompetence. Their assumed immaturity and social incompetence readily becomes the butt of humour. For example, people with mental health problems form easy targets for TV programmes, such as *Frasier* and the *Bob Newhart Show* (Sieff 2003).

This point can also be found in cartoon depictions and even in advertising, where the notion of 'nuts' is used to make a moral or humorous point about human failings (Wahl 1995). Cinematic portrayals of mental health problems have also been dominated by negative imagery, but Sieff (2003) points to some counter-examples recently, where films have been more sensitive about the seriousness of the patient's distress or have emphasized positive human attributes (e.g. the Oscar-winning *A Beautiful Mind*). Wahl (1995) historically analysed cinematic depictions of mental illness and found that these more sensitive and less stigmatizing portrayals have increased since the mid-1980s. Recently the question of the morality of the drug companies, the psychiatric profession and patients themselves has been explored in the film *Side Effects* (2013), reminding us that stigma and social rejection are entwined with other ethical considerations in our field of inquiry.

The literature summarized here suggests two processes in tension. The first is a self-reinforcing tradition of negative framing of mental health problems. Journalists and story-tellers play upon existing public prejudices (to entertain or to create a dramatic effect). They also use their own tried and tested frames of analysis and depiction from past stories. This first process is therefore a conservative vicious circle, with the assumed link between mental illness being rehearsed and reinforced by new events or storylines. The second process is about changing to more accurate and sensitive narratives or reporting. The depth of the inertia about negative media imagery is emphasized by the study of children's media. The latter provide negative stereotypes which both anticipate and reinforce adult media representations (Wahl 2000). And yet, some shifts into more balanced or sensitive reporting and narratives have occurred. Sieff (2003) suggests that sociological research in this area should concentrate on the cognitive sets of media producers in order to identify how these two processes in tension arise and are resolved.

Social exclusion and discrimination

Earlier we examined stereotyping and stigma. The literature about these has tended to focus on the personal and interpersonal aspects of creating a depersonalized and 'spoiled' identity. This emphasis has been criticized for being reductionist (reducing the field of inquiry to that of the characteristics and plight of the stigmatized individual). Critics have shifted the focus of attention away from those with a psychiatric diagnosis and towards the collective discriminatory response of others. This alters the field of sociological inquiry from the concept of stigma to that of social exclusion. Efforts to utilize an equivalent of 'racism' or 'sexism', such as 'sanism' or 'mentalism' have not been very successful (Sayce 2000), suggesting a failure of the required internal cognitive shift in individuals who constitute the 'sane' majority (whom psychiatric survivors sometimes call 'normies').

The fear and distrust of madness historically is deeply ingrained. Also, modern societies place a high value on rationality and so demonstrable irrationality may be used as a warranted basis for social rejection and invalidation. In most modern liberal democracies, racism and sexism are not seen as either rational or fair grounds for the distrust and dismissal of others, and a universal human rights framework is conceded by a majority of people about race and gender. This assumes that black people and women should have the same rights as white people and men. This can be contrasted with the fact that loss of reason is retained as an undeclared societal judgement for not allotting equal rights to the group we are discussing. If this conclusion is correct, then it would imply that psychiatric patients are still not viewed as deserving equal civil rights by most people in society. A universal corroborating factor supporting this interpretation is that some form of 'mental health' law exists in most societies, which permits the involuntary detention and coercive treatment of people who have committed no crime. This common legal feature points to a widespread legitimation (from voters and politicians) of the discriminatory treatment of people with mental health problems.

Sayce (2000) points out that although the frame of individual stereotyping needs to be widened to look at collective responses, the cognitive features of the latter are still an important starting point to understand a range of stances in society about the social inclusion or exclusion of people with mental health problems. She notes that different interest groups manifest different assumptions about three inter-related aspects of discrimination towards people with mental health problems:

- the nature of mental health problems;
- the causes of mental health problems;
- what should be done about discrimination.

If a psychiatrist or the relative of a patient considers that the latter is suffering from a genetically caused disturbance of brain biochemistry, then they will argue that discrimination will be reduced by campaigning for us all to accept mental illness to be like any other illness. Moreover, they would also demand more research into the (putative) genetic causes of mental illness, now framed as a brain disease, in order to reduce the prevalence of future 'sufferers'. The latter term is common within this approach because patients are seen as diseased victims of biological misfortune (being born with the wrong genes). By contrast, a service user who argues that psychological difference is caused by a variety of oppressive factors will argue for social change and the right to full citizenship and so the reduction or abolition of compulsory psychiatric treatment.

The first position about mental illness being a brain disease was taken up as an active campaign in the wake of 'anti-psychiatry' being accused of blaming parents for their children's madness. During the 1990s in the USA the National Alliance for the Mentally Ill led a campaign with a title that captures their assumptions about causation and anti-discrimination: 'Open your minds: mental illnesses are brain diseases'. The second position is more prevalent in critiques from disaffected patients (see Chapter 12).

There are overlaps between these contrasting positions about antidiscrimination (for example both argue for a greater public acceptance of people with a psychiatric diagnosis). However, apart from different assumptions operating about causality, there are also differences about the social policy demands. The relative lack of beds and inpatient treatment facilities have been pointed up by those committed to a bio-deterministic model of madness as evidence that 'sufferers' of 'schizophrenia' are being discriminated against by health services. This is the opposite of the demands of those focusing on citizenship, who want to minimize hospitalization and maximize community support and social inclusion. The latter refers to equal access to ordinary opportunities to work, housing and leisure facilities.

Thus the way in which mental health problems are represented shapes social policy preferences. For example, a biological view of depression might lead to an educational campaign to encourage patients to seek antidepressant treatment. For this reason the drug companies in some of their marketing strategies depict depression in a matter-of-fact way as a biological illness. Social inclusion in this context would be limited to an equal right to medical treatment. By contrast, an environmental aetiological view would lead to calls for reductions in social stressors (like poverty, work stress and so on) (Goldstein and Rosselli 2003). Social inclusion in this context would be about people with mental health problems having access to benign and supportive living environments and to satisfying work roles.

The representations of different diagnostic groups by others can also affect degrees of treatment equity within mental health services. For example, mental health workers tend to be paternalistic towards psychotic patients but distrusting and rejecting of those with a diagnosis of personality disorder (Markham 2003). Both are stigmatized groups but different attributions about personal 'fault' from professionals lead to differential levels of personal acceptance and support.

The micro-sociological emphasis upon labelling and prejudicial action perspective limits the debate about stigma and social disadvantage to empirical considerations about one-to-one interactions or the immediate social obligations of a social actor in a group of people directly around them (see earlier). The shift of emphasis by Sayce regarding the collective impact of acculturated assumptions about mental illness allows us to examine a different set of questions, which may be easier to answer. This is similar to the analytical advantage of shifting from a study of racial prejudice or the racism of an individual to that of studying institutional racism. Whether or not individuals reacted negatively to mental illness and whether or not those with the latter label feel rejected by this reaction, we can ask:

- What is their experience of life?
- What evidence is there about their role in the labour market?
- To what extent are psychiatric patients allowed to enjoy full citizenship?

With regard to the life experience of psychiatric patients, their principle concerns are in relation to various aspects of their social status (Rogers *et al.* 1993). They focus on oppressive and discriminatory features of community living, including poor physical health care, little informed choice about treatment, loss of employment, inability to return to paid work, poor community support services and poverty. The evidence on labour market disadvantage is unambiguous: patients with a diagnosis of psychosis have only a one in four chance of being employed; people with mental health problems are nearly three times as likely as physically disabled people to be unemployed (Labour Force Survey 1997–8). Moreover, being employed reduces the chances of relapse in psychotic patients (Warner 1985).

Although there is clear evidence that people with mental health problems suffer labour market disadvantage, for some problems cause and effect are ambiguous. For example, depression and anxiety may disable a person from coping at work but stress at work is an increasingly commonly cited cause of depression (Rogers and Pilgrim 2003). Evidence of a diverse range of discriminatory processes other than labour market disadvantage is also evident.

People with mental health problems are the target in most societies of a dedicated legal framework to remove their liberty without trial and to permit involuntary interference with their bodies and solitary confinement. This humiliating and degrading experience may be compounded by vulnerability to sexual assault during periods of detention of female patients. Mental patients have more limited social networks than others and these are more likely to be confined to those of mental health professionals and other patients (Pescosolido and Wright 2004). They are also more likely to be poor and housed in stressful, socially disorganized neighbourhoods. It is this cumulative list that demonstrates unequivocally that a person with a mental health problem experiences multiple disadvantages, which culminates recurrently in their social exclusion. The evidence discussed by those either supporting or criticizing labelling theory can be contrasted with this unambiguous picture of institutional discrimination against people with mental health problems.

Social capital, social disability and social exclusion

Social capital is often used in the social science literature to refer to social participation in the activities of the formal and informal networks of civil society and/or as generalized trust. Social participation and trust are two aspects of social capital that mutually affect each other. In this regard, as we have seen earlier, mental health users tend to have different ties as a result of their contact with services. Their social class position and marginalization in local communities mean that they are unlikely to have the advantages of 'weak ties' (Granovetter 1973).

'Strong ties' refer to kinship and peer group contacts. These are small in number and, although strong, generally have little instrumental value to the individual. 'Weak ties' refer to personal connections which are personally superficial but may be instrumentally powerful. For example, they might create employment opportunities and career progression. They may also create a general sense of safe civility and neighbourliness in a locality. Strong ties cannot easily serve larger community purposes, whereas weak ties can. For this reason Granovetter refers to the 'strength of weak ties'. This point applies to psychiatric patients in the community in particular because they are often both poor and socially avoided by non-patients. Indeed, psychiatric patients may, as a result of their primary psychological disability and the avoidance of others, lack both strong and weak ties.

Thus, while the concept of social capital has gained much popularity (particularly in social policy reforms), the distinction between weak and strong ties is important in order to place it in context. Those with multiple weak ties (i.e. those already financially and psychologically robust in a community), may be the very people who find it easier to contribute to, and gain from, social capital in a locality.

Sociologists of deviance introduced relevant concepts such as primary and secondary deviance in drawing attention to the social processes which lead to the creation of stigmatized identities. A criticism of labelling theory from those such as Walter Gove was that it was overly focused on secondary deviance (or 'deviance amplification') and that it denied the positive value of labelling. 'Disability' refers to the disadvantage and restriction of activity of people with impairments created by contemporary forms of social organization. Social disability theory traces the oppressive consequences of these restrictive and excluding forms of organization. A similar criticism to that about secondary deviance from Gove could also be levelled at the social model of disability because impairment (primary deviance) is downplayed. Nonetheless, it is a model which is popular with disabled people themselves, whether they are activists or academics (Barnes and Mercer 2004). It has also found some favour with mental health service users (Beresford 2005) and within academic analyses of the relationship between a psychiatric diagnosis and oppressive experiences (Mulvany 2000).

Stigma-sensitive management of mental health problems

Recent concerns regarding the persistence of negative attitudes to those with mental health problems have led to a range of new policy initiatives to combat stigma. Generously funded scientific evaluations of targeted campaigns concerned with changing knowledge about stigma as well as attitudes and behaviour seemingly fail in the same way that previous sociologically informed attempts to change the general orientation of the public did in the 1950s (Cumming and Cumming 1957). The effectiveness of anti-stigma campaigns, which have been scientifically evaluated, is evident in relation to the British 'Time to Change' initiative. The findings were in some respects disappointing for policy advocates: 'Some parameters showed a positive change, such as a small reduction in discrimination reported by service users and improved employer recognition of common mental health problems', implying a poor fit between well-intentioned efforts and ingrained rejection and intolerance (Smith 2013: 50). However, others (Corker et al. 2013) argue that a reduction in discrimination ratings by users of over 11 % in four years is 'remarkable', despite contrary evidence of experiences of discrimination being "extremely common".

The limited efficacy of these campaigns may relate to over-optimism in campaigns about the reversal of public ignorance. It is clear from wide-ranging evidence that information alone does not result in large changes of behaviour in most long-term conditions. Consequently, it is not likely to result in changes to stigma (Protheroe et al. 2009).

Psychiatric mental health professionals and the perpetuation of stigma

At times mental health professionals have proposed anti-stigma activities. But as Schulze (2007) points out they can simultaneously be stigmatizers, stigma recipients and powerful agents of de-stigmatization. What has been termed 'associative' stigma (stigma generated by association with a target group, in this case patients, in a defined work place (mental health settings)) perpetuated by mental health professionals towards users is related to the aspects of the role of being a mental health worker which include depersonalization, emotional exhaustion and low job satisfaction (Verhaeghe and Bracke 2012) The authors found that this leads to a vicious circle. Once workers are affected detrimentally by associative stigma, these aspects of 'burn out' can lead to them viewing their clients cynically, compounding their rejection and stigmatization. This 'pathological' version of professional action is different, though, from the routine and normal role of psychiatric theory and practice. Earlier we noted the routine and lawful labelling and control of people with mental health problems, and we turn to it again now. Psychiatrists (and in Britain specifically the Royal College of Psychiatrists) have shown an increasing interest in tackling stigma through media campaigns and, more generally, incorporating this as a part of their identity and work. While promoting a more inclusive and less discriminatory policy, these professional activities can be put in a wider sociological context. For example, stigma has been linked to a critique of the profession and has been discussed as a social phenomenon in sociology, whereas psychiatric authority is derived from its clinical knowledge claims.

In an examination of a major campaign endorsed and promoted by the Royal College of Psychiatrists, Pilgrim and Rogers (2005) noted that stigma has conveniently been 'carved at the same reified joints' as the diagnoses used by the profession. In that campaign, the College avoided a discussion of stigma as a wider social process and instead concentrated on the ways it was allegedly applied to one type of diagnosis and not another – they started at the other end of the telescope (the clinical domain, not society). Thus clinical categories (like 'schizophrenia') were the starting point, not stigma itself. Also, this campaign avoided any discussion of the contribution psychiatric diagnosis itself makes to the stigmatization of people receiving diagnostic labels (Royal College of Psychiatrists 1995). Campaigns like this, however well intentioned, are bound up with a re-professionalization strategy.

However, the role of psychiatry, in being part of the problem rather than the solution of stigma, is now being discussed within the public discourse about treatment and management in mental health services. A new emphasis on recovery and therapeutic optimism is now a counter-current to the criticism that psychiatric diagnosis and treatment are actually part of the problem of stigma. A more positive expectation that services should now play a role in engendering social inclusion runs counter to that traditional stigmatizing association of contact with mental health services. It is now evident in two main ways. First, lay management strategies of dealing with mental health problems have been given a higher priority than previously in mental health promotion and relapse (or 'tertiary') prevention. These include both proactive and reactive lay action, self-reliance, cognitive strategies (taking up a particular coping stance to everyday events) and stress-reducing activities, such as sport or regular exercise.

Second, there are new efforts by services to actively manage or 'treat' social exclusion and marginalization, which as we have seen above are tightly aligned with the impact of stigma. A focus on tackling poverty and deprivation, over-crowding and unemployment have become more visible in mental health policy. Delivering access to mainstream opportunities is seen as important in order to encourage 'hope, ambition and recovery'. Communities that substitute stigmatizing attitudes and discriminatory behaviours with reasonable housing arrangements and a 'realistic' view of mental health problems are prominent expectations in policies to reverse stigma and increase the chances of recovery. They focus on facilitating the employment and independent living opportunities of people with mental health problems. Such aspirations reflect the long-term ambitions from the WHO for the promotion of mental health and well-being. For example, the WHO proposed that: 'By the year 2000, people should have the basic opportunity to develop and use their health potential to live socially and economically fulfilling lives' (WHO 1986).

A focus on ordinary living, using housing arrangements as a springboard, in line with that aspiration of the WHO, can be found in the US initiative to promote recovery from mental health problems. 'Housing First' developed by Pathways to Housing, Inc. in New York City treats housing needs separately from any treatment expectations and provides independent housing to individuals regardless of their co-operation with treatment services (Padgett *et al.* 2006). The initiative includes service users in its governance arrangements and provides permanent housing. Tenancy rights and obligations are offered which are equivalent to any other housing arrangement. This model is explicitly recovery-oriented. We now turn more generally to this topic.

Recovery

The notion of recovery has become commonplace in recent discussions of mental health problems, though its precise definition and ownership are contested. It has been described as a 'polyvalent concept' (Pilgrim 2008b) and a 'working misunderstanding' (Hopper 2007). The latter author makes the point that the different meanings attached to it, by different (and within) communities of interest, enables a pragmatic form of politics to emerge, even if the parties 'at the table' are seeking different processes and outcomes at times.

A common starting point was the claim from within psychiatric rehabilitation that recovery was to be the 'guiding vision' for improving mental health services in the 1990s:

> Recovery is a deeply personal, unique process of changing one's attitudes, values, feelings, goals, skills, and/or roles. It is a way of living a satisfying, hopeful, and contributing life even with limitations caused by illness. Recovery involves the development of new meaning and purpose in one's life as one grows beyond the catastrophic effects of mental illness.
>
> (Anthony 1993: 527)

Pilgrim and McCranie (2013) note four discursive trends since then about recovery: a personal journey, critique of services, therapeutic optimism and a social model of disability. The first predominates in the literature because it is benign and readily agreed by all parties. It reflects the initial assertion from Anthony above and is endorsed particularly by service user researchers (Faulkner and Layzell 2000; Wallcraft *et al.* 2003). It should be noted though that some service users are suspicious of the recovery concept because it is potentially intolerant of those who do not change and so may remain, in their eyes, a source of oppression (Pilgrim and McCranie 2013).

The critique of the services approach to recovery reflects demands for benign alternatives to orthodox psychiatric care (Deegan 1996). This can be traced to some aspects of the service user opposition movement, which emphasized the replacement of offensive service models that were coercive and medication focused. It arose in other words from distressing experiences within services.

Therapeutic optimism was reflected in the range of professional initiatives associated with social psychiatry after the 1960s. Since then, professionally driven versions of therapeutic optimism can be found in Mosher's Soteria project (Spandler and Calton 2009) and in the Hearing Voices Network (Romme *et al.* 1992). Positive views about the helpful potential of service contact can be found now in recovery advocates in both psychiatry and clinical psychology.

The social disability model of recovery remains the most problematic. Attempts to transfer that model from physical disability to mental health problems have proved to be unpopular from both groups. Some physically disabled groups prefer not to be associated with those with mental health problems, and vice versa (Mulvany 2000; Beresford 2003).

The socio-ethical position of each group is different. Those with physical disabilities have complained that their expressed needs about social inclusion have been ignored and so they have demanded enabling changes from a society (i.e. the personal acceptance of abilities and investments in enabling environmental adaptations). However, it is not easy to identify precisely what a psychologically enabling society would look like, other than its demonstrating greater tolerance and compassion, than at present, about psychological difference or diversity (Pilgrim *et al.* 2011). Also, whereas people with physical disabilities were largely ignored in policy developments (the 'disability movement' arose in large part because of that neglect), those with mental health problems have been the persistent and careful focus of policy-makers, from the days of Victorian lunacy legislation to the present. People with mental health problems are far from ignored; they are under the recurrent scrutiny of professionals, and a whole legal apparatus exists to regulate their rule transgressions and role failures.

Discussion

This chapter has explored the ways in which people with mental health problems are understood, depicted and reacted to by others. With the loss of popularity of labelling theory in the 1970s, this type of sociological interest diminished. New frameworks incorporating broader elements of social structure have emerged recently. Scambler (2009) suggests that stigma reduction activities need to take into account a re-framing of notions of the relations of stigma which incorporates the changing dynamics between cultural norms of shame and blame. These dynamics are embedded in social structures of class, gender and ethnicity. Pescosolido *et al.* (2008) suggest, following Goffman, that several societal levels need to be understood concomitantly about stigma. The latter involves inner feelings, social psychological events and public settings. The latter are embedded in contexts influenced by media depictions and other social processes which shape particular cultural expectations about deviance. Thus multiple theorizing may be required to understand the various aspects of stigma (labelling theory, social network theory, the social psychology of prejudice and discrimination, and theories of the welfare state).

Thus, summing up this chapter, sociological debate about the role of lay views of mental health problems and their links to prejudicial action has now been revitalized in a number of ways linked to a broad and complex set of social processes:

- First, there has been a successful reassertion of the labelling theory approach (especially that associated with Bruce Link and his colleagues). This encourages us to revisit the work on stigma and mental health started by Erving Goffman in the 1950s and 1960s. Moreover, the tension with the competing body of knowledge created by Walter Gove and his colleagues, which emphasizes primary psychiatric disability, rather than social reactions to it, is useful to explore. Those who emphasize primary deviance (the patient is deemed to fail socially because they are mentally ill) will see labelling, especially that done diagnostically by professionals, as being positive not negative, as it warrants access to care and treatment. Labelling can be framed as a human right which gives the labelled person access to restorative interventions provided by others. By contrast, those who emphasize deviance amplification arising from labelling will view psychiatric diagnosis as a potential social disadvantage to its targets.

- Second, the role of the mass media in responding to, and reinforcing, public prejudices has now been well researched and has exposed important social processes, which maintain prejudice and stigma. A sociological research programme around media depictions and the thought processes of writers and journalists has been established.

- Third, it is now clear that there is no firm epistemological starting point about the nature of mental health problems and so any sociological inquiry must examine the ways in which different social groups depict this nature. Stigma and discrimination allow one way into this inquiry, because they encourage us to examine the interests being expressed by this rather than that way of depicting mental health problems. The study of social representations of mental health and illness then becomes an important area of sociological inquiry in its own right.

- Fourth, it may be that an individualistic focus on stigma is a necessary but not a sufficient way of understanding collective discrimination. Even if labelling theory in its modified or original form were proved to be empirically unfounded, what is not in doubt is the evidence about social disadvantage. The evidence about the social exclusion of people with mental health problems is unambiguous. They are more likely to live in poor localities and suffer the ecological consequences of this vulnerability. They encounter labour market disadvantage. They die early. They are shunned by others. They are detained without trial. This list (some of which we explore further in other chapters) provides a wide range of topics for sociological inquiry. Moreover, an emphasis on social exclusion can accept either of the positions described in the first point above, about the tension in emphasis between primary and secondary deviance. An emphasis on social exclusion is concerned less with the sources or causes of mental illness or residual deviance and more with the politics of discrimination and the constraints upon citizenship imposed upon people with a psychiatric diagnosis.

Questions

1 What are the similarities and differences between Scheff's original application of labelling theory to mental health problems and Link's modified labelling theory?
2 What contribution did Erving Goffman make to our understanding of mental abnormality?
3 Does labelling affect the lives of people with mental health problems?
4 What evidence is there that those with a diagnosis of mental illness are unintelligible?
5 How does an emphasis on social exclusion differ from one on stigmatization?
6 Can a social model of disability be applied to people with mental health problems?

For discussion

Stigma strikes like the Lernaean hydra of myth, a multi-headed serpent capable of attack and injury from many directions. Stigma robs people with mental illness of rightful opportunities in work, education, housing and healthcare

(Corrigan 2012: 7–8)

Consider the various ways in which people with mental health problems are affected by the individual and collective reactions of others.

12　Users of mental health services

Chapter overview

This chapter will explore the different ways in which those who are the recipients of mental health services can be understood sociologically. These are not merely different perspectives; they reflect the changing role of psychiatric patients in mental health services and in wider social life. A shift over a 30-year period, from patient to provider, highlights this point. As Speed (2006: 28) notes, 'notions of patients, consumers and survivors have entered the service users' discursive canon and they are actively utilized by service users to socially construct their perspectives on mental health.' The wider social and cultural influence of users, within and beyond health service provision, is also explored, particularly in relation to the (contested) formation of the mental health users' movement and its social impact.

The following topics will be discussed after the role of users' views in research is outlined:

- the diffuse concept of service use;
- the relatives or 'significant others' of psychiatric patients;
- users as patients;
- users as consumers;
- users as survivors;
- users as providers.

Users' views as evidence and user participation in service research

Work on users' experience of mental health services, with its roots in symbolic interactionism, has considered the experience of users to be worthwhile in its own right. This has been incorporated, to some extent, into a health outcomes approach to policy development, as has been pointed out by Godfrey and Wistow (1997).

In policy terms, great importance has been put on user-focused and evidence-based assessments and measurements of health outcomes. In a policy approach to audit and research, the accounts of users get transformed from narratives situated in their biographical context to a set of potential outcomes with which to measure the success, or otherwise, of a service. A more holistic approach to outcomes addresses users' perspectives, which consider the entire course and experience of mental illness – in other words, the meanings to users and significant others of 'becoming' and 'being ill'.

The utility of a more holistic approach to outcome work was confirmed by Felton and colleagues (1995). Their study examined whether employing mental health consumers as peer specialists in an intensive case-management programme could enhance outcomes for clients with a diagnosis of serious mental illness. They found that clients served by mental health teams with peer specialists demonstrated greater gains in several areas of quality of life and in an overall reduction in the number of major life problems experienced and reported. They also reported more frequent contact with their case managers, and the largest gains of all three groups in the areas of self-image and outlook and social support. Other research has illuminated the beneficial use of user perspectives, when informing future clinical governance strategies. For example, clinical practice guidelines now consider how to harness what users are already doing to manage risk, because they cannot always rely on staff to do this for them, particularly in volatile environments such as acute psychiatric wards. A set of identified contextual risks, which users manage, were found to include avoiding risky situations or individuals, seeking protection from staff, and seeking premature discharge.

Research funders have increasingly demanded evidence of user involvement as a prerequisite of a successful bid in health services research. The relatively advanced politicization and organization of users in this field of interest (see below) has meant that research into mental health users is more advanced than that into other health user groups. This can be seen in the institutional embeddedness of mental health user research. For example, the setting up of dedicated service user research units, such as the Service User Research Enterprise (SURE) as part of the Institute of Psychiatry in London, indicates the success of getting recognition for user-focused priorities. The aim of routinely involving users in research is premised on an ethos of collaboration. The latter should apply to every aspect of the process of research, from design to dissemination.

The introduction of user research has brought with it new considerations about ethical practice. For example, it has been suggested that a focus of ethical practice should be to carry out research which addresses and counteracts the stigma experienced by users (Faulkner 2004). Thus, by placing demands for adopting an emancipatory and value-full (rather than value-free) approach to research, this now reinforces the view that the perspectives of service users differ from mental health service workers and from those who have a purely academic interest in the field, and requires recognition.

Finally in this section, we can note that user-led research on service contact has been central to the development of recovery-orientated service development. We discussed this point more in Chapter 11. We now turn to the conceptual challenges surrounding the term 'users of mental health services'.

The diffuse concept of service use

The term 'user' of mental health services has generally been accepted. In the past, the term has been eschewed in the USA because of its narrow connotation of drug misuse. There, user groups tend to prefer the term 'patient', 'ex-patient' or 'survivor'. The last of these is also preferred sometimes in the UK, when some service recipients object to the term 'user'. Policy-makers and service managers in the USA and Australia tend to favour the term 'consumer' but that term implies voluntarism and choice, which is compromised at times. Legal powers of compulsion, enacted or threatened, inevitably affect service styles and weaken the true connotation of the word 'choice'.

Notwithstanding these problems with the notion of 'consumer', it is also true that the simple term 'service user' is far from self-evident in its meaning. Social groups, other than designated patients, benefit from the existence of mental health services. If many parties, including but not only 'identified patients', use mental health services then there are many parties that might reasonably be called 'service users'. Although currently the latter term is typically limited to patients, here we still need to clarify the conceptual ambiguity. Thus not only is the notion of 'user' rendered ambiguous, but so is the notion of 'service': a service to or for whom?

Mental health legislation has traditionally been split into two broad parts to permit the lawful coercive control of some but not all psychiatric patients: one concerns civil sections and the other, mentally disordered offenders. This separation implies, and at times spells out, that mental health services will serve a range of statutory and civil groups in wider society: the criminal justice system, social services, the immigration service, primary health care and relatives of people entering the psychiatric patient role. Even strangers in public places are served indirectly because the police can detain people reported to them who are thought to be mentally disordered. Commissioners of mental health services, purchasing the latter on behalf of local communities, can also be construed as 'users'. Commissioners attempt to ensure the quality of services. Providers of the latter are accountable to the former via institutional processes of 'clinical governance' (Gask *et al.* 2008). These examples highlight the diverse range of groups who in one sense or another 'use' mental health services.

Thus notions of 'user involvement' in service governance are now commonplace. This can be distinguished from service *utilization*, which is an individualized way in which users are involved in services. User involvement has largely been linked to statutory specialist services but this is virtually non-existent in primary care settings, where initiatives to offer psychological therapy emphasize ensured individual *access*. Thus individual user access and collective user governance arrangements are quite distinct in meaning and occur separately in the two service sectors. While more overt statutory powers shape the conditional access to services in secondary care inpatient services, there are also restrictions of a different sort operating in primary care. This type of involvement becomes more relevant as access is rationed according to contingencies and capacities. For example, according to Gask and colleagues (2012), access and utilization by users of primary care are contingent upon three distinct, but overlapping, domains:

- the world beyond primary care, the conditions that occur before service contact (e.g. candidacy, navigation, appearance);
- the interface with primary care, the processes by which services and those that use them are able to agree on appropriate access to care (categorization, adjudication and offer);
- the acceptability of interventions available in that setting and the likelihood that they will be attended, used and benefited from (receipt).

The variegated administrative arrangements and contingencies surrounding access and use indicate that many groups, other than identified patients, effectively constitute users of mental health services in practice. Some of these parties and relationships have been discussed in earlier chapters. Here we will focus on those close to psychiatric patients (as blood relatives or through emotional bonds) before considering patients themselves in the next section.

Relatives or 'significant others'

Whether or not psychiatric patients enter the role voluntarily or involuntarily, it is not unusual for their relatives (or 'significant others') to be interested parties with regard to service contact. Not only might they be involved in formal decision-making about hospital admission, they might have previously been involved in engendering, coping with, and eventually informally labelling the incipient patient's mental abnormality, prior to formal psychiatric diagnosis. As Coulter (1973) noted in his ethnomethodological account of psychiatric labelling, the latter begins in the lay arena. Also, once professional interventions are triggered, relatives may have service contact as visitors. Sometimes they act as advocates for patients (demanding improved services) and they certainly act as lay referrers (Owens *et al.* 2009). Sometimes they might express concern that services are *not* being coercive enough in ensuring treatment compliance or about the insufficient treatment or premature discharge of their relative.

The concept of the 'betrayal funnel', first put forward by Goffman (1961), suggested that psychiatric coercion was used as a solution for those immediately around mad people to resolve a shared social crisis. This implied some sort of conscious or unconscious alliance of professionals and relatives against the patient. The prospect of this oppressive collusion triggered an unresolved debate about whether a relative should be construed as a 'carer', always acting beneficently for the patient, or as a beneficiary of actions that might be against the patient's interest (or even a variable mixture from case to case). The ambiguity is made more acute when the impact on the mental health of 'carers' is taken into consideration. This has sometimes been conceptualized as 'burden'. However, it is clear that 'burden' and therefore the likelihood of a carer developing a mental health problem themselves is more likely in the presence of significant unmet needs of the 'patient' (Cleary *et al.* 2006).

Within some treatment rationales, relatives are framed by professionals as implicit or adjunct service clients (in part but not only as having mental health needs themselves), in order to engender change in the patient or minimize the chances of relapse in their condition. Because of wide-ranging powers of professional discretion within services, this imputed role is variegated and relatives may not always be informed of the assumptions operating about them in a particular service setting. A number of examples of this point can be given.

- *Family role in aetiology.* In the contested model of 'schizophrenia' being intelligible within mystifying and dysfunctional family communication patterns, some professionals sought to engage with relatives to render the patient's behaviour and experience intelligible or to trace causal antecedents. A critical review of this strand of therapeutic work is provided by Howells and Guirguis (1985). Longitudinal research on intra-familial adversity is now demonstrating that it does indeed increase the risk of symptom presentation in later life (Read *et al.* 2003; Varese *et al.* 2012) though it is linked more to adversity in early family life for the incipient patient than current family tensions (see below).
- *Family role in relapse.* A less controversial model relates to relapse. Here, professionals do not necessarily question either the validity of psychiatric diagnosis or the role of genetic factors in causality. Instead they argue that relatives who are intrusive and emotionally labile (high on 'expressed emotion') place stress upon mentally ill people, which increases the probability of *relapse* in those diagnosed as depressed or schizophrenic. Within this model, relatives may be contacted in a process of 'psycho-education' in order to reduce levels of 'expressed emotion' during their contact with the identified patient. This work is summarized by Jenkins and Karno (1992). It has been critiqued by Johnstone (1993).
- *Relatives as risk assessors.* A paradoxical effect of the above two therapeutic approaches is that they may have changed professional norms about the credibility and involvement of family members. However, involving families by asking their views about risk in their relative-patient increases the accuracy of risk assessment and efficiency of risk management (Klassen and O'Connor 1987). This reflects the philosophical shift towards an actuarial approach in services (see Chapter 10). It also highlights that risk rather than assumptions about diagnosis or aetiology drives service decisions.
- *Relatives as perpetrators and victims of abuse.* Leaving aside the particular controversy noted above about family aetiology in 'schizophrenia', the families of people with a psychiatric diagnosis may be sites of victimization. In Chapter 5 we discussed the raised levels of diagnosis in survivors of childhood sexual abuse. The 'schizophrenia' literature may be contested about causal antecedents, but the long-term post-traumatic effects of childhood abuse are clear. In the other direction, some relatives may at times become the victims of violence at the hands of children who are psychiatric patients (Estroff and Zimmer 1994). This highlights that families are sites of multi-directional risk.

Over and above these variable professional assumptions operating about the antecedent and current role of relatives for psychiatric patients, family members have also become an important self-organizing lobby. For example, they have been highly influential in the 'third sector' developments of mental health charities in Britain.

In Britain the amalgam phrase of 'users and carers' has been common in the discourse of mental health service management and government policy forming part of the National Service Framework for Mental Health produced by the Department of Health in 1999. Such an amalgam phrase, preferred for now by politicians and services managers, could be misleading to students in the field, because it lumps together social groups with potentially different interests. In particular the assumptions about the word 'carer', and its conceptual and practical conflation with near blood relatives, need to be checked carefully in this field for a number of reasons.

- Relatives may or may not *subjectively* care for their patient relative; the notion of 'care-as-emotion' cannot be taken for granted in a family relationship. They may dislike the identified patient or they have even made a contribution to the development of their mental health problem.
- Relatives may or may not offer *practical* care – shelter, tangible support and domestic tending.
- *Patients themselves* may, when not in hospital, be the carer of their non-mentally ill relatives (e.g. their children or elderly parents).
- Sometimes those offering a caring role to someone who is mentally distressed are *not family members*. A natural experiment in whether or not users define a close family member as the person most likely to look after them is provided in the enactment of the Mental Health (Care and Treatment) Scotland Act 2003. The latter removed the role of the nearest relative, allowing service users to nominate instead a 'named person'. In research exploring who users nominated, it was found that service users often did not want to nominate their nearest relative, with many choosing to nominate a friend instead. Trust and the ability to carry out the service user's wishes were paramount in making a nomination (Berzins and Atkinson 2009). This suggests that those close to patients in their family system or social network vary in the confidence they inspire when someone has a mental health crisis.
- Relatives of patients may want to *preserve a different identity* as a partner, wife or husband and may not feel comfortable with the ascribed role of 'carer' (Forbat 2002; Forbat and Henderson 2003).

For these reasons, caution needs to be exercised, on logical grounds, about conflating the term 'carer' and 'relative', or assuming that the role of carer is accepted by those it is applied to. Despite this complexity, there is a literature which has used the term 'carer' simplistically to mean 'family relatives', who are assumed to clearly be acting in the interests of patients. For example, there is the review book of *Family Caregiving in Mental Illness* (Lefley 1996). The extensive literature it contains depicts relatives singularly as victims of 'care burden' created by (a presumed genetically caused) mental illness. Thus, not only is the logical problem of conflating 'family member' with 'care-giver' logically problematic, it can also obscure sociological and psychological complexity.

Another conceptual problem with this 'burden'-focused literature is the tendency to see mental illness as creating similar political demands for relatives and patients alike. As a consequence, the self-advocacy movements of patients and their relatives have not properly been separated for academic analysis. They are assumed to arise for similar reasons and to have the same interests (see for example, Watkins and Callicutt 1997).

Elsewhere (Rogers and Pilgrim 1996) we have argued that social scientists should avoid stereotypical assumptions about the role of family members. Sociologically we deciphered two dominant currents of professional discourse – one which tends to blame relatives for their aetiological role and the other which tends to sympathize with the martyrdom created by 'care burden'. It may be that relatives can be *both* victims of circumstance when, for example, struggling to cope with a disruptive and distressing son or daughter, *and* a causal source of distress when, for example, they abused an incipient patient in childhood. A whole range of other contingent styles of relating can exist between prospective and current patients and their relatives.

The stress of living with people who have severe mental health problems can itself lead to distress in relatives (see above). For this reason, it is not unusual for relatives to seek professional help for their own emotional difficulties and thus become patients themselves (Perring *et al.* 1990). It is little surprising that relatives, when asked, will express the need for services to support them as well as the primary identified patient. Within the mental health field, this image of the 'carer' is slowly changing, with some concessions to the arguments we raise here about complex and diverse scenarios, implicating patients and their intimate relationships.

For example, a survey of different stakeholders illuminated the value placed on different aspects of primary mental health care (Campbell *et al.* 2004). Overall, GPs rated a low number of practice-level indicators as valid (e.g. access, information, treatment effectiveness) while 'carers' rated the highest number valid. The reason for the differences in what was seen to count as high-quality mental health care is likely to be an expression of different interests. GPs are likely to want to restrict the demand placed on their services to manage mental health. The high number of items mentioned by carers is likely to be an expression of the extent to which needs associated with mental health, from their perspective are not being met.

Similarly, another study exploring the commitment to various models of mental disorder (psychotherapeutic, medical, social, cognitive, behavioural and so on) indicated that, compared to users and other practitioners, 'informal carers' were non-committal. A slight preference was shown for the medical and family models (Colombo *et al.* 2003).

Having discussed the wider notion of service use and looked at patients' relatives, we will now discuss the specific question of what services might describe as the 'identified patients' – people who formally enter the sick role voluntarily or against their will. We will examine the different ways in which the psychiatric patient's voice has been portrayed or conceptualized. We concentrate on four views of mental health service users, which reflect different discourses and interests:

* users as patients;
* users as consumers;
* users as survivors;
* users as providers.

Users as patients

One (still common) way in which users of psychiatric services have been portrayed is as objects of the clinical gaze of mental health professionals. This is clearly seen in the academic literature, which forms the basis of most psychiatric and psychological knowledge. In the former case, psychiatrists still place a high professional priority on 'getting the diagnosis right'; from the outset the emphasis is on a traditional doctor–patient role (Blackman 2010). The patient is ill and it is the doctor's responsibility to offer a clear diagnosis of what is wrong. This monologue of diagnostic power thus defines patienthood. Even in the case of clinical psychology, their professional research concerns reflect the same monologue of power. For example, the editorial policy of the *British Journal of Clinical Psychology* is to only publish studies of patient samples (Pilgrim 2008c). And although clinical psychology practitioners often argue for idiosyncratic, context-specific formulations, rather than de-contextualized diagnoses, this is not always the case. Many practitioners simply reproduce uncritically the use of medical categories used by their psychiatric colleagues (Pilgrim and Carey 2010).

Clinical research in the area of mental health has tended either to exclude the views of patients or to portray them as the passive objects of study (the example given above about clinical psychology research). Their individual characteristics and feelings are mostly variables to be 'controlled out' in order to ensure valid results. For example, up until fairly recently the Medical Research Council prioritized the funding of 'schizophrenia' research, with an emphasis on promoting genetic and biological studies. Evaluation of services to patients and user evaluation of services and treatment were given little mention. Explicitly or implicitly, 'mental patients' are still portrayed in a way which emphasizes their pathology. Here we mention four forms in which patients have traditionally been denied a valid viewpoint.

The disregarding by researchers of those users' views that do not coincide with the views of mental health professionals

In an early attempt at providing a genuine user perspective, Mills (1962) found some interesting results. The study, which mainly used the accounts of patients and their relatives, found that users of services preferred contact with non-professionals to contact with social and health services personnel. When the latter were 'from a different social class [they] were often received with hostility'. The greatest forms of support were regarded as coming from people such as the local publican, the secretary of the local darts club and home helps, who were seen to provide 'down to earth common sense'. However, a reviewer of this work appeared to dismiss this errant view of services on the grounds that it could not be cross-validated.

> It is hard to believe that there were no sympathetic and sensible social workers in the area . . . The material is taken very largely from patients and their relatives, and no attempt at validation appears to have been made. Since some of the patients were suffering from paranoia and others from depression, it would have been a basic precaution to check the objective value of statements with the medical records or the responsible psychiatrist.
>
> (Jones 1962: 343)

This criticism insists that patients' views are to be treated with inevitable suspicion and that a professional view inevitably carries a greater claim to validity or truth.

The notion that psychiatric patients are continually irrational and so incapable of giving a valid view

Discussions around informed consent, which are relevant to the administration of treatments and participation in research programmes, also tend to invalidate the views of users. 'Schizophrenics' are a particular group thought inherently incapable of giving genuine informed consent. This is not infrequently linked to the high rate of 'non-compliance' to prescribed medication:

> Since the majority of clients with schizophrenia deny their illness, special difficulties are encountered in the criteria for understanding the nature of the psychiatric condition . . . Denial is a major psychopathological mechanism which can impair appreciation.
>
> (Davidhazar and Wehlage 1984: 385)

Why those labelled as schizophrenic should 'deny' their 'illness' is left unexplored. There is an assumption that this is due to a lack of 'insight'. That is, patients fail to agree with the opinion of their treating psychiatrist, which in itself is viewed as a symptom of mental illness. In the example given, the diagnostic label of 'schizophrenia' is taken as a neutral one that can only be of benefit to patients.

Assumptions about the inability of patients to hold valid opinions are held by therapists of all kinds. This is summarized in a literature review of consumer satisfaction with mental health treatment by Lebow (1982: 254), who notes that therapists often suggest that the consumer cannot adequately judge the treatments they are given:

> Distortion is seen as inherent in consumer evaluation because of the client's intensity of involvement in treatment and impaired mental status, and the client is viewed as lacking the requisite experience to assess treatment adequately. Consumer satisfaction is regarded as

principally determined by transference projections, cognitive dissonance, unconscious processes, *folie à deux*, client character, and a naivety about treatment, rather than an informed decision process reflecting the adequacy of treatment.

Patients and relatives are assumed to share the same perspective, and where they do not, the views of the former are disregarded by researchers

Another tendency in clinical work that superficially gives credence to the consumer voice is the conflation of the patient's view with that of their relatives. This is evident in a study which set out to examine the impact of the Mental Health Act 1959 (Hoenig and Hamilton 1969). The authors of the study conclude that: 'On the whole, [therefore] the general picture given here is of a large degree of satisfaction on the part of patients and their relatives' (1969: 130). However, if one scrutinizes their results in detail, there are some important contradictions. While 84 per cent of the relatives' group was favourably disposed to the admission of the patient, only 47 per cent of the patients were content to be admitted, with 43 per cent being reluctant. Yet, the implication of these findings, which seem to suggest, on close reading, that the interests of these two groups may at times be divergent, was not noted by the researchers. Moreover, disquieting results were glossed over and excused by referring to patient pathology. For instance, complaints made by patients about services were dismissed thus: 'Their complaints referred to rough handling by nursing staff. It must be remembered that they were rather sick patients, and it was also not within our brief to verify individual complaints' (Hoenig and Hamilton 1969: 126).

Framing patient views in terms which suit professionals

Often, lay conceptions of mental health problems are researched in such a way that there is little room for people to express their own views about the subject in hand. One example, from a psychologist's perspective (Furnham 1984) involved a research design aimed at examining lay people's conceptions of 'neuroticism'. Leaving aside the problem of representativeness (the experimental group was 'a fairly homogeneous, young, well-educated sample'), such questionnaires leave little room for self-expression, since all the items are predetermined as standardized items by the researcher, with no open-ended questions.

Even where credence is given to the freely expressed views of patients, there is a tendency on the part of some researchers who are also mental health practitioners to adopt a 'victim-blaming' approach. This approach tends to leave practitioners' own role and that of their service unquestioned. One example of this is a study which found that clients attending a psychiatric day unit found it stigmatizing (Teasdale 1987). Patients preferred to 'hide' the reasons for attendance, because a label of 'mental illness' was experienced as being unhelpful. The analysis focused on the need for clients to be helped 'to arrive at unambiguous personal interpretations and management of the stigmatizing reaction of the local community' (Teasdale 1987: 345). It was suggested that this might be achieved 'if they [the patients] are supported in their attempts to understand and manage the resulting stigma, then the social and therapeutic effectiveness of the service should increase'. The professional's signal role in alleviating stigma was outlined as the 'need to encourage clients to be open about their fears and to help them demystify the idea of psychiatric care'.

A shift to incorporate users' perspectives

A recent shift in the credence given to users' perspectives about treatment and experience as patients is evident in the growing research not only about expressed needs but also about desirable outcomes. The latter is most evident in comparative research of constructs and aspects of care over which there is an 'on the face of things' consensus. For example, both patients and clinicians identify 'continuity of care' to be an aspect of good service quality. However, the meaning associated with this concept might be very different for users. Compared to professionals, who tend to focus on the continuity of aspects of *treatment*, service users place more emphasis on relational aspects of continuity. For example, patients complain of discontinuity (seeing different clinicians in subsequent consultations) and depersonalized care, as well as their social vulnerability and communication gaps. For patients the emphasis is not on 'treatment compliance' but on the personal supportive aspects experienced during service contact and the particular difficulties to be dealt with in their daily lives (Jones *et al.* 2009). We noted this in Chapter 11 in relation to expectations of 'recovery'.

Since the early 2000s there has been more opportunity for the priorities of users to be heard in services aspiring to be increasingly 'patient-centred' under policy directives from government and in relation to the consensus on a 'recovery-orientated' approach to care. This is has led to an emerging evidence base of user research about service quality. Research priorities identified by users differ from professionals. They want more user-defined research, research that is social or psychological rather than bio-medical in nature and a greater focus on alternative and complementary therapies (Rose *et al.* 2008).

Users as consumers

An alternative way of conceptualizing psychiatric patients is not as the objects of clinical interventions but as consumers of services. The term 'consumerism' implies the existence of choice between products, and an active insistence on value for money. Consumerism in one form or another has informed health policy-making in Britain since the beginning of the 1980s. It is often linked to the introduction of general management principles in the NHS, which tended, when it was first introduced, to modify the clinical view of services.

The administration of the health services by consensus decision-making among different clinical groups was replaced by the concentration of responsibility for services and management in the general manager. Part of this trend towards general management has involved what Offe (1984) has referred to as the 'commodification' of welfare services. This has introduced the logic of the wider economic system into the health service. An example of this is the tendering out of health service catering and laundry services (Pilgrim 2012).

Another example can be seen in government attempts to introduce an internal market for services by creating 'purchasers' and 'providers' of services, originally under the NHS and Community Care Act 1990 and then under subsequent legislation. One of the effects of this philosophy has been a growing acknowledgement of the importance of consumer satisfaction dating back to the late 1980s (DHSS 1988), the importance of the health service being accountable to the patient has been emphasized. The importance of consumer choice has continued to be stressed since then and to the present day in government consultative documents on primary care and community care.

Thus, there is now a clear acceptance within health policy circles that more credence and authority should be given to a user perspective. The expectation that consumer choice and opinion in health settings are valid (operationalized through national patient experience surveys) has itself generated a response, which indicates a more critical consumerist stance. For example, in the British NHS there is evidence of less tolerance for delays in responsiveness of services and the quality of some services (e.g. out-of-hours GP care). In the past, attention given to psychiatric patient views and levels of satisfaction with services tended to lag behind other client groups using health service facilities. This is likely to have been a result of the assumption that the accounts of psychiatric patients lacked credibility. However, this has changed, in no small part due to the impact of users' voices in the mental health field. Three UK examples are illustrative:

- The involvement of service users is now viewed as essential for high-quality services in the National Service Framework for Mental Health (Department of Health/Home

Office 1999) and for the contracting of community mental health services (Department of Health 2009).

- In 2003 there was the formation of the Commission for Patient and Public Involvement in Health, and all NHS trusts now have a duty to carry out a range of activities related to service user involvement, under section 11 of the Health and Social Care Act 2001.
- The National Institute of Mental Health for England has incorporated the agenda of users as 'experts by experience' and invited the input of user/survivor experience in a discussion forum. It was launched for people who use services to discuss the future of mental health services and other important issues in a safe, non-judgemental environment.

There are a number of difficulties associated with viewing patients as consumers. Although, since the 1980s, general management in the NHS has shaped up a market-influenced system, permitting consumer choice, the extent to which the health service has actually achieved this has been restricted by the 'clinical autonomy' exercised by the medical profession in treating patients. Britten (1991) showed that consultants who adhered to a bio-medical, rather than psycho-social, model of illness were less likely to agree with a proposed policy of patient access to their own records. Professionals sometimes claim that patients do not wish to know that they are ill.

There are also doubts about whether users of health services are currently in a position to make informed choices. Customers of health care do not have the same access to clinical knowledge as health care professionals, who have many years of training and experience on which to base their choices. Informed consent, in which the benefits and negative effects of treatment are made available to patients, has only recently been acknowledged as an area which needs attention. As we noted in Chapter 8, patients do not routinely have access to information about their treatment, whereas professionals do. In particular, there is the bias set up by professionals selectively withholding information which might alarm or demoralize the patient.

There are also objections to the notion of 'consumer' being used specifically in relation to psychiatric patients. 'Consumer' tends to denote a positive choice from a range of alternatives. As one user representative put it:

Consumer implies you are getting something of value. The majority of people in the users' movement do not feel that they have consumed anything of value and many say quite clearly that the real consumers of mental health services are relatives, the police and the state.

(cited in Rogers and Pilgrim 1991: 136)

Since this research, the British government has changed but the connotation of patients as consumers has been retained within health policy. Clearly, then, being a 'consumer' of health services is a complex affair. In order to understand the health care consumer's position, and in particular that of the psychiatric patient, we also require an analysis in terms of their relationship to market forces on the one hand, and professional power on the other. Figure 12.1 provides a way of

	Market forces	Professional Power
	−	+	
Psychiatric patient	Private patient	+
Acute medical/surgical NHS patient	Complementary medicine user	−

Figure 12.1 Typology of health consumers.

conceptualizing these variables, putting psychiatric patients in a context of other medical service users. It can be seen that there are some areas of health care to which the term 'consumer' seems more applicable than others.

Complementary medicine (bottom right) provides a service predominantly in the private sector where market forces operate most freely. (There is little provision for alternative medicine within the NHS.) This allows for free competition between individual practitioners, who compete for patients. Prices charged for therapies take place in a competitive environment. The necessity for social control on the part of professionals is also minimized. The typical person who chooses alternative medicine is middle class and articulate, and consults for non-life-threatening illness, under a voluntary contract which involves regular but limited service contact. Here the term 'consumer' seems to be highly appropriate.

The private patient using conventional medicine (top right) can choose health care according to the range of private hospitals available. However, professional control is greater than in the case of the complementary medicine user. General practitioners control access to specialist medical services, so the patient is not totally free of professional constraints. Moreover, in terms of professional power, in the private sector the internal constraints (such as complaints procedures and health authority policies) which govern clinical practice in the NHS are absent. Here the term 'consumer' is plausible, but the power of professionals to impede or dictate consumer choice renders it problematic.

Professional power is still influential in relation to NHS acute patients. However, this is arguably not as strong as in the private sector given the constraints placed on professional dominance through policy-making and fiscal arrangements determined by the State. For example, as well as the gate-keeping function of GPs, the NHS acute medical patients' free choice is constrained by the rationing of health services made available by health authority funds (see Figure 12.1, bottom left). If demand outstrips supply (clinical resources of manpower and technology), access to public health care is usually rationed according to the notion of a waiting list. In other instances, such as kidney dialysis, other selection criteria may also apply. In the case of fertility treatment, for example, sexual orientation, marital status, socio-economic status and number of existing children are factors that may be taken into consideration in permitting the uptake of services. Thus, the term 'consumer' becomes more dubious in this group of service recipients, given limited resources and mechanisms to filter out 'unworthy' cases.

Users of psychiatric services (top left) experience professional power even more acutely, while being denied the freedom to choose their therapist or service (compare this with the consumer of alternative medicine). Psychiatric patients can be forced into the sick role by means of compulsory admission. Even though this relates to only a small minority of patients, the fact that a person may be forced to enter hospital or receive treatment makes any notion of free positive choice tenuous. Being excluded from employment in the main, psychiatric patients are also a group with very little 'buying power' and so they penetrate little into either of the boxes on the right of the figure. By the time we reach the top left box, the term 'consumer' hardly appears to be apposite at all.

In measuring satisfaction in the area of mental health, there appear to be a number of other differences between patients who use services for acute physical problems and those who receive psychiatric services:

1   Contact with services for those with mental health problems is far more extensive than for most others who use the health and social services, although they have this in common with some groups of physically disabled people. Those who enter hospital for acute physical problems, such as appendicitis, are patients for a short time only, whether or not they experience their hospitalization as positive or negative.

2   The consequences of being labelled 'ill' are often greater for a person who is given a psychiatric diagnosis. For the majority of those with physical problems, the diagnosis itself is often only temporary and is often not stigmatizing. Since the diagnosis of a person as 'mentally ill' is done primarily on the basis of a judgement about a person's conduct, there is always a risk of invalidating their whole identity or sense of self. Again, certain physical disabilities (such as epilepsy) may carry with them stigma, and so the mental patient is not unique.

3   There are social and economic consequences of contact with psychiatric services, which apply much less often when acute medical services are used. Those labelled as being mentally ill are discriminated against by present and prospective employers and, as a result, are often subjected to a life of poverty. Educational opportunities are curtailed, family and intimate relationships affected and making social contact with people is fraught with difficulties. Again, some of these impediments to citizenship often apply to people with long-term physical disabilities.

Users as survivors

There has been some analysis of the users' views of services from those who do not work directly with people in service settings either as clinicians or as managers. The position of psychiatric users in a wider social context is the object of these analyses. Two perspectives can be identified in this regard. The first has adopted a phenomenological approach to understanding the social position of the mental patient. The second has tried to analyse the structural position of users as a social group within wider society. In particular there is an interest in users campaigning collectively as a 'new social movement' (see below).

The phenomenology of surviving the psychiatric system

An example of the expansion of the felt-need approach to users described earlier is provided by a phenomenological study. This is concerned with understanding the subjective meaning that people give to their experience of the social world. An example of this is the work of Barham and Hayward (1991), who made use of personal accounts of mental patients to explore their experiences of trying to live outside of hospital. The aim of this study was:

> To attempt to bring people with mental illness under the concept of personhood, required of us will be what Bernard Williams terms an 'effort at identification', in which the person 'should not be regarded as the surface to which a certain label can be applied, but one should try to see the world (including the label) from his point of view'.
>
> (Barham and Hayward 1991: 12)

In adopting this approach, their work takes us beyond the measuring of consumer satisfaction. Rather, the concern is with the mental patient's identity and social position in everyday life. The themes identified from the subjects themselves were:

- exclusion from participation in social life;
- burden, which 'refers to the cultural freight which agents are obliged to carry';
- reorientation, which refers to 'coping' with their vulnerabilities.

Everyday encounters reported by subjects in the study by Barham and Hayward (1991) suggested the continuing marginalization of people labelled as schizophrenic, as illustrated by this quote from one respondent who struck up a conversation in a pub: 'I said I was schizophrenic and he said "You don't want to tell people things like that, they might take you out and beat you up outside". Anyway, I just got up and left because I didn't want any trouble'. Participants in the study were also reluctant to enter or re-enter patienthood. Most of them wanted to establish their credibility as ordinary people with rights of citizenship, such as adequate employment and housing. The participants were only marginally more willing to be incorporated into community services than the old custodial regime. This suggests a fundamental questioning of the utility of services from the perspective of users themselves. Such a questioning is not acknowledged by the other two views (of patient and consumer) discussed earlier. Phenomenological analysis gives primacy to the individual experience of the patient in relation to the mental hospital or community. The wider collective role of mental health consumers, as a group within civil society, is also an aspect which is important in understanding the contemporary position of mental patients.

Survivors as a type of new social movement

The growth in the collective activities of mental health users since the early 1980s has been noted by a number of commentators (Haafkens *et al.* 1986; Burstow and Weitz 1988; Chamberlin 1988; Rogers and Pilgrim 1991; Crossley and Crossley 2001). During the 1970s, the Dutch and US survivors' movements gained national and State recognition. By 1977, 35 organizations were represented in the Netherlands. Organized mental patient pressure in the USA resulted in funding for research and for mental health services to be run exclusively by patients (Campbell and Schraiber 1989). From the 1980s onwards similar developments took place in the UK. User dissatisfaction reached such a point that, in terms of numbers and organizations, it arguably constituted a mature 'new social movement'.

Social movements can be defined as loose networks of people that actively resist established dominant forms of power or pursue cultural or social change (Toch 1965). Tactics of civil disobedience, which were built into a strategy for social change, were typified in the non-violent movements led by Mahatma Gandhi and Martin Luther King. Social movements are characterized by mass mobilization (e.g. demonstrations) and for the most part act outside of formal organizations and bureaucratized pressure and charity groups. 'New' social movements can be distinguished conceptually from 'old' social movements in that they are further removed from the arena of production than the latter. Additionally, rather than seeking to defend existing social and property rights from erosion by the State, new social movements seek to establish new agendas and conquer new territory (Habermas 1981). Many, but not all, are built upon a shared oppressed identity (e.g. the women's movement, gay liberation). Some are not built on a common identity but on a common cause (animal tights, the ecology movement).

Scott (1990) contrasts new social movements with the labour (or workers') movement (the focus of the Marxian tradition in sociology). This movement has become a part of the political process through organized industrial action and negotiation (e.g. the Trades Union Congress and the Labour Party in the UK). Its organization has become formalized or bureaucratized and its aims have been economic and political. By contrast, the new social movements have mainly had social and cultural aims and have emphasized direct action and non-hierarchical forms of organization. Some social scientists have gone as far as arguing that the absorption of the Labour movement into the established political process, in capitalist society, leaves the new social movements as the only remaining radical challenge to the status quo (Marcuse 1964; Brown and Zaverstoski 2004). The mental health service survivors' movement arguably fits broadly conceptually within this new political pattern of radicalism. It is characterized by opposition to expert medical knowledge and a form of politics based on an identity derived from their mental health problems and contact with specialist services. However, the formulation of a clear and sustained users' movement does not always find favour with all survivor activists.

For example, Campbell (2009, personal communication) questions whether the more cautious notion of 'survivor action' might better capture what has happened in the UK. He queries whether a true social movement has arisen from disaffected patients, though he has used the term in his own writing (Campbell 1987; 1996). Another interpretation is that, between 1970 and 1990, UK survivor activity did indeed for a while truly constitute an identifiable movement but that user involvement in services subsequently subverted its energy, coherence and sustainability (Pilgrim 2005b). What is agreed is that a range of user-led organizations emerged in this period, which argued either for the abolition of psychiatry or for its radical reform. These included the British Network of Alternatives to Psychiatry, PROMPT (Protection of the Rights of Mental Patients in Therapy), CAPO (Campaign Against Psychiatric Oppression) and Survivors Speak Out. Irwin *et al.* (1972) stimulated the formation of the Mental Patients' Union arguing in their campaigning pamphlet that 'psychiatry is one of the most subtle methods of repression in advanced capitalist society' (see Crossley 1999).

One way of discussing this ambiguity about the existence or otherwise of the British mental health service user movement is instead to consider the actions constituted by the term 'advocacy'. Sang (1989) pointed out that the term was co-opted by professionals and used loosely by them to include 'meeting clinical needs'. He distinguished this professional discourse from two separate notions from service users themselves: citizen advocacy and self-advocacy. In the first of these, ordinary citizens (i.e. not professionals) form a relationship with a psychiatric patient to represent their interests as if they were their own. In the second case, psychiatric patients work together to represent their individual and collective interests independently of non-patients. Examples of self-advocacy since the 1980s in Britain are given in Box 12.1.

Box 12.1 The emergence of the collective voice of the user: examples of direct action from the British survivors' movement after 1980

Example 1

In 1988, a campaign was launched by users in London to oppose changes being advocated by the Royal College of Psychiatrists to the Mental Health Act 1983. The proposed Community Treatment Order (CTOs) would have allowed doctors to treat patients in the community on a compulsory basis. This hostility to CTOs culminated in over a hundred users and their allies marching from Hyde Park to Belgrave Square. There, a wreath was laid at the steps of the Royal College of Psychiatrists, in honour of the deceased recipients of ECT and major tranquillizers. Speeches were made (including one from a Labour MP) and patients read poems critical of psychiatric treatment.

Example 2

An organized opposition to the poster campaign, in the south of England, of SANE (Schizophrenia A National Emergency). This advertising campaign enjoyed the patronage of Prince Charles and the pop singer Sting. It was heavily financed by, amongst others, Rupert Murdoch and P&O ferries. The posters depicted psychiatric patients as frenziedly dangerous and called for a halt to the hospital closure programme. In response, London-based users' groups lobbied the Advertising Standards Authority about the offending posters.

Example 3

Just before the election of the first Blair government, there was a lobbying of the then opposition (Labour Party) spokespeople in Parliament by a national network of 56 different users' groups. This network was dispersed throughout the country. The MPs agreed to meet the groups, to hear their complaints about existing services and their recommendations for changes in mental health policy.

Example 4

In 2002 the NO Force movement organized a march through London which was attended by over three hundred people wishing to voice their opposition to government proposals to make it easier to detain people with a diagnosis of 'dangerous personality disorder' and compulsory treatment in the community.

Example 5

In 2013 a lobby from the Hearing Voices Network demonstrated outside the Royal College of Psychiatrists in London, following the publication of DSM-5. This was to focus attention on the need for people to be treated uniquely (rather than being reduced to a diagnosis).

Example 6

International recognition and uptake of user demands and involvement in every aspect of mental health achieved through the engagement and operationalization of a World Psychiatric Association Task Force. The *Partnerships for Better Mental Health Worldwide* (Wallcraft *et al.* 2011) illuminates how powerful the users' movement has been in lobbying for change. It reflects the culmination of user involvement in advocacy, research self-help, social inclusion, The task ('best practices in working with service users and family carers') was established in 2008 with the explicit aim to:

> support international and national programmes aiming to protect the human rights of persons with mental disorders; to promote the meaningful involvement of these persons in the planning and implementation of mental health services; to encourage the development of a person-centred practice in psychiatry and medicine; and to promote equity in the access to mental health services for persons of different age, gender, race/ethnicity, religion and socioeconomic status.
>
> (Wallcraft *et al.* 2011)

The 10 recommendations published in 2011 included the global aim that:

> The international mental health community should promote and support the development of service users' organizations and carers' organizations.

Survivors' groups have shared several concerns highlighted first by critical professionals during the 1960s (the so called 'anti-psychiatry' movement). While that critique was highly intellectual and came from professionals themselves, the more recent movement has come from service users directly and is less theoretically orientated. Instead, practical direct action characterizes its form. However, the 'clinical' group described in the USA clearly draws upon the therapeutic alternatives, which the 'anti-psychiatrists' themselves developed and advocated at an earlier point.

Box 12.1 indicates types of survivor action which emerged, and which transformed previously atomized voices of lone mental patients. The transformation led briefly to a collective voice of shared resistance and demands for change. The latter emerged as a result of a dialectical relation to wider public and collective movements, which in turn connected to broader transformations in the social, economic and health arenas. The notion of 'habitus' has been used as a basis for understanding this transformation (Crossley and Crossley 2001). The notion combines the phenomenology (the survivors' personal experience) and historical features of social life. Thus, collective experience and action are viewed as being structured by the residue of previous experience, and this 'habitus' in turn contributes to the further structuration of further experience and action.

From this perspective, the current activities and success of the survivors' movement can be related to the existence of audiences, relations of symbolic power and to the historical activity of service-user protest and resistance. Changes in the 'personal' voice of the mental patient changed significantly in the post-war period (Crossley and Crossley 2001). In the face of a discreditable identity of the mental patient, which prevailed in the 1950s and 60s, the Mental Patients Union in the 1970s and the subsequent survivor organizations noted above were concerned with 'pleas' to be assigned an authentic personal voice. This enduring core drive of survivor action to regain a voice denied to them by professionals and other non-patient groups is a feature still evident, even if the notion of a 'survivors movement' is now open to question.

Survivor action in the post-1980s period focused on broader social groupings and issues (e.g. gender and sexual abuse). Their agenda of activism contributes explicitly to the discourse of political activism and resistance on the one hand and the development of alternative ways of managing madness on the other. The 'lived experience' and voice of users is combined in a way which produces an emancipatory form of dealing with madness and distress. This combination is evident, for example, in the way in which the Hearing Voices Network embraces and makes the connections between the social and the therapeutic:

> People who hear voices and their families and friends can gain greater benefits from de-stigmatizing the experience, leading to a greater tolerance and understanding. This can be achieved through promoting more positive explanations, which give people a more positive framework for developing their own ways of coping and raising awareness about the experience in society as a whole.

More broadly in the articulation of their preferred narratives of recovery, which closely align with their lived experiences, survivor activists do not only reframe the meaning of their experiences (away from a defect or pathology construction). They also construct an alternative notion of the 'good life'. They offer counter-cultural communities, aim for social justice and demand human rights in the mental health system; they engage in political activism (Adame and Knudson 2008). One aspect of the latter has been the construction of the Survivors History website, which is open to all comers but is numerically dominated by survivors, who exchange their views and experiences (see http://studymore.org.uk/mpu.htm). This sort of initiative combines an incipient collective oral history with strategic discussions about political activism in relation to a range of topics, including recovery and compulsory treatment in the community (Campbell and Roberts 2009).

Users as providers

Mental health work is only partly undertaken by health professionals. The notion of user 'work' or 'labour' is one way of conceptualizing the mental health work which is undertaken by patients (Figure 12.2). This differs from the support and treatments 'delivered' by professionals. Notions of co-production have arisen to acknowledge a shift in the way in which the professional–patient relationship has been conceptualized, by some, to include shared decision-making, self-management and expectations of greater participation than expected in previous more passive role conceptualizations (Protheroe et al. 2012). Some users have identified the interface between co-production and recovery as centred around four aspects:

1   reducing/eliminating control and restraint on wards;
2   shared decision-making around medication;
3   developing real advance directives and joint crisis plans;
4   co-produced structures for service user involvement.

A three-dimensional view of illness work recently subjected to modification in a number of studies looking at user involvement in long-term conditions (see Corbin and Strauss 1985) identified

Types of chronic illness work (Corbin and Strauss 1985)	Types of work
Illness work (concerned with symptom management)	Delegated work; Redistributive work; Surveillance work; Diagnostic work; Emotional work; Invisible work ('work that gets things back on track'); Interactional work; Information work; Adherence work; Body projects; Sentimental work; Articulation work
Everyday life work (the practical tasks such as housework, caring, paid employment)	
Biographical work (the reconstruction of the ill person's biography)	

Figure 12.2   Types of work.

three types of inter-related domains of chronic illness work which are of use. When applied to ana-lysing the activities of the work of users from a secondary analysis of transcripts of the experience of 'depression', the types of work that are undertaken by users can be easily seen in Figure 12.3.

Thinking

Ruminating

Coping/self-management

Taking tablets

Seeing a counsellor

Negotiating/agreeing problem with self/others/health professionals

Sense making

Accounting for/explaining

Discovery (Balint flash)

Managing announcement and transition

Working or not working

Role

Managing others

Retreating/isolating/withdrawal (all = active work)

Somatic camouflage

Drowning in sorrows

Survival work/hard work of living

Beckoning silence – mountain top – risk of death

Figure 12.3   The work of being depressed: towards a taxonomy of activity.

Some effort can involve what could be termed 'useless work' or 'negative work'. This is the type of work equated with the 'Sysyphus syndrome' (Sysyphus was condemned by the gods to roll a boulder up to the top of the hill only to see it roll back down again). For some people this could be work associated with treatments that turn out to be ineffective or indeed may cause iatrogen-esis, but which involve a lot of invested physical and emotional effort around their condition (e.g. periods in hospital or trying different medications despite the adverse effects that accrue). (see for example Kokanovic *et al.* (2008) Chew-Graham *et al.* (2013))

User work and provision also manifests itself collectively

For some time now services have been provided by users of services (Chamberlin 1988; Lindow 1994; Wallcraft 1996). User-led safe houses and drop-in day centres reflect the users' movement's priorities of voluntary relationships, alternatives to hospital admission, crisis intervention and personal support. Between the diffuse self-care strategies and mutual support occurring spontaneously between patients in statutory services and funded user-led services, there is another layer of user involvement. In recent years, service providers have, to various degrees in different localities, sought the collaboration of users to support service developments. Minimally this has entailed surveys or consultation exercises about local-need identification (an extension of the role of user as consumer). It has also included: the formal acceptance by professional providers of innovations, such as patients' councils; users being paid to train mental health staff (Crepaz-Keay *et al.* 1998) and users' and carers' groups being called upon to improve services in collaborative experiments in service development (Carpenter and Sbaraini 1997; Pilgrim and Waldron 1998).

User-led services have also introduced an alternative philosophical base to the management and treatment of mental health problems. At times this has had a feedback impact on traditional services. The Hearing Voices Network, informed by the work of Romme, works positively with people's experiences of hearing voices. Rather than attempting to obliterate the voices, as a traditional symptom-based approach might do, this user-led initiative attributes meaning to voice hearing. This offers alternative means of coping with voices that may at times cause their recipients distress.

The limits of the user as provider are essentially set by the willingness (or lack of it) to encroach upon the care and social control role, which professionals have traditionally adopted. Professional norms have included State-delegated powers to detain and forcibly intervene in the lives of people who are socially deviant or incompetent (under the paternalistic guise of the 'treatment' of illness). Not only do user-led projects not include this function currently, because of the absence of legal powers, it is unlikely that they would want to accrue this traditional psychiatric professional service role, given that one main stimulus for the development of the service users' movement internationally was the civil libertarian objection to the coercive role of psychiatry in society. This point is made in a critical way by an academic psychiatric nurse:

> What matters here is that such services can show that they can provide safe and effective care to a high standard. The fact that all such services so far have had to institute rules that enable difficult people to be excluded indicates that such services are developing in a way that is supplementary rather than alternative to psychiatry.

> (Bowers 1998: 138)

However, what user-led projects do provide is an alternative to the readiness of psychiatry to coercively control those who are not 'difficult' (in the sense of being dangerous rule-breakers) but who are harmlessly unintelligible to their fellows (e.g. voice hearers and those with inoffensive delusions).

User-led projects offer more benign alternatives grounded in the experience of this group of people and in so doing provide a redefinition of who is difficult, by showing how this latter group can be helped where traditional services have failed as well as incorporating strategies of management that users themselves have found to be beneficial.

The tension between advising, providing and campaigning

Survivor groups have sought to assert both the legitimacy of experiential knowledge and their positions as citizens in the face of official responses, which have not always been supportive (Lewis 2009). These survivor concerns have converged with the interests of health service managers, and relate to the development of user-led service innovations. For example, user-led services can be found in the voluntary sector in Britain and occasionally they are supported by statutory authorities. User-controlled facilities and activity varies from the latent role of patients being self-caring and mutually supportive in professionally led services and self-help groups, right through to funded projects which are managed and staffed by users themselves.

The State and its paid providers have now responded to and incorporated user-based approaches to care and support. Within mainstream health policy there has been a gradual shift in the design and delivery of services from viewing users as patients to their being 'partners'. The notion of 'expert by experience' has gained gradual acceptance and been established and implemented as part of mainstream health policy. This is encompassed in the 'recovery' notion, which has US origins but is being adopted as a strand within British mental health services. The proliferation of the recovery emphasis in the UK has given rise to a proliferation of user-led services incorporating these values. For example, Working Towards is a Scottish community development project established in 2008 to develop user-centred services. The focus is on allowing people to have more choices in their lives (www. scottishrecovery.net/Latest-News/can-mental-health-services-as-we-know-them-really-support-recovery.html).

User and patient involvement in the planning and delivery of adult mental health services has been increasingly promoted. There is some evidence that this has resulted in greater inclusivity and the dismantling of power differentials between users and professionals. Users have been able to position themselves as active citizens, not merely as individual consumers, by drawing on a broad range of networks (Bolzan and Gale 2002). These shifts suggest possibilities for greater inclusivity. However, barriers have also been noted. Despite the rhetoric of partnership and user involvement, which accompanies new policies, such as the co-ordination of care, there is an absence of a corresponding involvement of users (Rose *et al.* 2003). The practical implementation of government rhetoric about user involvement has been patchy: a mixture of local successes and failures.

User involvement for the most part remains in the gift of provider managers, in so far as they retain control over decision-making and may expect users to address the organization-set agendas and conform to their management practices. Pressures to accommodate to the structure and assumptions of mental health services organizations have been interpreted as the need for organizations to adapt and for users to acquire new skills (Truman and Raine 2002). While users' involvement may have brought about changes in services and policies, the demands of the survivors' movement for improvements in the status and social conditions of people with mental health problems is still marginalized (Rutter *et al.* 2004).

A question remains over whether this incorporation of users within the structures of health services might undermine the strength of the very new social movement which facilitated the State response to increase user involvement in the first place. Smelser (1962), an early commentator on new social movements, noted that conservative interest groups might make concessions to the demands of social movements in order to defuse their more radical demands for social change. State incorporation and diversion into service structures may be another way to diffuse the strength of demand for changes in status and social inclusion in civil society.

Discussion

The four ways of viewing service users described in the second part of this chapter illustrate the construction of the mental patient from different vantage points. The first, of patient, has a narrow clinical conception of the user of services – as an extension or carrier of the mental illness he or she is deemed to be suffering. The conceptualization of the user as consumer defines the user of services as a whole person, who has needs over and above those defined from a diagnostic viewpoint. This approach tends still to be professionally defined and is limited to the parameters of the provision and delivery of existing or achievable services. It also contains the contestable assumption that service users 'consume' products that are aligned with their expressed needs. The third approach takes those expressed needs as the main reference point of analysis, along with the collective structural position of mental patients within a wider social context.

The implications that stem from these conceptualizations are consequently different. The first accepts that professionally led services are most appropriate, given the paternalism that mental illness is deemed to necessitate. The second modifies this by recognizing the (contestable) notion of the positive choice that the ideology of consumerism implies. The third position marks a departure from a professionally defined discourse. By giving a voice to user demands, professionally delivered services are brought into question or are rendered problematic.

The clinical conception points to a traditional therapist–patient relationship. Consumerism envisages a larger role for mental health users in health care. There is an implicit assumption that views and participation should be in relation to existing services, whether some of these are expanded or diminished as a result of feedback on the basis of 'felt need'. The survivor view, in eschewing or distrusting professional interventions, emphasizes that the fundamental needs of patients reflect rights of citizenship rather than a desire for specialized services. This would imply an increase in material and social resources, for example, improved access to housing and employment opportunities. A further requirement might be legislation aimed at ensuring that people with a psychiatric label are not discriminated against in civil society, along the lines of that already existing for race and sex. It might even imply the political demand to abolish coercive 'mental health law' as a condition of that assured position in civil society.

These divergent implications of the three conceptions of the mental patient outlined earlier suggest that, rather than being neutral or value free, each is imbued with, or reflects, a set of competing interests and ideologies related to the three groups central to contemporary mental health services: clinicians, managers and users. The power of each of these interest groups interact to determine the types of priorities that come to prevail in the organization, distribution and delivery of services and resources to those with mental health problems in society. The interaction is also affected by media portrayals of psychiatric patients and by the influence of groups of their relatives. Thus, any social understanding of the role, status and credibility of people who use mental health services needs to be reached after an appraisal of the relative salience of a number of dynamic processes and disparate actors which surround and inscribe a set of identities upon them.

This chapter has highlighted some basic problems about defining who exactly is a user of mental health services. Although the term 'user' (in Britain) has become a proxy term for 'psychiatric patient', we drew attention to the other parties being served by, and thus arguably 'using', these services. If a variety of parties use services then it is inevitable that they are a source of disappointment, as the different interest groups often seek different ends or their requirements might vary over time. Both the relatives of psychiatric patients and patients, arguably, have themselves become involved in important social movements, which have shaped the character of mental health services. The emergence of user-led mental health provision has also highlighted the shortcomings of professional work (from a patient perspective), defined the social control role of psychiatry more clearly and suggested new models of care based on mutuality and recovery. The recent production of user knowledge and research and its use to shape the direction of resources and service provision is just one indicator of the success and power of users to change the face of mental health services.

Finally we can offer a caution about the overview in this chapter: its applicability is limited overwhelmingly to Western Europe, North America and Australia and New Zealand. We have little or no knowledge of the application, or presence, of these debates about service users in other parts of the world. For example, they are inherently only pertinent where a) there is an extensive welfare state apparatus, which includes 'mental health services' and b) where civil rights have become part of the polity of a particular country.

In the case of Eastern Europe and the old Soviet Union, the first conditions applied but not the second. Indeed, since the transition in those countries to neo-liberal capitalism, participation in social movements and informal civil organizations has actually been lower than in other liberal Western democracies (Brown 2001; Howard 2003). The economic transition did not encourage participatory democracy and the growth of strong new social movements. The latter have not been entirely absent, but they have not been as extensive as in the countries considered in relation to the content of this chapter.

The implications of this may be reflected in the continuing criticisms of the quality of mental health services in post-Communist countries, which remain under-developed, authoritarian and relatively untouched by human rights debates, common in the West since the period of 'antipsychiatry' and reinforced by service user activism (Jenkins *et al.* 2005). This final point is made to remind readers that any topic of interest within mental health debates tends to be dominated by research from some parts of the world but not others. This book generally reflects the limitations of a Western developed world discursive focus. This is not to invalidate our explorations in the chapters of this book but it is simply to note its limitations and focus.

Questions

1 Describe the reasons for the rise of the mental health service users' movement.
2 Compare and contrast the expectations which patients and their relatives are likely to have about mental health services.
3 How do the mass media shape our views of psychiatric patients?
4 What have 'survivors' of the psychiatric system 'survived'?
5 What do user-led services tell us about mainstream mental health provision?
6 Why is the term 'carer' problematic in the field of mental health?

For discussion

If you were the relative of a person who became psychotic what would you want from services? Now consider what you would want if you were the patient. Compare and contrast both parts of the exercise.

13 Prevention, public mental health and the pursuit of happiness

Chapter overview

Definitions of public mental health broadly follow the contours of public health as a discipline. It has been described by the Mental Health Foundation as 'the art, science and politics of creating a mentally healthy society'. The pursuit of a public mental health agenda is concerned with how individuals, families, organizations and communities think and feel, individually and collectively, and the attendant impact that this may have on overall mental health and well-being in society. Evidence of the structural determinants of mental health, the flow of happiness and unhappiness through social networks and the presence of socially derived responses to mental health such as stigma have all reinforced the need for a focus on 'public' rather than a purely individualized response or approach to mental health problems.

Public mental health more than any other area of mental health has become part of a global mental health movement which is a perspective that includes the ambition of improving mental health and achieving equity worldwide (Patel and Prince 2010). Nowhere is this more apparent than in public health where the WHO definition of mental health has been widely adopted as an aspirational goal for health policy. The WHO defines mental health as a 'a state of well-being which every individual realizes his or her own potential, can cope with the normal stresses of life, can work productively and fruitfully, and is able to make a contribution to her or his community' (www.who.int/features/qa/62/en).

The link to mental health promotion in the aspirational project of the field of global health also relates to the idea that mental health can be promoted through the provision of information about the mental health profile of different countries, identifying and comparing needs with a view to developing interventions with the capacity to meet different and specific needs. Implicitly tackling inequalities which are illuminated through comparing rich with poor countries and across gender and cultures forms an agenda of organizations like the WHO. A global approach also draws attention to common problems associated with public and institutional responses to mental health. An issue discussed earlier in relation to stigma.

The interest in public mental health more specifically has emerged as a response to government policies and the need for evidence and cost-effectiveness (www.mentalhealth.org.uk/our-work/policy/public-mental-health). In the twenty-first century the pursuit of happiness (or at least the contented life) has also emerged as a salient cultural theme taken up by policy-makers. This is a somewhat paradoxical position, given that happiness is arguably a form of mental abnormality: 'it is statistically abnormal, consists of a discrete cluster of symptoms, is associated with a range of cognitive abnormalities, and probably reflects the abnormal functioning of the central nervous system' (Bentall 1992: 94). Bentall (1992) notes that realistic predictions about life arise from a slightly depressive rather than happy personal outlook.

This final chapter explores this emergent trend in the context of re-visiting some basic sociological points introduced in Chapter 1 about the importance of causes and meanings. Public mental health will then be examined under the following headings:

- preventing mental disorder and promoting mental health;
- the consequences of desegregation;
- the new emphasis on well-being and happiness;
- the interaction of physical and mental health;
- health, illness and societal norms.

Introduction

Throughout this book we have drawn attention to the double significance of the social, when we consider the topic of mental health and illness. On the one hand, for those interested predominantly or wholly in *causal* arguments, there is an overwhelming case that past and present social conditions are strong determinants of mental health status. For example, being poor, black, old or a woman alters one's chances at the individual level of well-being, madness or distress. This is also the case when we consider the proven role of childhood neglect and abuse in predicting diagnosed mental disorder (which we discussed in Chapter 5). These arguments about social determination can be located strongly in the structuralist and materialist traditions of sociology (especially derived from Marx and Durkheim).

On the other hand, for those more interested in *constructivist* arguments, the social is also important because of the relationship between language and power. Beginning with symbolic interactionism, rooted in the work of Weber, and culminating in the interest since the early 1980s in post-modern or post-structuralist social science (underpinned philosophically by Foucault, Derrida, Rorty and Lyotard), mental health has been usefully opened up or 'deconstructed'. It is in this work that we encounter the importance of meaning and values rather than causation.

These orientations, one causal in emphasis and the other constructivist, which as we argued in Chapter 1 can be viewed as compatible or incommensurable, are pertinent when we come to consider the topic of this final chapter. From our perspective, both causes and meanings are important. No more is this point relevant than when we come to address public mental health or, put differently, mental health as a public health matter. For example, what do we mean when talking of 'the burden of schizophrenia'? Or what do we mean if we say that Denmark is currently the happiest country in the world? For convenience, and in line with this introductory logic, in this chapter we address the topic of public mental health in a way in which both causes and meanings are considered.

Preventing mental disorder and promoting mental health

This section explores the conceptual and practical overlap between the promotion of mental health and the prevention of mental disorder (Pilgrim 2009). Mental health promotion has been defined in a variety of ways but tends to include recurring strands: happiness, the right to freedom and productivity, the absence of mental illness, and the fulfilment of an individual's emotional, intellectual and spiritual potential. The promotion of psychological well-being is closely linked to the primary prevention of mental health problems. However, in the former case, positive mental health has to be defined as one or more desired outcomes. By contrast, in the latter case there needs to be a demonstration that the probability of diagnosed mental illness is reduced. Tudor (1996) notes that the danger of conflating mental health promotion with the primary prevention of mental illness is that it may maintain a medical focus on a limited clinical population and not address the population's needs as a whole. The WHO (1986) advocates mental health promotion in terms of the ability of individuals to 'have the basic opportunity to develop and use their health potential to live socially and economically productive lives'. Later the Organization went on to argue that 'the concept of health potential encompasses both physical and mental health and must be viewed in the context of personal development throughout the life span' (WHO 1991).

Types of prevention

The primary prevention of mental illness can be distinguished from secondary and tertiary forms. Secondary prevention refers to nipping mental health problems 'in the bud' following early diagnosis or when symptoms have been clearly manifested (e.g. a first episode of psychosis or early indications of phobic anxiety). Tertiary prevention refers to lowering the probability of

$$\text{Incidence of mental illness} = \frac{\text{stress} + \text{exploitation} + \text{organic factors}}{\text{support} + \text{self-esteem} + \text{coping skills}}$$

$$\text{Promotion of mental health} = \frac{\text{coping skills} + \text{benign environment} + \text{self-esteem}}{\text{stress} + \text{exploitation} + \text{organic factors}}$$

Figure 13.1 Distinguishing the incidence of mental illness from the promotion of mental health using common factors (modified from Albee (1993)).

relapse in those with chronic mental health problems and so is close to ongoing treatment. The distinction, but also the relationship, between promotion and primary prevention is conceived as the differing relationship between common factors (see Figure 13.1).

The factors in the two equations in Figure 13.1 can be addressed one by one.

Stress

We address this elsewhere (Chapter 2) when accounting for some of the differences in diagnosis between poorer and richer people. While both groups have adverse and positive experiences, the richer group has more buffering positive experiences. Those exposed to lower levels of personal and environmental stress are more likely to remain mentally healthy. Conversely, the higher the level of stress, the higher the probability a person will develop a mental health problem. Thus we can think of any social context as providing a range of types and quantities of 'stressors', which impinge on those in its midst.

Exploitation

The exploitation of individuals, whether it is economic or related to physical, sexual or emotional abuse or oppression, increases the risk of mental health problems. Conversely, a person not exposed to these versions of exploitation is more likely to remain mentally healthy. This notion of exploitation disrupts the more traditional 'scientific' approach to mental health found in psychiatry and psychology (Sartorius and Henderson 1992). The two disciplines tend to avoid the language of politics, which might bring accusations of unscientific bias and risk undermining professional credibility. However, a problem for the human sciences is that they are intrinsically about human relationships and values. Efforts on the part of psychiatry and psychology to adopt a disinterested stance thus are doomed to failure but the stance is attempted in order to make claims of objectivity (a rhetorical requirement in both professions). Also, exploitation is beyond their immediate control and their scope of interventions is limited to the micro level.

Organic factors

These refer to environmental toxins and stressors and to biological susceptibility and are easily overlooked or even eschewed by social science but they are part of the social landscape. For example, environmentally present poisons (such as lead and petrochemicals) damage the nervous system. Other organic factors with social linkages relate to behavioural stressors, which are then mediated by physiological mechanisms to produce brain damage. The most common example of this is in relation to raised blood pressure. This increases the risk of stroke and vascular dementia. Stressors that affect blood pressure levels include insecure work conditions, noisy and dangerous living environments and lifestyle habits such as quality of diet and exercise levels.

Social support

This is discussed later and is an important and well-proven buffer against mental health problems. Chronic personal isolation increases the risk of symptoms and these are reduced in probability in those people who are part of a supportive social network (be it close friends or family).

Self-esteem building

This refers to early family life and schooling and their capacity for developing (or undermining) confidence in the growing child. It also refers to the presence of benign and affirming *current* relationships and so links back to the previous point about social support.

Coping skills

People vary in their ability to cope with adversity and this probably links back to personal styles learned in the family and at school. Much of the work of psychotherapists is devoted to enabling patients lacking these coping skills normally to learn new ones. Therapy thus provides an offer of compensation at the individual level for group or social adversity. These factors indicate that positive mental health and the primary prevention of mental illness implicate a wide range of factors, which are political, social, psychological and biological. With such a wide range of factors operating, mental health promotion implicates both public policies and public education (Tones and Tilford 1994).

The economic as well as social case for mental health promotion and prevention

Societal norms about the benefits of attempts to improve mental health and well-being are shaped by the resources available to health systems and adjacent social systems, such as housing, employment and education. Economic rationales are now a key focus of advanced welfare societies. In this case, to what extent is an investment in prevention and promotion policy strategies a worthwhile use of available resources? In a major recent report addressing this question, Knapp and colleagues (2011) examined returns on investment in interventions which focused on economic pay-offs (for every pound spent). They concluded that not all interventions are likely to produce cost-effective solutions. Interventions with the three highest pay-offs (set against investment) were identified as the prevention of dysfunctional conduct through social and emotional learning programmes, suicide prevention through bridge safety barriers and suicide training in primary care. The three poorest interventions, in terms of cost-effectiveness, were early intervention for depression in diabetes, befriending of older adults, and health visitor interventions to reduce post-natal depression. The interventions reviewed, with costs implications, are presented in Table 13.1.

These conclusions drawn from Table 13.1 about public policy are sufficiently open-textured for us to recognize that, from a broad social perspective, virtually everything that happens to us from conception onwards can affect our mental health. In the next section we examine another public policy topic related to the citizenship of those where mental health problems have developed.

The consequences of desegregation

In Chapter 10, where we discussed legalism, we argued that some diagnoses (of 'personality disorder' and 'schizophrenia') remain linked to dis-valued and distrusted patient groups. They are strongly associated with the perceived or actual threat and nuisance of patients with these diagnoses. Patients, including many of those with these diagnoses, are now living outside of hospital settings. Post-institutional societies in Europe, North America and Australasia contain people with a range of problems that previously would have been shut away out of sight and out of mind. In this sense, mental disorder has become much more a *public* matter. As governments, professionals and mental health charities now readily emphasize, one in four in the population will have a mental health problem at some point in their lives (though as our chapters on race, class and gender showed, this is not a random one in four but is socially patterned).

Table 13.1 Economic estimates of mental health promotion interventions (adapted from Knapp *et al.* 2011)

Context	Intervention	Cost impact
Health visiting to reduce post-natal depression	Post-natal screening + psychologically informed sessions	No cost savings. Benefits outweighed by training and higher staff costs
Parenting to prevent persistent conduct disorders	Parenting style programmes targeted parents of children at risk of conduct disorders	Cost savings of 8:1 over 25 years to mainly the criminal justice system and NHS
School-based social and emotional learning programmes	Programmes to help children recognize and manage, emotions and relationships, and to set goals for decision-making	Lower conduct problems drives net savings from crime- and NHS-related impact and wider benefits
Reducing bullying	Anti-bullying programmes in schools	Good value for money based on improved future earnings
Early detection and intervention for psychosis	Early detection and treatment service (CBT, medication)	NHS cost savings initially from avoidance of suicide and psychotic episodes but reduced savings over time
Primary care screening for prevention of alcohol misuse	Screening by GPs and 5-minute advice session	Robust economic case for intervention increased savings by use of practice nurses rather than GP and by targeting
Workplace screening for anxiety and depression	Screening and six sessions of CBT for those at risk	Cost saving for business relates to reduction in absenteeism
Promoting well-being in the work place	Well-being programmes including risk appraisal, personalized information advice, and online and workshop resources	Costs reduced for business and public-sector employers and NHS
Debt and mental health	Mixture of debt reduction advice models, and telephone, Internet and face-to-face advice	Better outcomes compared to no action
Population-level suicide awareness	GP suicide prevention education	Highly cost-effective for the health care system
Bridge safety measures for suicide prevention	Construction of bridge safety barriers	Substantial cost savings but risk of diversion to other lethal means
Primary care collaborative care for depression in type 2 diabetes	Case management by nurse and liaison with GP over and above routine care	Cost effective after 2 years but high net additional costs due to implementation
Tackling medically unexplained symptoms	CBT for somatoform conditions	Cost saving estimated for the long term from reduced utilization
Befriending of older adults	Weekly befriending contact for an hour for isolated and lonely people	Unlikely to be cost-effective to public purse but improved quality of life at low cost

With an ageing population, the prevalence of dementia is increasing (see Chapter 5) and so the care of older people now increases the visibility of these patients in community, not hospital, settings. In the case of psychotic patients, the increasing expectation is that alone or with service support, most will now live outside of hospital. Even if they remain symptomatic, such patients may represent the move towards *recovery in* rather than recovery from mental illness (see Chapter 11).

Thus our current discussion of public mental health in its broad sense refers to two aspects. The first, which we deal with in the next section, is about the increased public presence of mental abnormality and the distinctions within that presence made by those giving and receiving labels. The second is about positive mental health and we deal with this in a later section.

Here are two general points that can be made about a post-institutional world in summary.

- Although mental disorder is more visible than it was at the beginning of the twentieth century, segregation has not completely disappeared. However, social capital is important in relation to public mental health because it lowers the rates of first episodes and prevents relapse for many forms of madness and distress.
- A conceptual distinction can be made between the social inclusion of *individuals* and forces of social exclusion, such as discrimination in the workplace and stigma in neighbourhoods. The former is about working with patients to enable them to re-enter society; hence the consensus on a social recovery model now in mental health services. By contrast social exclusion is about discriminatory social forces that exist independent of the success, or otherwise, of recovery or rehabilitation strategies to promote social inclusion. This point is emphasized because social exclusion may be re-framed politically as simply the aggregate of successfully socially included individuals, arguably a mystification created by the logical and sociological conflation of different processes.

The new emphasis on well-being and happiness

In the light of all of the above we now find an increasing political consensus that a true mental health policy should be directed towards maximizing happiness in the population and minimizing misery. Miserable people make poor workers and they are thus an impediment to socio-economic efficiency. This position was pushed to its logical conclusion by the labour economist Richard Layard, who argued that it is *cost-effective* for governments to treat mental illness in order to remove the burden it creates in lost productivity, poor fitness for work and the costs of long-term health care access (Layard 2005). As Teghtsoonian (2009) has pointed out, this response has been part of a recent neo-liberal pattern of policies in North America and Europe, which individualizes mental health, especially 'common mental health problems' like depression. This is a de-socialized pattern, as it shifts the focus from the social determinants of unhappiness to the unhappy individual.

However, Layard's work, and that of others like Wilkinson (2005), is more than an argument about the downstream rescuing of society's psychological casualties. It also points up some important upstream social determinants. The first of these is about hyper-consumerism in late modernity. For example, Layard talks of the 'Hedonic Treadmill' (Layard 2005). In a similar vein, James (2008) writes about 'Affluenza', when material possessions and consumption have taken precedence in modern societies over low-cost and low-striving forms of social affiliation. This point returns us to the importance of social capital or social support for well-being, discussed above and in Chapter 2. If kith and kin are relegated in importance compared to the role of consumer in our societal norms, then distress is generally not far behind.

This form of critique chimes with the findings of the longitudinal study of happiness worldwide which has found that the happiest countries are those in which 'post-materialist values' predominate

(Inglehart *et al.* 2008). As the latter authors note, the relationship between gross domestic product and happiness is not linear but curvilinear. That is, poverty causes misery (see Chapter 2) but once any society reaches a point where the great bulk of its population is not in a state of absolute poverty, then it does not follow that being richer makes people happier – it does not.

For example, even with dramatic negative changes in economic circumstances after years of growth in the 'noughties', there were only slight declines measured in self-rated happiness amongst those in Ireland (Doherty and Kelly 2013). However, in a European context there remain variations between nation states and a strong correlation between countries. The European Social Survey, for example, shows that individuals in one of the richer countries, Denmark, report the highest level of happiness, with individuals in Bulgaria (which has the lowest per capita income in Europe) reporting the lowest levels (Doherty and Kelly 2010). In these relatively rich countries, in a global context what starts to come into play are two major factors. One has already been mentioned (that of post-materialist values). The other, which is related to this, is the degree of status envy created by socio-economic competition. The adverse mental health consequences of the latter are greater, the more that there is internal inequality in a particular society. Thus the richest country in the world, the USA, is not the happiest.

The pattern of relationships just described also produce another interesting effect: the blurring of the boundary between physical and mental health (see later section). In societies with high social capital, lower inequalities, strong income maintenance policies and low-cost childcare, we find more happy citizens than in those with the inverse of this pattern. The impact on both physical and mental health then becomes evident from these social and political arrangements.

We noted in Chapter 2 that social support affects health in a number of ways. Social capital predicts morbidity of most kinds and it also is correlated with rates of recovery from illness. Also, social isolation and status envy are similarly predictive, which is confirmed by evidence on social support (e.g. Cassel 1976; Cobb 1976). Indeed, some studying social support go further and point out that the mere absence of relationships *is* the reason people are depressed, even without other evidence of past or current social adversity (Henderson 1992). The latter reported 35 separate studies of the relationship between social support and depression. The great majority found a significant (inverse) relationship between level of perceived social support and frequency of reported depressive symptoms.

The chances of a person enjoying the mental health advantages of social support increase with their marital status and their socio-economic status, as we noted in Chapters 2 and 3. This suggests a virtuous circle, in which the rich get richer in two senses. Those with an intimate partner enjoy more social contact than single people and those with more disposable income have richer social networks (Ross and Mirowsky 1995; Turner and Marino 1994). This suggests that lower levels of income provide fewer opportunity structures for people to develop social contact and thereby experience personal support (House *et al.* 1988). These opportunity structures include the access to paid social events, as well as the increased confidence to interact with others with increasing socio-economic status.

Economic inequality sets up *relative* disadvantage, even in developed societies, where very few are starving from absolute poverty, in a number of ways based around consumption, self-confidence and social status. Relative disadvantage creates envy and insecurity (De Botton 2004; Wilkinson 2005). When we combine this point with Layard's point noted above about the 'Hedonic Treadmill' of consumerism, it becomes obvious why materialism, especially conspicuous consumption, is a source of mental ill-health. The consensus across these writers on the paradoxical presence of much unhappiness in rich societies is that it is the quality of relationships, not buying power, which predicts well-being.

Studies of happy people suggest that domestic intimacy, religious affiliation and employed status are all predictive (Myers 2000). All three domains are potential sources of social support. Wilkinson (2005) adds that low socio-economic status brings with it shame and insecurity. In turn this makes the low-status person more disinclined to make social contact, leading to the next and complementary point about social affiliation. This is the vicious circle of insecurity, depression and social isolation.

Low levels of social support *ipso facto* bring increasing social isolation. Social isolation predicts the emergence of mental health problems and relapse in those who have had them in the past. Durkheim's original theorizing about the antecedents of suicide pointed up *inter alia* the integrative and protective impact of marriage, parenthood, religious affiliation and employment. Subsequent research of the ecological wing of the Chicago School of sociology and beyond confirmed that the incidence of mental health problems is correlated directly with social integration (Faris and Dunham 1939; Leighton 1959; Srole *et al.* 1962).

In more recent times, this ecological picture has been confirmed in relation to the incidence of psychosis, suicide and psychiatric admissions in ethnic minority patients living in areas with low numbers of those from their background (Boydell *et al.* 2001). While this point about 'ethnic density' specifically helps us to understand mediating processes about ethnic disadvantage, it also helps more generally to understand the importance for mental health of 'social belonging'.

Taken together, the above findings suggest two important aspects of the connection between personal relationships and mental health. First, the social integration findings suggest that people have a need for *group* belonging. A lack of group membership predicts the emergence of mental health problems and relapse. Second, embedded in group belonging is the opportunity for *particular intimate* relationships (some of which is expressed in long-term sexual bonding). These intimate and 'close confiding' relationships provide conditions of stable existential security.

The notion of group belonging and membership is also a theme taken up by the study of social networks. Rather than focusing on changes in relation to individual behaviour, social network analysis focuses on collective behaviours: for example, in answering the question as to whether happiness can spread from individual to individual to form 'niches' of 'happiness'. Fowler and Christakis (2008) found in a longitudinal analysis that people who find themselves surrounded by other and many happy people are more likely to become happy in the future. Clusters of people who are happy emanate from the spread of happiness rather than simply the desirability for people to associate with people like themselves. The fact that the health and well-being of one person impact on the mental well-being of others provides what Christakis and Fowler refer to as a 'conceptual justification' for the discipline of public health.

The interaction of physical and mental health

The relationship between physical and mental health highlights the two approaches, one causal and the other conceptual, that we noted in the introduction to this chapter. From a causal perspective, materialist explanations can be collapsed into unitary models, including the biomedical assumptions of neo-Kraepelinian psychiatry, with its emphasis on biological and especially genetic determination. From this strong position of hoped-for-reductionism we explained in Chapter 1, mental illness and physical illness are both assumed to be products of bodily dysfunction, with the brain being the organ of main relevance in the former case. This biological monism is at odds with Western Cartesian dualism, which has traditionally separated mind and body. Moreover, psychological and social explanations for mental ill health have often emerged in large part as a reaction to biological reductionism (again see Chapter 1).

The challenge now for social science is to develop unitary models of health, which build upon this legitimate reaction to biological reductionism but avoid dualism or the temptation of sociological reductionism. Currently, one option in this regard is to view individual and population measures of health as multi-factorial (to include a mixture of somatic, behavioural, cognitive and emotional indicators). This allows the possibility of multiple forms of interaction, requiring a flexible and concurrent consideration of biological, psychological and social variables (some add spirituality and spiritual fulfilment to this mix).

For example, in the case of vascular dementia, its sources include untreated hypertension but its consequences are largely psychological (about memory and orientation). In turn these psychological changes alter the person's capacity to fulfil adult roles and comply with rules expected of them – a social outcome. Because those who fail role and rule expectations are dis-valued, this increases the risk of people with dementia being treated poorly in society. They are outside the labour market (as is the case with older people generally) *and* they are mentally abnormal *and* they place demands for their survival on others. This leaves them exposed to the vagaries of the degree of caring commitment or paternalism of those around them.

At the population level the importance of understanding multi-factorial interactions is now fairly obvious. For example, psychiatric patients receive poor health care and die significantly younger than non-patients (Harris and Barraclough 1998; Danner *et al.* 2001). Or, in another example, widowers and male divorcees cope less well than their female equivalents. Their unhappiness can lead to poor self-care and a greater risk of alcohol abuse (Mental Health Foundation 2006). In turn, this psychological pattern alters the probability of developing physical health problems (Keyes 2004). To understand a depressed widower who turns to drink and then dies of cirrhosis of the liver, some form of flexible bio-psycho-social formulation is implied. Liver functioning and gender relations are equally important to consider case by case.

If we invert this picture about pathology and look at people with positive indicators of mental health, we find that this multi-factorial picture predicts global health scores (Benyemanini *et al.* 2000), stroke incidence and survival (Ostir *et al.* 2001), blood pressure and cortisol levels (physiological measures of stress) (Steptoe *et al.* 2007), and the lower age-linked incidence of physical illness (Keyes 2007). Variations on these findings include those that demonstrate that positive mental health is associated with improved diet, exercise and sleep (Mental Health Foundation 2006). The fact that this association leaves the direction of causality an open question signals a circular, not a linear, argument (or in this case a 'virtuous circle' of health).

Linear arguments can be developed though from the findings that improvement in mental health *predicts* lower alcohol consumption and smoking (Graham 2004). In turn, these predictions indicate a next level of outcome (alcohol and smoking lead to poor health outcomes which will then have *psychological* consequences for patients). Thus the relationship in models of health between linear predictions and circular or interactive process need to be borne in mind; they imply the need to develop monistic multi-factorial models of health. Moreover, they bring into question our acculturated and misleading neat separation between physical and mental health. At the same time, the conceptual similarities and differences between them are likely to remain contentious for the following reasons:

- Bio-medical models provoke competition from social determinism, with the latter tending to take biological reductionism as a signal of biological irrelevance. The risk then is of sociological reductionism in the field of health research. Put differently, sociologists (and some psychologists) have a disciplinary bias to dismiss the relevance of biology (see Benton (1991) for a discussion of this caution).
- With the exception of dementia and drug-induced psychosis, most psychiatric diagnoses are social judgements, justified as medical descriptions on weak grounds; they deal only with symptoms (what people say and do), with measurable somatic signs being absent. At its most extreme this leads to the judgement that mental illness is a myth and that it is just about value judgements (see Chapter 1).
- Notwithstanding the previous point, it is also the case that social, especially stigmatizing, judgements are by no means limited to mental health problems. They have also been applied historically and in different social contexts, for example, to sexually transmitted disease, epilepsy, tuberculosis and even cancer (see Chapter 11 on stigma).

Finally in this section, it is important to mention the rise in interest in the coalescence of physical and mental health via the notion of 'multiple' or 'co-morbidities'. The complexity in identifying the variety of relationships between the psychological and physical are illuminated when depression and diabetes are considered. People with diabetes suffer from much higher levels of depression than other groups in the population. The experience of poor mental health is affected by the dual reduction in illness burden, each is labelled with different facets of stigma which in turn have implications for the presentation of self in everyday life (Gask *et al.* 2012).

Health, illness and societal norms

In the light of arguments in previous sections, if it is the case that public mental health and public health more generally are difficult to clearly distinguish, what does this say about causes and meanings? This question can be answered partially in social science by some sort of philosophical inquiry about ontology (what is deemed to exist) and epistemology (what form of knowledge it is legitimate to generate). Broadly three positions are evident in the sociology of health and illness in relation to ontology and epistemology (see Chapter 1). Naïve realists take the current naming of causes and outcomes for granted (confusing reality with what we currently opt to call reality, the 'epistemic fallacy'). Radical constructivists consider that reality is always socially constructed and so we cannot get beyond representations to understand reality in, and of, itself. Critical realists argue that reality exists, is only partially known to date and is forceful in its impact on health but that social interests shape and constrain how we can come to know it, so we must approach knowledge claims sceptically. Our arguments, because they adopt this third position – which starts with ontology but concedes that epistemology is also important – emphasize the following.

- First, distress, madness and dysfunction have occurred in all societies and are determined by many factors, some known and some still mysterious, but what they are called and how they are valued varies over time and place.
- Second, distress (fear and sadness) is easier to understand than madness because it has many stable elements across contexts and even species. Fear in particular has predictable and measurable physical signs in all mammals. And most of us know what it is to feel sad in the face of loss and can even spot it with some confidence in other animals. This regularity of observation is not the case with madness or 'personality disorder', which arise from context-specific norms about rationality, mutual recognition and obligations, and intelligibility. These forms of deviance are peculiarly human and so must be understood in the normative contexts of our forms of social organization. At the same time, we find it difficult to think of a past, present or future society in which most people would be indifferent to unintelligibility or recurrent personal dysfunction. We cannot escape from this normative starting point – the fourth point below.
- Third, any notion of positive mental health necessarily subsumes hedonic and eudemonic aspects (about mood and meaning respectively).
- Fourth, judgements about illness or health thus are inherently social. Ultimately they are value judgements about what it is to act, or be capable of acting, in a good way (connoting implicitly or explicitly some version of Aristotle's 'eudaimonia' or 'good life'). Put differently, terms like 'mental disorder' or 'mental abnormality' always imply other forms of action and emotion, which are mentally 'ordered' or 'normal'; the way that people *ought* to think, feel and act as part of an ideal moral order.

These arguments about how we understand illness be it physical or mental have not been discussed in sociology alone. They have also taxed physicians and epidemiologists. For example, Smith (2002) (then the editor of the *British Medical Journal*) reports a number of studies in which doctors and lay people were given long lists of phenomena and then asked to decide whether

1	Ageing
2	Work
3	Boredom
4	Bags under eyes
5	Ignorance
6	Baldness
7	Freckles
8	Big ears
9	Grey or white hair
10	Ugliness
11	Childbirth
12	Allergy to the 21st century
13	Jet lag
14	Unhappiness
15	Cellulite
16	Hangover
17	Anxiety about penis size/penis envy
18	Pregnancy
19	Road rage
20	Loneliness

Figure 13.2   Top 20 non-diseases (voted on www.bmj.com by readers), in descending order of 'non-diseaseness'.

each item was or was not a disease. This 'non-disease' approach to understanding lay and professional discourses about pathology is very revealing. Not surprisingly, medical practitioners ascribe pathology more often than lay people. However, they do not pathologize *all* deviations from norms. They also disagree with one another about what is a disease and how important diagnosis is in principle (compared for example to negotiating a desired outcome with and for the patient). In Figure 13.2 Smith shows how the 'top 20' non-diseases identified by the readership of the *British Medical Journal* were ranked in order.

It is worth noting how many of these items are psycho-social phenomena of interest to mental health researchers and practitioners (e.g. work, road rage, boredom, unhappiness and loneliness). Indeed even the ones which are somatic indicators (e.g. freckles, baldness and big ears) imply that it is merely the way that people *think* about bodily variations that is at issue, not the variations themselves. This may suggest that from a general medical perspective at least, somatically based judgements of true diseases persevere and there is a bias towards the exclusion of the new public mental health agenda of happiness, as we discussed earlier.

This was a self-selected general medical sample. A targeted survey of physicians involved in treating or researching, say, pregnancy or childbirth would probably yield a different result. Their medical management (obstetrics) constitutes a high status specialism, which claims a superior medical authority over what others might deem to be 'non-diseases'. Thus, current general medical scepticism about non-diseases is not neatly aligned with the enthusiasm of specialist clinical gazes, such as obstetrics and psychiatry. The latter might diagnose bodily dysmorphoric disorder to account for a patient's obsession with their big ears or baldness.

Also experiences, such as jet lag or a hangover, may not be called 'diseases' but they still may be ameliorated by remedies. Something that is not called a disease may still be an uncomfortable state; a form of experienced dis-ease. Moreover, some forms of disease may have no functional expression – they are 'clinically silent', as when a person is HIV+ but feels very healthy. Ageing was at the top of the list of non-diseases. However, given a range of 'normal changes' in functioning in old age from loss of sensory acuity and memory to benign enlargement of the prostate and weaker bones, when do any of these phenomena become diseases inviting medical expertise and intervention? This complexity permits plenty of scope for argument about what any of us mean by 'pathology' and 'normality'.

The point here is not to arbitrate about which group in society is more correct in those arguments. Rather it is to highlight that ultimately it is a matter of judgement. Disease and health are socially contested, not self-evident in their appearance. For example, the 'happiness' agenda is essentially a socio-political one, which appeals to economists and politicians (because it implicates such matters as productivity, fiscal burden and even voting behaviour). Psychiatrists, clinical psychologists and psychotherapists have been keen to support and reinforce this discourse because it raises their status and expands their jurisdiction. However, orthopaedic surgeons may be more opposed to the pathologization, rather than the normalization, of misery, and so too might Buddhists. The latter consider that suffering is part of the human condition and dealing with it is a recurring human challenge, not an abnormal state inviting professional expertise or understanding.

At this point we encounter a contestable assumption in the professional literature, particularly about mental health: the drive to improve 'mental health literacy'. This has emerged as one attempt, mainly by social psychiatrists, to reduce stigma in community settings of workplaces and neighbourhoods by increasing lay people's understanding of 'knowledge and beliefs about mental disorders, which aid their recognition, management and prevention' (Goldney *et al.* 2001: 278). The argument advanced is that the more that the general public understands about the nature of mental illness, then the less that stigma and discrimination will occur.

The problem with the cogency of this type of campaigning, as an aspect of a public mental health policy, is that it assumes that the nature of mental illness or mental health has been resolved, when clearly it has not. The phrase 'knowledge and beliefs', from Goldney and colleagues above, denoted a separation between professionals (knowledgeable) and lay people (driven more by ignorance and prejudicial beliefs). This simple division can be challenged when we overview the contestation involved in the topic of this book. The professional view about our topic has been a source of constant dispute and controversy (see Chapter 1). In this light, what precisely is 'mental health literacy'?

To offer 'mental health literacy' (and indeed 'health literacy' generally), as an assured public-information campaign ignores or denies the lack of *professional* consensus in the field. Of course, to argue as a general principle that we should be more trusting and accepting of those different from us might be a worthy injunction in most situations in society. However, to *justify* that moral appeal on grounds of a form of knowledge that is highly contested is less compelling. At present, there is simply too much uncertainty about both ontology and epistemology in our field of interest to make clear distinctions between 'knowledge and beliefs'. Moreover, stigma is not just linked to lay views: for many patients, psychiatric diagnosis and service contact are themselves stigmatizing, a point overlooked at times by the psychiatric profession (Pilgrim and Rogers 2005).

Discussion

As far as the debates about mental health are concerned, in this book we have encountered a number of arguments.

- The first implied by the emphasis on the determination and thus potential prevention of madness and misery is that a good society would be one in which these expressions of psychological difference should be eliminated or minimized. Social measures from poverty reduction to birth control could be used to ensure the latter. Psychological deviance is seen as a problem to be solved and dealt with, not accepted.
- The second is that we should be more concerned with some deviations than others. For example, maybe the 'major mental illnesses' are true diseases warranting professional

expertise but other labelled mental disorder is simple residual deviance to be coped with or ignored or dealt with as a point about variations on our well-being. In other words, categories are warranted about madness but continua are implied about misery. This position implies the need to offer treatment services for the mentally abnormal and forms of social organization which would maximize happiness for the rest of us.

- The third is that madness and misery simply exist and that they are potential sources of meaning. We know something of the origins of mental abnormality but still much is a matter of debate and supposition; the work of the 'anti-psychiatrists' (drawing on existentialism) and 'post-psychiatrists' (drawing on post-structuralism) had this emphasis. For example, David Cooper argued that madness and true sanity are very near to one another and they are equidistant from 'normality' in capitalist societies (Cooper 1968). Michel Foucault pointed up the loss of meaning, when there was a breakdown in communication between sanity and madness, after the Enlightenment, and historians have noted that in antiquity madness was considered to be a gift from the gods (Screech 1985).

In more recent times organizations such as 'Mad Pride' exemplify this position, which resonates with that from activists in the disability movement (that they do not want to be made 'normal'). Madness might be liberated not cured. But if so, how would a diverse range of moral orders, in which the balance of rationality and non-rationality was permitted, alter the look of our current form of social organization? The latter is mainly based upon the premise of a single moral order for the majority, who are sane by common consent, which then in progressive mode seeks to 'socially include' those who are not and, when not, stigmatizes and excludes them. This single-majority-moral-order position may have seen rationality predominate but it has also witnessed recurring warfare, ongoing ecological degradation and socio-economic collapse. What then is a 'rational' society? Is it what Fromm (1944) called the 'pathology of normalcy'?

These three positions are clearly different options or political ambitions to consider and return us to different views about eudaimonia and what we might mean by 'public mental health'. The first is broadly eugenic, i.e. we might eliminate by prevention or treatment that which offends our current view of a more efficient and less troublesome society. The second is broadly paternalistic, offering treatment for the sick and well-being for the rest. The third is broadly libertarian: it seeks to maximize the right to be different. Given these discrepant value positions, currently there is no single platform from which to launch a campaign for improved 'mental health literacy', noted earlier, or to set out a single blueprint for a public mental health policy.

Questions

1 Should happiness be classified as a psychiatric disorder?
2 What is the relationship between material wealth and well-being?
3 What contribution does social capital make to public mental health?
4 What is 'mental health literacy' and what problems are associated with the term?
5 Is the truism of 'healthy body, healthy mind' well founded?
6 What role does alcohol use have in limiting public mental health?

For discussion

If you were in government what policies would you develop to improve the mental health of the population? Consider this question from the perspective of different social groups.

References

Abel, B. (1988) *The British Legal Profession*. Oxford: Blackwell.

Abel, G., Becker, J., Mittleman, M. *et al.* (1987) Self-reported sex crimes of nonincarcerated paraphiliacs. *Journal of Interpersonal Violence*, 2(1): 3–25.

Abraham, J. and Sheppard, J. (1998) International comparative analysis and explanation in medical sociology: demystifying the Halcion anomaly. *Sociology*, 32(1): 141–62.

Abramson, M. (1972) The criminalisation of mentally disordered behaviour: possible side effects of a new mental health law. *Hospital and Community Psychiatry*, 23(3): 101–5.

Adame, A.L. and Knudson, R.M. (2008) Recovery and the good life: how psychiatric survivors are revisioning the healing process. *Journal of Humanistic Psychology*, 48(2): 142–64.

Addis, S., Davies, M., Greene, G. *et al.* (2009) The health, social care and housing needs of lesbian, gay, bisexual and transgender older people: a review of the literature. *Health and Social Care in the Community*, 17(6): 647–58.

Adorno, T.W., Frenkel-Brunswik, E., Levinson, D.J. and Sanford, R.N. (1950) *The Authoritarian Personality*. New York: Harper and Brothers.

AGE UK (2010). *Loneliness and Isolation Evidence Review*. London: AGE UK.

Ahmad, W. and Bradby, H. (eds) (2005) *Ethnicity, Health and Health Care*. London: Blackwell.

Ahmad, W.I.U. and Bradby, H. (2007) Locating ethnicity and health: exploring concepts and contexts. *Sociology of Health and Illness*, 29(6): 795–810.

Ahmad, W.I.U., Atkin, K. and Jones, L. (2002) (Re) constructing multiracial blackness: women's activism, difference and collective identity in Britain. *Social Science and Medicine*, 5(10): 1757–69.

Albee G.H. (1996) Revolutions and counter revolutions in prevention. *American Psychologist*, 51(11): 1130–3.

Albrecht, G., Walker, V. and Levy, J. (1982) Social distance from the stigmatized: a test of two theories. *Social Science and Medicine*, 16: 1319–27.

Alemi, F., Mosavel, M., Stephens, R. *et al.* (1996) Electronic self-help and support groups. *Medical Care*, 34(10): 32–44.

Alexander, L.A. and Link, B.G. (2003) The impact of contact on stigmatizing attitudes toward people with mental illness. *Journal of Mental Health*, 12(3): 271–90.

Alexander, M.J., Haugland, G., Ashenden, P. *et al.* (2009) Coping with thoughts of suicide: techniques used by consumers of mental health services. *Psychiatric Services*, 60(9): 1214–21.

Al-Issa, I. (1977) Social and cultural aspects of hallucinations. *Psychological Bulletin*, 84: 570–87.

Al-Issa, I. (1987) Gender roles, in L. Diamant (ed.) *Male and Female Homosexuality: Psychological Approaches*. New York: Hemisphere.

Allison, T.R., Symmons, D.P., Brammah, T. *et al.* (2002) Musculoskeletal pain is more generalised among people from ethnic minorities than among white people in Greater Manchester. *Annals of Rheumatic Disorders*, 61(2): 151–6.

Allsop, J. (2002) Regulation and the medical profession, in J. Allsop and M. Saks (eds) *Regulating the Health Professions*. London: SAGE.

Almog, M., Curtis, S., Copeland, A. *et al.* (2004) Geographical variation in acute psychiatric admissions within New York City 1990–2000: growing inequalities in service use? *Social Science and Medicine*, 59(2): 361–76.

Alston, M. and Kent, J. (2008) The big dry: the link between rural masculinities and poor health outcomes for farming men *Journal of Sociology*, 44(2): 133–47.

Althusser, L. (1971) *Lenin and Philosophy and Other Essays*. London: New Left Books.

American Psychiatric Association (APA) (1994) *Diagnostic and Statistical Manual of Mental Disorders*. Washington, DC: APA.

Angermeyer, M.C. and Schulze, B. (2001) Reinforcing stereotypes: how the focus on forensic cases in news reporting may influence public attitudes towards the mentally ill. *International Journal of Law and Psychiatry*, 24(4–5): 469–86.

Anthony, W.A. (1993) Recovery from mental illness: the guiding vision of the mental health system in the 1990s. *Psychosocial Rehabilitation Journal*, 16: 11.

Appelbaum, P.S., Robbins, P.C. and Roth, L.H. (1999) A dimensional approach to delusions: comparisons across delusion type and diagnoses. *American Journal of Psychiatry*, 156: 1938–43.

Appelbaum, P.S., Robbins, P.C. and Monahan, J. (2000) Violence and delusions: data from the

MacArthur Violence Risk Assessment Study. *American Journal of Psychiatry*, 157(4): 566–72.

Araya, R., Dunstan, F., Playle, R., Thomas, H., Palmer, S. and Lewis, G. (2006) Perceptions of social capital and the built environment and mental health. *Social Science and Medicine*, 62: 3072–83.

Arber, S. and Ginn, J. (1991) *Gender and Later Life*. London: SAGE.

Archer, M. (1995) *Realist Social Theory: The Morphogenetic Approach*: Cambridge: Cambridge University Press.

Armstrong, D. (1980) Madness and coping. *Sociology of Health and Illness*, 2(3): 393–413.

Armstrong, S. (2002) The emergence and implications of a mental health ethos in juvenile justice. *Sociology of Health and Illness*, 24: 599–620.

Atkinson, P. (1983) The reproduction of the professional community, in R. Dingwall and P. Lewis (eds) *The Sociology of the Professions*. London: Macmillan.

Audit Commission (1986) *Making a Reality of Community Care*. London: HMSO.

Babiak, P. and Hare, R.D. (2007) *Snakes in Suits: When Psychopaths go to Work*. New York: Harper Collins.

Backett, K. and Davison, C. (1995) Lifecourses and life style: the social and cultural location of health behaviour. *Social Science and Medicine*, 40(5): 629–38.

Backett-Milburn, K., Cunningham-Burley, S. and Davis, J. (2003) Contrasting lives, contrasting views? Understandings of health inequalities from children in differing social circumstances. *Social Science and Medicine*, 57(4): 613–23.

Badesha, J. and Horley, J. (2000) Self-construal among psychiatric outpatients: a test of the golden section. *British Journal of Medical Psychology*, 73(4): 547–51.

Baker, A.W. and Duncan, S.P. (1985) Child sexual abuse: a study of prevalence in Great Britain. *Child Abuse and Neglect*, 9: 457–67.

Baker, M. and Menken, M. (2001) Time to abandon mental illness. *British Journal of Medicine*, 322: 937.

Baldwin, D. and Thompson, C. (2003) The future of antidepressant pharmacotherapy. *World Psychiatry*, 2(1): 3–8.

Bannister, D. (1968) The logical requirements of research into schizophrenia. *British Journal of Psychiatry*, 114: 1088–97.

Bannister, D. and Fransella, F. (1970) *Inquiring Man*. Harmondsworth: Penguin.

Barbato, A., D'Avanzo, B., Rocca, G., Amatulli, A. and Lampugnani, D. (2004) A study of long-stay patients resettled in the community after closure of a psychiatric hospital in Italy. *Psychiatric Services*, 55(1): 839–50.

Barham, P. and Hayward, R. (1991) *From the Mental Patient to the Person*. London: Routledge.

Barker, C. and Pistrang, N. (2002) Psychotherapy and social support: integrating research on psychological helping. *Clinical Psychology Review*, 22(3): 361–79.

Barnes, C. and Mercer, G. (eds) (2004) *Implementing the Social Model of Disability: Theory and Research*. Leeds: Disability Press.

Barr, M. and Rose, D. (2008) The great ambivalence: factors likely to affect service users and public acceptability of the pharmacogenomics of antidepressant medication. *Sociology of Health and Illness Special Issue. Pharmaceuticals and Society: Critical Discourses and Debates*, 30: 944–58.

Barrett, M. and Roberts, H. (1978) Doctors and their patients, in H. Smart and B. Smart (eds) *Women, Sexuality and Social Control*. London: Routledge and Kegan Paul.

Bartley, M., Davey Smith, G. and Blane, D. (1997) Vital comparisons: the social construction of mortality measurement, in M.A. Elston (ed.) *The Sociology of Medical Science and Technology*. Oxford: Blackwell.

Bartley, M., Blane, D. and Davey Smith, G. (1998) Beyond the Black Report. *Sociology of Health and Illness*, 20(5): 563–77.

Barton, W.R. (1959) *Institutional Neurosis*. Bristol: Wright and Sons.

Baruch, G. and Treacher, A. (1978) *Psychiatry Observed*. London: Routledge and Kegan Paul.

Basaglia, F. (1964) *The Destruction of the Mental Hospital as a Place of Institutionalisation: Thoughts Caused by Personal Experience with the Open Door System and Part Time Service*. London: First International Congress of Social Psychiatry.

Bassuk, E., Rubin, L. and Lauriat, A. (1984) Is homelessness a mental health problem? *American Journal of Psychiatry*, 141: 1546–50.

Bateson, G. (1980). *Mind and Nature: A Necessary Unity*. New York: Bantam Books

Bayer, R. and Spitzer, R.L. (1985) Neurosis, psychodynamics and DSM-III: a history of the controversy. *Archives of General Psychiatry*, 42: 187–96.

Bean, P. (1980) *Compulsory Admissions to Mental Hospital*. Chichester: Wiley.

Bean, P. (1986) *Mental Disorder and Legal Control.* Cambridge: Cambridge University Press.

Bean, P., Bingley, W., Bynoe, I. *et al.* (1991) *Out of Harm's Way: MIND's Research into Police and Psychiatric Action Under Section 136 of the Mental Health Act.* London: MIND.

Bebbington, P.E., Hurry, J. and Tennant, C. (1981) Psychiatric disorders in selected immigrant groups in Camberwell. *Social Psychiatry,* 16: 43–51.

Beck, A.T. (1970) Cognitive therapy: nature and relation to behaviour therapy. *Behaviour Therapy,* 1: 184–200.

Beck, U. and Beck-Gersheim, E. (1995) *The Normal Chaos of Love.* Oxford: Polity Press.

Becker, J.V. (1988) The effects of child sexual abuse on adolescent sexual offenders, in G.E. Wyatt and G.J. Powell (eds) *Lasting Effects of Child Sexual Abuse.* Thousand Oaks, CA: SAGE.

Beck-Sander, A. (1998) Is insight into psychosis meaningful? *Journal of Mental Health,* 7(1): 25–34.

Beecham, J., Ramsay, A., Gordon, K., Maltby, S., Walshie, K., Shaw, I., Worrall, A. and King, S. (2010). Cost and impact of a quality improvement programme in mental health services. *Journal of Health Services Research & Policy,* 15(2): 69–75.

Beliappa, J. (1991) *Illness or Distress? Alternative Models of Mental Health.* London: Confederation of Indian Organizations.

Bendelow, G. (2009) *Health Emotions and the Body.* Cambridge: Polity Press.

Bendalow, G. and Williams, S. (1998) *Emotions in Social Life: Critical Themes and Contemporary Issues.* London: Routledge.

Bentall, R.P. (1992) A proposal to classify happiness as a psychiatric disorder. *Journal of Medical Ethics,* 18(2): 94–8.

Bentall, R.P. (2003) *Understanding Madness: Psychosis and Human Nature.* London: Penguin.

Bentall, R.P. and Morrison, A.P. (2002) More harm than good: the case against neuroleptics to prevent psychosis. *Journal of Mental Health,* 11: 351–6.

Bentall, R.P. and Pilgrim, D. (1993) Thomas Szasz, crazy talk and the myth of mental illness. *British Journal of Medical Psychology,* 66: 69–76.

Bentall, R.P. and Slade, P. (1985) Reality testing and auditory hallucinations: a signal detection analysis. *British Journal of Clinical Psychology,* 24: 159–69.

Bentall, R.P., Jackson, H. and Pilgrim, D. (1988) Abandoning the concept of schizophrenia: some impli-
cations of validity arguments for psychological research into psychotic phenomena. *British Journal of Clinical Psychology,* 27: 303–24.

Benton, T. (1991) Biology and social science: why the return of the repressed should be given a (cautious) welcome *Sociology* 25(1): 1–29.

Benyemanini, Y. *et al.* (2000) Positive affect and function as influences on self-assessment of health. *Journal of Gerontology,* 55(8): 107–16.

Benzeval, M., Green, M.J. and Macintyre, S. (2013) Does perceived physical attractiveness in adolescence predict better socioeconomic position in adulthood? Evidence from 20 years of follow up in a population cohort study. *PLoS ONE,* 8(5): e63975.

Beresford, P. (2003) *Its Our Lives: A Short Theory of Knowledge, Distance and Experience.* London: Citizen Press in association with Shaping Our Lives.

Beresford, P. (2005) Developing self-defined social approaches to distress, in S. Ramon and J. Williams (eds) *Mental Health at the Crossroads: The Promise of the Psychosocial Approach.* London: Ashgate.

Bergin, A.E. (1971) The evaluation of therapeutic outcomes, in A.E. Bergin and S. Garfield (eds) *Handbook of Psychotherapy and Behavior Change.* New York: Wiley.

Bergin, A.E. and Lambert, M. (1978) The evaluation of therapeutic outcomes, in S. Garfield and A. Bergin (eds) *Handbook of Psychotherapy and Behavior Change,* 2nd edn. Chichester: Wiley.

Berrios, G.E. (1985) Obsessional disorders during the nineteenth century: terminological and classificatory issues, in W.F. Bynum, R. Porter and M. Shepherd (eds) *The Anatomy of Madness* (Volume 1). London: Tavistock.

Berzins, K. and Atkinson, J. (2009) Service users' and carers' views of the Named Persons Provisions under the Mental Health (Care and Treatment) Scotland Act 2003. *Journal of Mental Health,* 18(3): 207–15.

Bhaskar, R. (1978) *A Realist Theory of Science.* Hassocks: Harvester.

Bhaskar, R. (1989) *Reclaiming Reality.* London: Verso.

Bhui, K. and Bhugra, D. (2001) Transcultural psychiatry: some social and epidemiological research issues. *International Journal of Social Psychiatry,* 47(3): 1–9.

Bhui, K., Stansfeld, S., Hull, S., Preibe, S., Mole, T. and Feder, G. (2003) Ethnic variations in pathways to and use of specialist mental health services in the UK. *British Journal of Psychiatry*, 82: 105–16.

Biafora, F. (1995) Cross cultural perspectives on illness and wellness: implications for depression. *Journal of Social Distress and the Homeless*, 4(2): 105–29.

Biddle, L., Donovan, J., Sharp, D. *et al.* (2007) Explaining non-help-seeking amongst young adults with mental distress: a dynamic interpretive model of illness behaviour. *Sociology of Health and Illness*, 29(7): 983–1002.

Biddle, L., Brock, A., Brookes, S.T. *et al.* (2008) When things fall apart: gender and suicide across the life-course. Suicide rates in young men in England and Wales in the 21st century: time trend study. *British Medical Journal*, 336: 539–42.

Bifulco, A., Harris, T.O. and Brown, G.W. (1992) Mourning or inadequate care? Reexamining the relationship of maternal loss in childhood with adult depression and anxiety. *Development and Psychopathology*, 4: 119–28.

Bion, W.R. (1959) *Experiences in Groups*. New York: Basic Books.

Birmingham, L. (1999) Prison officers can recognise hidden psychiatric morbidity in prisoners. *British Medical Journal*, 319: 853.

Birmingham, L. (2002) Doctors working in prisons. *British Medical Journal*, 324: 440.

Blackburn, R. (1988) On moral judgements and personality disorders: the myth of psychopathic disorder re-visited. *British Journal of Psychiatry*, 153: 505–12.

Blackman, J. (2010) *Get the Diagnosis Right!* New York: Routledge.

Blashfield, R. (1982) Feighner et al: invisible colleges and the Mathew Effect *Schizophrenia Bulletin*, 8: 1–12.

Blaxter, M. (1990) *Health and Lifestyles*. London: Routledge.

Blaxter, M. (1997) Whose fault is it? People's own conceptions of the reasons for health inequalities. *Social Science and Medicine*, 44(6): 747–56.

Blom-Cooper, L., Brown, M., Dolan, R. and Murphy, E. (1992) *Report of the Committee of Inquiry into Complaints about Ashworth Hospital*, Cm2028. London: HMSO.

Blumenthal, S. and Lavender, T. (2000) *Violence and Mental Disorder: A Critical Aid to the Assessment and Management of Risk*. London: Zito Trust.

Bolam, B., Murphy, S. and Gleeson, K. (2004) Individualisation and inequalities in health: a qualitative study of class identity and health. *Social Science and Medicine*, 59(7): 1355–65.

Bolton, P. (1984) Management of compulsorily admitted patients to a high security unit. *International Journal of Social Psychiatry*, 30: 77–84.

Bolzan, N. and Gale, F. (2002) The citizenship of excluded groups: challenging the consumerist agenda. *Social Policy and Administration*, 36(4): 363–75.

Borsch-Supan, A. and Schuth, M. (2013) Early retirement, mental health and social networks, in D.A. Wise (ed.) *Discoveries in the Economics of Aging*. Chicago: University of Chicago Press, available at www.nber.org/chapters/c12982.pdf (accessed 21 January 2014).

Bourdieu, P. (1997) The forms of capital, in J. Richardson (ed.) *Handbook of Theory and Research for the Sociology of Education*. New York: Greenwood Press.

Bowen, A., Rogers, A. and Shaw, J. (2009) Medication management and practices in prison for people with mental health problems: a qualitative study. *International Journal of Mental Health Systems*, 3: 24.

Bowers, L. (1998) *The Social Nature of Mental Illness*. London: Routledge.

Bowl, R. (1996) Legislating for user involvement in the United Kingdom mental health services and the NHS and Community Care Act. *International Journal of Social Psychiatry*, 42(3): 165–80.

Bowlby, J. (1951) *Maternal Care and Mental Health*. Geneva: World Health Organization.

Boydell, J., van Os, J., McKenzie, K. *et al.* (2001) Incidence of schizophrenia in ethnic minorities in London: ecological study into interactions with environment. *British Medical Journal*, 323: 1336.

Boyle, M. (1991) *Schizophrenia: A Scientific Delusion*. London: Routledge.

Boynton, J. (1980) *Report of the Review of Rampton Hospital*, Cmnd 8073. London: HMSO.

Bracken, P. and Thomas, P. (2001) Post psychiatry: a new direction for mental health, *British Journal of Psychiatry*, 322: 724–7.

Bradley K. (2009) *The Bradley Report: Lord Bradley's Review of People with Mental Health Problems or Learning Disabilities in the Criminal Justice System*. London: Department of Health.

Braginsky, B.M., Braginsky, D.D. and Ring, K. (1973) *Methods of Madness: The Mental Hospital as a Last Resort*. New York: Holt, Rinehart and Winston.

Braithwaite, J. (1989) *Crime, Shame and Reintegration*. Cambridge: Cambridge University Press.

Brakel, J., Parry, J. and Weiner, B. (1985) *The Mentally Disabled and the Law*. Chicago: American Bar Foundation.

Brayne, C. and Ames, D. (1988) The epidemiology of mental disorders in old age, in B. Gearing, M. Johnson and T. Heller (eds) *Mental Health Problems in Old Age*. London: Wiley.

Breeding, J. and Bauman, F. (2001) The ethics of informed parental consent to the psychiatric drugging of children. *Ethical Human Science Services*, 3(3): 175–88.

Breggin, P. (1993) *Toxic Psychiatry*. London: HarperCollins.

Breggin, P.R. (1994) Should the use of neuroleptics be severely limited? in S.A. Kirk and S.D. Einbinder (eds) *Controversial Issues in Mental Health*. Cambridge: Cambridge University Press.

Bresnahan, M., Begg, M.D., Brown, A., Schaefer, C., Sohler, N., Insel, B., Vella, L. and Susser E. (2007) Race and risk of schizophrenia in a US birth cohort: another example of health disparity? *International Journal of Epidemiology*, 36: 751–8.

Briere, J. and Runtz, M. (1987) Post-sexual abuse trauma: data implications for clinical practice. *Journal of Interpersonal Violence*, 2: 367–79.

British Psychological Society. (2011) Response to the American Psychiatric Association: DSM–5 development. Retrieved from http://apps.bps. org.uk/_publicationfiles/consultation-responses/ DSM-5%202011%20-%20BPS%20response.pdf (accessed 21 January 2014).

Britten, N. (1991) Hospital consultants' views of their patients. *Sociology of Health and Illness*, 13(1): 83–97.

Brooker, C., Sirdifield, C., Blizard, R., Denney, D. and Pluck, G. (2012) Probation and mental illness. *Journal of Forensic Psychiatry and Psychology*, 23(4): 522–37.

Broverman, D., Clarkson, F., Rosenkratz, P. *et al.* (1970) Sex role stereotypes and clinical judgements of mental health. *Journal of Consulting and Clinical Psychology*, 34: 1–7.

Brown, G.W. (1959) Experiences of discharged chronic schizophrenic patients in various types of living group. *Millbank Memorial Fund Quarterly*, 37: 105.

Brown, G.W. (1996) Onset and course of depressive disorders: summary of a research programme, in C. Mundt, M. Goldstein, K. Hahlweg and P. Fiedler (eds) *Interpersonal Factors in the Origin and Course of Affective Disorders*. London: Gaskell.

Brown, G.W. and Harris, T.O. (1978) *The Social Origins of Depression*. London: Tavistock.

Brown, G.W. and Moran, P.M. (1997) Single mothers, poverty and depression. *Psychological Medicine*, 27(1): 21–33.

Brown, G.W. and Wing, J.K. (1962) A comparative clinical and social survey of three mental hospitals. *The Sociological Review Monograph*, 5: 145–71.

Brown, G.W., Harris, T.O. and Bifulco, A. (1986) Long term effects of early loss of parent, in M. Rutter, C. Izard and P. Read (eds) *Depression in Childhood: Developmental Perspectives*. New York: Guilford Press.

Brown, G.W., Harris, T.O. and Hepworth, C. (1995) Loss, humiliation and entrapment among women developing depression: a patient and non-patient comparison. *Psychological Medicine*, 25: 7–21.

Brown, J.F. (2001) *The Grooves of Change: Eastern Europe at the Turn of Millennium*. Durham, NC: Duke University Press.

Brown, P. (1995) Naming and framing: the social construction of diagnosis and illness. *Journal of Health and Social Behaviour*, Extra Issue: 34–52.

Brown, P. and Funk, S.C. (1986) Tardive dyskinesia: barriers to the professional recognition of iatrogenic disease. *Journal of Health and Social Behaviour*, 27: 116–32.

Brown, P. and Zaverstoski, S. (2004) Social movements in health. *Sociology of Health and Illness*, 26(6): 679–94.

Brown, T.N. (2003) Critical race theory speaks to the sociology of mental health: mental health problems produced by social stratification. *Journal of Health and Social Behavior*, 44(3): 292–301.

Browne, A. and Finklehor, D. (1986) Impact of child sexual abuse: a review of the research. *Psychological Bulletin*, 99: 66–77.

Browne, D. (1990) *Black People, Mental Health and the Courts*. London: NACRO.

Browning, C.R. and Cagney, K.A. (2003) Moving beyond poverty: neighborhood structure, social processes and health. *Journal of Health and Social Behavior*, 44(4): 552–71.

Bullough, V.L. (1987) The first clinicians, in L. Diamant (ed.) *Male and Female Homosexuality: Psychological Approaches*. New York: Hemisphere.

Burstow, B. and Weitz, D. (eds) (1988) *Shrink Resistant: The Struggle Against Psychiatry in Canada*. Vancouver: New Star.

Burns, T., Rugkåsa, J., Molodynski, A. *et al.* (2013) Community treatment orders for patients with psychosis (OCTET): a randomised controlled trial. *The Lancet*, 381 (9878): 1627–33.

Bury, M. (1986) Social constructionism and the development of medical sociology. *Sociology of Health and Illness*, 8: 137–69.

Bury, M. and Gabe, J. (1990) Hooked? Media responses to tranquillizer dependence, in P. Abbott and G. Payne (eds) *New Directions in the Sociology of Health*. London: Falmer Press.

Buss, A.H. (1966) *Psychopathology*. New York: Wiley.

Cahill, C., Llewelyn, S.P. and Pearson, C. (1991) Long term aspects of sexual abuse which occurred in childhood: a review. *British Journal of Clinical Psychology*, 30: 117–30.

Calton, T., Ferriter, M., Huband, N. and Spandler, H.(2007) A systematic review of the Soteria paradigm for the treatment of people diagnosed with schizophrenia. *Schizophrenia Bulletin*, 34(1): 181–92.

Cameron, E. and Bernardes, J. (1998) Gender and disadvantage in health: men's health for a change. *Sociology of Health and Illness*, 20(5): 673–93.

Camp, D.L., Finlay, W.M.L. and Lyons, E. (2002) Is low self-esteem an inevitable consequence of stigma? An example from women with chronic mental health problems. *Social Science and Medicine*, 55(5): 823–34.

Campbell, J. and Schraiber, R. (1989) *In Pursuit of Wellness: The Well-Being Project*. Sacramento: The California Department of Mental Health.

Campbell, P. (1987) Giants and goblins: a description of Camden Consortium's campaign to change statutory plans, in I. Barker and E. Peck (eds) *Power in Strange Places: User Empowerment in Mental Health Services*. London: Good Practices in Mental Health.

Campbell, P. (1996) The history of the User Movement in the United Kingdom, in T. Heller, J. Reynolds, R. Gomm, R. Muston and S. Pattison (eds) *Mental Health Matters: A Reader*. Buckingham: Open University Press.

Campbell, P. and Roberts, A. (2009) Survivors' history. *A Life In the Day*, 13: 3 August.

Campbell, T. and Heginbotham, C. (1991) *Mental Illness, Prejudice, Discrimination and the Law*. Aldershot: Dartmouth.

Campbell, S.M., Shield, T., Rogers, A.E. and Gask, L.L. (2004). How do stakeholder groups vary in a Delphi technique about primary mental health care and what factors influence their ratings. *Quality & Safety in Health Care*, 13(6): 428–34.

Cantor-Grae, E., Zolkowska, K. and McNeill, T.F. (2005) Increased risk of psychotic disorder in Malmo: a 3-year first contact study. *Psychological Medicine* 35: 1155–63.

Carchedi, G. (1975) On the economic identification of the new middle class. *Economy and Society*, 4(1): 1–85.

Carlezon, W.A. and Konradi, C. (2004) Understanding the neurobiological consequences of early exposure to psychotropic drugs: linking behavior to molecules. *Neuropharmacology*, 47(1): 47–60.

Carpenter, J. and Sbaraini, S. (1997) *Choice, Information and Dignity: Involving Users and Carers in Care Management in Mental Health*. London: Policy Press.

Carpenter, L. and Brockington, I. (1980) A study of mental illness in Asians, West Indians and Africans living in Manchester. *British Journal of Psychiatry*, 137: 201–5.

Carpenter, M. (1980) Asylum nursing before 1914: a chapter in the history of nursing, in C. Davies (ed.) *Re-writing Nursing History*. London: Croom Helm.

Carpenter, M. (2000) 'It's a small world': mental health policy under welfare capitalism since 1945. *Sociology of Health and Illness*, 22(5): 602–19.

Carrick, R., Mitchell, A., Powell, R.A. and Lloyd, K. (2004) The quest for well-being: a qualitative study of the experience of taking antipsychotic medication. *Psychology and Psychotherapy: Theory Research and Practice*, 77: 19–33.

Carstairs, G.M. and Kapur, R.C. (1976) *The Great Universe of Kota: Stress, Change and Mental Disorder in an Indian Village*. London: Hogarth Press.

Cassel, J. (1976) The contribution of host environment to host resistance. *American Journal of Epidemiology*, 14: 107–23.

Castel, F., Castel, R. and Lovell, A. (1979) *The Psychiatric Society*. New York: Columbia Free Press.

Castel, R. (1983) Moral treatment: mental therapy and social control in the nineteenth century, in S. Cohen and A. Scull (eds) *Social Control and the State*. Oxford: Basil Blackwell.

Chadwick, P. (1997) *Schizophrenia: The Positive Perspective*. London: Routledge.

Chamberlin, J. (1988) *On Our Own*. London: MIND Publications.

Chang, C.-K., Hayes, R.D., Perera, G. *et al.* (2011) Life expectancy at birth for people with serious mental illness and other major disorders from a secondary mental health care case register in london. *PLoS ONE*, 6(5): e19590.

Chatzitheochari, S. and Arber, S. (2012) Gender, class and time poverty: a time use analysis of British workers' free time researches. *British Journal of Sociology*, 63(3): 451–71.

Chen, E., Harrison, G. and Standen, P. (1991) Management of first episode psychotic illness in Afro-Caribbean patients. *British Journal of Psychiatry*, 158: 517–22.

Cheshire, K. and Pilgrim, D. (2004) *A Short Introduction to Clinical Psychology*. London: Sage.

Chesler, P. (1972) *Women and Madness*. New York: Doubleday.

Chew-Graham, C., Kovandžic, M., Gask, L. *et al.* (2012) Why may older people with depression not present to primary care? Messages from secondary analysis of qualitaive data. *Health & Social Care in the Community*, 20(1): 55–60.

Chew-Graham, C.A., Mullin, S., May, C.R., Hedley, S. and Cole, H. (2008) Managing depression in primary care: another example of the inverse care law? *Family Practice*, 9: 632–7.

Ciompi, L. (1984) Is there really a schizophrenia? The long term course of psychotic phenomena. *British Journal of Psychiatry*, 145: 636–40.

Clare, A. (1976) *Psychiatry in Dissent*. London: Tavistock.

Clausen, J.A. and Kohn, M.L. (1959) Relation of schizophrenia to the social structure of a small city, in B. Pasamanick (ed.) *Epidemiology of Mental Disorders*. Washington, DC: American Association for the Advancement of Science.

Cleckley, H. (1941) *The Mask of Sanity*. St Louis, MS: C.V. Mosby.

Cleary, M., Feeeman, A., Hunt, G.E. and Walter, G. (2006) Patient and Carer Perceptions of Need and Associations with Care-Giving Burden in an Integrated Adult Mental Health Service. *Social Psychiatry and Psychiatric Epidemiology*, 40(3): 208–14.

Clegg, S.R. (1990) *Modern Organisations*. London: Sage.

Cobb, S. (1976) Social support as a moderator of life stress. *Psychosomatic Medicine*, 8: 300–14.

Cochrane, R. (1983) *The Social Creation of Mental Illness*. London: Longman.

Cohen, D. (1989) *Soviet Psychiatry*. London: Paladin.

Cohen, D. (1997) A critique of the use of neuroleptic drugs in psychiatry, in S. Fisher and R.P. Greenberg (eds) *From Placebo to Panacea*. New York: Wiley.

Cohen, D. and Prusak, L. (2001) *In Good Company: How Social Capital Makes Organizations Work*. Boston: Harvard Business School Press.

Cohen, D., McCubbin, M., Collin, J. and Perodeau, G. (2001) Medications as social phenomena. *Health*, 4: 441–69.

Cole, M.G. and Bellavance, F. (1997) Depression in elderly inpatients: a meta-analysis of outcomes. *Canadian Medical Association Journal*, 15(157): 1055–60.

Colletta, J.J. and Cullen, M.L. (2000) *Violent Conflict and the Transformation of Social Capital*. Washington, DC: International Bank for Reconstruction and Development/World Bank.

Collins, P.Y, von Unger, H. and Armbrister, A. (2008) Church ladies, good girls, and locas: stigma and the intersection of gender, ethnicity, mental illness, and sexuality in relation to HIV risk. *Social Science and Medicine*, 67(3): 389–97.

Collins, P.Y., Patel, V., Joestl, S. *et al.* (2011) Grand challenges in global mental health. *Nature*, 475(7354): 27–30.

Colombo, T., Bendelow, G., Fulford, B. and Williams, S. (2003) Evaluating the influence of implicit models of mental disorder on processes of shared decisions making within community based multi-disciplinary teams. *Social Science and Medicine*, 56: 1557–70.

Comas-Herrera, A., Wittenberg, R., Pickard, L. and Knapp, M. (2007) Cognitive impairment in older people: future demand for long-term care services and the associated costs. *International Journal of Geriatric Psychiatry*, 22: 1037–45.

Commander, M.J., Cochrane, R., Sashidaran, S.P., Akilu, F. and Wildsmith, E. (1999) Mental health care for Asian, black and white patients with non-affective psychoses: pathways to the psychiatric hospital, in-patient and after-care. *Social Psychiatry and Psychiatric Epidemiology*, 32(9): 484–91.

Cooper, D. (1968) *Psychiatry and Anti-Psychiatry*. London: Tavistock.

Cooperstock, R. (1978) Sex differences in psychotropic drug use. *Social Science and Medicine*, 12: 179–86.

Cope, R. (1989) The compulsory detention of Afro-Caribbeans under the Mental Health Act. *New Community*, 15(3): 343–56.

Copeland, J., Dewey, M., Wodd, N. *et al.* (1987) Range of mental illness among the elderly in the community. *British Journal of Psychiatry*, 150: 815–23.

Corbin, J. and Strauss, A. (1985) Managing chronic illness at home: three lines of work. *Qualitative Sociology*, 8: 224–7.

Corher, E., Hamilton, S., Wenderson, C. *et al.* (2013) Experiences of discrimination among people using mental health services in England (2008–2011). *The British Jornal of Psychiatry* 2000: 558–63.

Corrigan, P.W. (1998) The impact of stigma on severe mental illness. *Cognitive and Behavioral Practice*, 5(2): 201–22.

Corrigan, P. (2012) Research and the elimination of the stigma of mental illness. *The British Journal of Psychiatry*, 201: 7–8.

Corrigan, P.W. and Mathews, A.K. (2003) Stigma and disclosure: implications for coming out of the closet. *Journal of Mental Health*, 12(3): 235–48.

Coulter, J. (1973) *Approaches to Insanity*. New York: Wiley.

Craddock N., Antebi D., Attenburrow, M.J. *et al.* (2008) Wake-up call for British psychiatry. *British Journal of Psychiatry*, 193: 6–9.

Craib, I. (1997) Social constructionism as a social psychosis. *Sociology*, 31(1): 1–15.

Craib, I. (1998) *Experiencing Identity*. London: Sage.

Crawford, D. (1989) The future of clinical psychology: whither or wither? *Clinical Psychology Forum*, 20: 29–31.

Crawford, M.J., de Jonge, E., Freeman, G.K. and Weaver, T. (2004) Providing continuity of care for people with severe mental illness: a narrative review. *Social Psychiatry and Psychiatric Epidemiology*, 39(4): 265–72.

Crepaz-Keay, D., Binns, C. and Wilson, E. (1998) *Dancing With Angels: Involving Survivors in Mental Health Training*. London: CCETSW.

Crocetti, G., Spiro, H. and Siassi, I. (1974) *Contemporary Attitudes Towards Mental Illness*. Pittsburgh: University of Pittsburgh Press.

Crompton, R. (1987) Gender, status and professionalism. *Sociology*, 21(3): 413–28.

Crossley M.L. and Crossley, N. (2001) 'Patient' voices, social movements and the habitus: how psychiatric survivors 'speak out'. *Social Science and Medicine*, 52(10): 1477–89.

Crossley, N. (1999) Fish, field, habitus and madness: the first wave mental health users' movement. *British Journal of Sociology*, 50(4): 647–70.

Crow, T.J., MacMillan, J.F., Johnson, A.L. and Johnstone, E.C. (1986) The Northwick Park study of first episodes of schizophrenia II: a controlled trial of prophylactic neuroleptic treatment. *British Journal of Psychiatry*, 148: 120–7.

Cuffe, S.P., Waller, J.L., Cuccaro, M.L., Pumariega, A.J. and Garrison, C.Z. (1995) Race and gender differences in the treatment of psychiatric disorders in young adolescents. *Journal of the American Academy of Child and Adolescent Psychiatry*, 34(11): 1536–43.

Cullen, F.T. (1994) Social support as an organizing concept for criminology: presidential address to the Academy of Criminal Justice Science. *Justice Quarterly*, 11(4): 527–60.

Cullen, F.T. (1997) Can a prison be a therapeutic community? The Grendon template, in E. Cullen, L. Jones and R. Woodward (eds) *Therapeutic Communities for Offenders*. Chichester: Wiley.

Cumming, E. and Cumming, J. (1957) *Closed Ranks: An Experiment in Mental Health Education*. Cambridge, MA: Harvard University Press.

Currer, C. (1986) Concepts of well- and ill-being: the case of Pathan mothers in Britain, in C. Currer and M. Stacey (eds) *Concepts of Health, Illness and Disease*. Leamington Spa: Berg.

Curtis, S. and Jones, I. (1998) Is there a place for geography in the analysis of health inequality? *Sociology of Health and Illness*, 20(5): 645–72.

Danner, D.D., Snowdon, D.A. and Friesen, W.V. (2001) Positive emotions in early life and longevity: findings from the nun study. *Journal of Personality and Social Psychology*, 80: 804–13.

Das, A. and Rao, M. (2012) Universal mental health: re-evaluating the call for global mental health. *Critical Public Health*, 22(4): 383–9.

Das-Munshi, J., Goldberg, D., Bebbington, P.E. and Brugha, D.K. (2008) Public health significance of mixed anxiety and depression: beyond current classification. *British Journal of Psychiatry*, 192: 171–7.

Davidhazar, D. and Wehlage, D. (1984) Can the client with chronic schizophrenia consent to nursing research? *Journal of Advanced Nursing*, 9: 381–90.

Davis, A., Llewellyn, S.P. and Parry, G. (1985) Women and mental health: a guide for the approved social worker, in E. Brook and A. Davis (eds) *Women, the Family and Social Work*. London: Tavistock.

Davis, D. (2004) Dementia: sociological and philosophical constructions *Social Science & Medicine*, 58: 369–78.

Davey Smith, G., Shipley, M.J. and Rose, G. (1990) The magnitude and causes of socio-economic differentials in mortality: further evidence from the Whitehall studies. *Journal of Epidemiology and Community Health*, 44: 265–70.

Day, D.M. and Page, S. (1986) Portrayal of mental illnesses in Canadian newspapers. *Canadian Journal of Psychiatry*, 31: 813–17.

De Boer, F. (1991) Sex differences in the construction of mental health care problems. Paper presented at the British Sociological Association Medical Sociology Conference, York.

De Botton, A. (2004) *Status Anxiety*. London: Hamilton.

de la Cuesta, C. (1993) Fringe work: peripheral work in health visiting. *Sociology of Health and Illness*, 15(5): 665–82.

Dean, G., Walsh, D., Downing, H. and Shelly, P. (1981) First admission of native-born and immigrants to psychiatric hospitals in South-East England 1976. *British Journal of Psychiatry*, 139: 506–12.

Deegan, P. (1996) Recovery as a journey of the heart. *Psychiatric Rehabilitation Journal*, 19(3): 91–7.

DelVecchio Good, M.J., Hyde, S., Pinto, S. and Good, B. (2008) *Postcolonial Disorders*. Berkeley: University of California Press.

Dennis, D.L. and Monahan, J. (eds) (1996) *Coercion and Aggressive Community Treatment.* New York: Plenum Press.

Department of Health (1998) *Our Healthier Nation.* London: Department of Health.

Department of Health (2000) *The NHS Plan.* London: Department of Health.

Department of Health (2004) *Draft Mental Health Bill.* London: Department of Health.

Department of Health (2007) *Mental Health Act 2007.* London: HMSO.

Department of Health (2009) *Delivering 'Our Vision for Primary and Community Care'.* London: Crown Publishers.

Department of Health (2013) *Independent review into delegation of approval functions under the Mental Health Act 1983,* www.gov.uk/government/publications/independent-review-into-delegation-of-approval-functions-under-the-mental-health-act-1983 (accessed 25 November 2013).

Department of Health/Home Office (1999) *National Service Framework for Mental Health.* London: Department of Health.

De Swaan, A. (1990) *The Management of Normality.* London: Routledge.

DHSS (1980) *Inequalities in Health: Report of a Working Group* (the Black Report). London: HMSO.

DHSS (1988) *Community Care: Agenda for Action* (the Griffiths Report). London: HMSO.

Diala, C., Muntaner, C., Walrath, C., Nickerson, K.J., LaVeist, T.A. and Leaf, P.J. (2000) Racial differences in attitudes towards professional mental health care and in the use of services. *American Journal of Orthopsychiatry,* 70(4): 455–64.

Diamont, L. (1987) *Male and Female Homosexuality: Psychological Approaches.* New York: Hemisphere.

Dimock, P.T. (1988) Adult males sexually abused as children: characteristics and implications for treatment. *Journal of Interpersonal Violence,* 3: 203–21.

Dingwall, R., Tanaka, H. and Minamikata, S. (1991) Images of parenthood in the United Kingdom and Japan. *Sociology,* 25(3): 423–46.

Dinos, S., Lyons, E. and Finlay, W.M. (2005) Does chronic illness place constraints on positive construction of identity? Temporal comparisons and self evaluations in people with schizophrenia. *Social Science and Medicine,* 60: 2239–48.

Doherty, A.M. and Kelly, B. (2010) Social and psychological correlates of happiness in 17 European countries. *Irish Journal of Psychological Medicine,* 27(3): 130–4.

Doherty, A.M. and Kelly, B.D. (2013) When Irish eyes are smiling: income and happiness in Ireland 2003–2009. *Irish Journal of Medical Science,* 182(1): 113–19.

Dohrenwend, B.P. (2006) Inventorying stressful life events as risk factors for psychopathology. *Psychological Bulletin,* 132: 477–95.

Dohrenwend, B.P. and Dohrenwend, B.S. (1977) Sex differences in mental illness: a reply to Gove and Tudor. *American Journal of Sociology,* 82: 1336–41.

Dohrenwend, B.P., Brice, P., Levar, I. *et al.* (1992) Socio-economic status and psychiatric disorders: the causation selection issue. *Science,* 255: 946–51.

Dolan, B. and Coid, J. (1993) *Pychopathy and Antisocial Personality Disorders.* London: Gaskell.

Donat, J.G. (1988) Medicine and religion: on the physical and mental disorders that accompanied the Ulster Revival of 1859, in W.F. Bynum, R. Porter and M. Shepherd (eds) *The Anatomy of Madness* (Vol. III). London: Tavistock.

Donnelly, M. (1983) *Managing the Mind.* London: Tavistock.

Donzelot, J. (1979) *The Policing of Families.* London: Hutchinson.

Dooley, D., Prause, J. and Ham-Rowbottom, K.A. (2000) Underemployment and depression: longitudinal relationships. *Journal of Health and Social Behavior,* 41: 421–36.

Double, D. (1990) What would Adolf Meyer have thought about the neo-Kraepelinian approach? *Psychiatric Bulletin,* 14: 472–4.

Dover, S. and McWilliam, C. (1992) Physical illness associated with depression in the elderly in community based and hospital patients. *Psychiatric Bulletin,* 16: 612–13.

Dowrick, C. (2004) *Beyond Depression: A New Approach to Understanding and Management.* Oxford: Oxford University Press.

Dowrick, C. (2009) When diagnosis fails: a commentary on McPherson and Armstrong. *Social Science and Medicine,* 66: 1–3.

Dowrick, C., May, R., Richardson, M. and Bundred, P. (1996) The biopsychosocial model of general practice: rhetoric or reality? *British Journal of General Practice,* 46: 105–7.

Drapeau, A., Boyer, R. and Lesage, A. (2009) The influence of social anchorage on the gender difference in the use of mental health services. *Journal of Behavioral Health Services and Research,* 36(3): 372–84.

Drentea, P. and Reynolds, J.R. (2012) Neither a borrower nor a lender be: the relative importance of debt and SES for mental health among older adults. *Aging Health*, 24(4): 673–95.

Dudley, M., Cantor, C. and Demoore, G. (1996) Jumping the gun: firearms and the mental health of Australians. *Australian and New Zealand Journal of Psychiatry*, 3: 370–81.

Dunham, H. (1957) Methodology of sociological investigations of mental disorders. *Journal of Social Psychiatry*, 3: 7–17.

Dunham, H. (1964) Social class and schizophrenia. *American Journal of Orthopsychiatry*, 34: 634–46.

Eastman, N.L.G. (1994) Forensic Psychiatric Services in Britan: a current review. *International Journal of Law and Psychiatry*, 16(1–2): 1–26.

Edge, D. (2013 'Why are thou cast down, o my soul?' Exploring intersections of ethnicity, gender, depression, spirituality and implications for Black British Caribbean women's mental health. *Critical Public Health*, 23(1): 39–48.

Edge, D. and Rogers, A.E. (2005) Dealing with it: Black Caribbean women's response to adversity and psychological distress associated with pregnancy, childbirth and early motherhood. *Social Science And Medicine*, 61(1): 15–25.

Edge D., Baker, D. and Rogers, A. (2004) Perinatal depression among Black Caribbean women. *Health and Social Care in the Community*, 12(5): 430–8.

Eichenbaum, L. and Orbach, S. (1982) *Outside In Inside Out*. Harmondsworth: Penguin.

Elias, N. (1978) *The Civilising Process*. Oxford: Blackwell.

Elliot, A. (1992) *Social Theory and Psychoanalysis in Transition*. Oxford: Blackwell.

Ellis, A. (1970) *The Essence of Rational Psychotherapy*. New York: Institute for Rational Living.

Emerson, R.M. and Pollner, M. (1975) Dirty work designations: their features and consequences in a psychiatric setting. *Social Problems*, 3: 243–54.

Engel, G.L. (1980) The clinical application of the biopsychosocial model. *American Journal of Psychiatry*, 137: 535–44.

Ennis, B. and Emery, R. (1978) *The Rights of Mental Patients: An American Civil Liberties Union Handbook*. New York: Avon.

Estroff, S. and Zimmer, C. (1994) Social networks, social support and violence among persons with severe and persistent mental illness, in J. Monahan and H. Steadman (eds) *Violence and Mental Disorder: Developments in Risk Assessments*. Chicago: Chicago University Press.

Ettema, E.J., Derksen, L.D. and van Leeuwen, E. (2010) Existential loneliness and end of life care: a systematic review. *Theoretical Medicine and Bioethics*, 21(2): 141–69.

Eysenck, H.J. (1952) The effects of psychotherapy: an evaluation. *Journal of Consulting Psychology*, 16: 319–24.

Eysenck, H.J. (1955) Psychiatric diagnosis as a psychological and statistical problem. *Psychological Reports*, 1: 3–17.

Eysenck, H.J. (1975) *The Future of Psychiatry*. London: Methuen.

Fabrikant, B. (1974) The psychotherapist and the female patient: perceptions and change, in V. Franks and V. Burtle (eds) *Women in Therapy*. New York: Brunner Mazel.

Farina, A. and Felner, R.D. (1973) Employment interviewer reactions to former mental patients. *Journal of Abnormal Psychology*, 82: 268–72.

Faris, R.E.L. (1944) Ecological factors in human behavior, in R.E.L. Farris and H.W. Dunham (eds) *Mental Disorders in Urban Areas: An Ecological Study of Schizophrenia*. Chicago: Chicago University Press.

Faris, R.E.L. and Dunham, H.W. (1939) *Mental Disorders in Urban Areas*. Chicago: University of Chicago Press.

Faulkner, A. (1997) 'Strange bedfellows' in the laboratory of the NHS? An analysis of the new science of health technology assessment in the United Kingdom, in M.A. Elston (ed.) *The Sociology of Medical Science and Technology*. Oxford: Blackwell.

Faulkner, A. (2004) *The Ethics of Survivor Research: Guidelines for the Ethical Conduct of Research Carried Out by Mental Service Users and Survivors*. Bristol: Policy Press.

Faulkner, A. and Layzell, S. (2000) *Strategies for Living*. London: Mental Health Foundation.

Fazel, S. and Danesh, J. (2002) Serious mental disorder in 23000 prisoners: a systematic review of 62 surveys. *The Lancet*, 359: 545–50.

Felton, C., Stansty, P., Shern, D. *et al.* (1995) Consumers as peer specialists on intensive case management teams: impact on client outcomes. *Psychiatric Services*, 46(10): 1037–44.

Fennell, G., Phillipson, C. and Evers, H. (1988) *The Sociology of Old Age*. Milton Keynes: Open University Press.

Fennell, P. (1991) Diversion of mentally disordered offenders from custody. *Criminal Law Review*, 1: 333–48.

Fenton, S. and Sadiq, A. (1991) *Asian Women and Depression*. London: Commission for Racial Equality.

Fenton, S. and Sadiq-Sangster, A. (1996) Culture, relativism and mental distress. *Sociology of Health and Illness*, 18(1): 66–85.

Fernandez, F., and Lézé, S. (2011) Finding the moral heart of treatment: mental health care in a French prison. *Social Science and Medicine*, 72(9): 1563–9.

Fernando, S. (1988) *Race and Culture in Psychiatry*. London: Routledge.

Fernando, S., Ndegwa, D. and Wilson, M. (1998) *Forensic Psychiatry, Race and Culture*. London: Routledge.

Field Institute (1984) *In Pursuit of Wellness: A Survey of California Adults*. Sacramento: California Department of Mental Health.

Finkelhor, D. (1979) *Sexually Victimized Children*. New York: Free Press.

Finkelhor, D. (1984) *Child Sexual Abuse: New Theory and Research*. New York: Free Press.

Finkelhor, D. and Russell, D. (1984) Women as perpetrators: review of the evidence, in D. Finkelhor (ed.) *Child Sexual Abuse: New Theory and Research*, pp. 171–87. New York: Free Press.

Finn, S.E., Bailey, M., Schultz, R.T. and Faber, R. (1990) Subjective utility ratings of neuroleptics in treating schizophrenia. *Psychological Medicine*, 20: 843–8.

Fish, F. (1968) *Clinical Psychopathology*. Bristol: John Wright.

Fisher, S. and Greenberg, R.P. (eds) (1997) *From Placebo to Panacea: Putting Psychiatric Drugs to the Test*. New York: Wiley.

Fitzpatrick, M. and Newton, J. (2005) Profiling mental health needs: what about your Irish patients? *British Journal of General Practice*, 55(519): 739–40.

Forbat, L. (2002) 'Tinged with bitterness': re-presenting stress in family care. *Disability and Society*, 17(7): 759–68.

Forbat, L. and Henderson, J. (2003) The professionalisation of informal carers, in C. Davies (ed.) *The Future of the Health Workforce*. Basingstoke: Palgrave.

Forsythe, B. (1990) Mental and social diagnosis and the English Prison Commission 1914–1939. *Social Policy and Administration*, 24(3): 237–53.

Foucault, M. (1961) *Folie et Déraison: Histoire de la Folie à L'âge Classique*. Paris: Plon.

Foucault, M. (1965) *Madness and Civilisation*. New York: Random House.

Foucault, M. (1975) *Discipline and Punish: The Birth of the Prison*. New York: Random House.

Foucault, M. (1978) About the concept of the 'dangerous individual' in 19th century legal psychiatry.

International Journal of Law and Psychiatry, 1: 1–18.

Foucault, M. (1980) Power/knowledge, in C. Gordon (ed.) *Selected Essays and Other Writings*. Brighton: Harvester Press.

Foucault, M. (1981) *The History of Sexuality* (Vol. 1). Harmondsworth: Penguin.

Foucault, M. (1988) Technologies of the self, in L. Martin (ed.) *Technologies of the Self*. London: Tavistock.

Fowler, J.H. and Christakis, N.A. (2008) The dynamic spread of happiness in a large social network: longitudinal analysis over 20 years in the Framingham Heart Study. *British Medical Journal* 337: a2338.

Francis, E. (1989) Black people, dangerousness and psychiatric compulsion, in A. Brackx and C. Grimshaw (eds) *Mental Health Care in Crisis*. London: Pluto.

Francis, E., Pilgrim, D., Rogers, A. and Sashidaran, S. (1989) Race and 'schizophrenia': a reply to Ineichen. *New Community*, 17: 161–3.

Franks, C.M. (1993) Cognitive-behavioural assessment and therapy with adolescents. *Psychotherapy*, 30(4): 698–9.

Freckleton, I. and Keyzer, P. (2010) Indefinite detention of sex offenders and human rights: the intervention of the human rights committee of the United Nations. *Psychology, Psychiatry and Law*, 17(3): 345–54.

Frederick, J. (1991) *Positive Thinking for Mental Health*. London: The Black Mental Health Group.

Fredriksen-Goldsen, K., Emlet, C. and Hyan, J. (2013) The Physical and Mental Health of Lesbian, Gay Male, and Bisexual (LGB) Older Adults: The Role of Key Health Indicators and Risk and Protective Factors. *The Gerontologist*, 53(4): 664–75.

Freidson, E. (1970) *Profession of Medicine*. New York: Harper and Row.

Freud, S. (1920) Beyond the pleasure principle, in the *Standard Edition of the Complete Psychological Works of Sigmund Freud* (Vol. 18). London: Hogarth Press.

Freud, S. (1930) *Civilisation and Its Discontents*. London: Hogarth Press.

Freund, P. (1988) Understanding socialised human nature. *Theory and Society*, 17: 839–64.

Fromm, E. (1942) *Fear of Freedom*. New York: Routledge and Kegan Paul.

Fromm, E. (1944) Individual and social origins of neurosis. *American Sociological Review*, 4(4): 10–15.

Fromm, E. (1955) *The Sane Society*. New York: Holt, Rinehart and Winston.

Fryers, T., Brugha, T., Morgan, Z. *et al.* (2004): Prevalence of psychiatric disorder in Europe: the potential and reality of meta-analysis. *Social Psychiatry and Psychiatric Epidemiology*, 39(11): 899–905.

Fujiwara, T. and Kawachi, I. (2008) A prospective study of individual-level social capital and major depression in the United States. *Journal of Epidemiology and Community Health*, 62: 627–33.

Fullagar, S. and O'Brien, W. (2013) Problematizing the neurochemical subject of anti-depressand treatment: the limits of biomedical responses to women's emotional distress. *Health*, 17(1): 57–74.

Furnham, A. (1984) Lay conceptions of neuroticism. *Personality and Individual Difference*, 5(1): 95–103.

Gabe, J. and Bury, M. (1996) Halcion nights: a sociological account of a medical controversy. *Sociology*, 30(3): 447–71.

Gabe, J. and Lipshitsz-Phillips, S. (1982) Evil necessity? The meaning of benzodiazepine use for women patients from one general practice. *Sociology of Health and Illness*, 4(2): 201–11.

Gabe, J. and Thorogood, N. (1986) Prescribed drug use and the management of everyday life: the experiences of black and white working class women. *Sociological Review*, 34: 737–72.

Gamarnikow, E. (1978) Sexual division of labour: the case of nursing, in A. Kuhn and A. Wolpe (eds) *Feminism and Materialism: Women and Modes of Production*. London: Routledge and Kegan Paul.

Gask, L., Dowrick, C., Dixon, C. *et al.* (2000) A pragmatic cluster randomized trial of an educational intervention for general practitioners in the assessment and management of depression. *Psychological Medicine*, 34: 63–72.

Gask, L., Rogers, A., Campbell, S. *et al.* (2008) Beyond the limits of clinical governance? The case of mental health in English primary care. *BMC Health Services Research*, 8:63.

Gask, L., Bower, P., Lamb, J. *et al.* (2012) Improving access to psychosocial interventions for common mental health problems in the United Kingdom: narrative review and development of a conceptual model for complex interventions. *BMC Health Services Research*, 13(12): 249.

Gater, R., Amaddeo, F., Tansella, M., Jackson, G. and Goldberg, D. (1995) A comparison of community based care for schizophrenia in Verona and South Manchester. *British Journal of Psychiatry*, 166: 344–52.

Gelder, M., Mayou, R. and Cowen, P. (2001) *Shorter Oxford Textbook of Psychiatry*. Oxford: Oxford University Press.

Gelinas, D. (1983) The persisting negative effects of incest. *Psychiatry*, 46: 312–32.

Gerard, D.L. and Houston, L.G. (1953) Family setting and the ecology of schizophrenia. *Psychiatric Quarterly*, 27: 90–101.

Gergen, K. (1985) The social construction movement in modern psychology. *American Psychologist*, 40: 266–75.

Giddens, A. (1992) *Sociology*. Cambridge: Polity Press.

Gilbert, P. (1992) Depression: *The Evolution of Powerlessness*. Hove: Lawrence Erlbaum.

Gilbody, S., Whitty, J., Grimshaw, J. *et al.* (2003) Educational and organizational interventions to improve the management of depression in primary care: a systematic review. *Journal of the American Medical Association*, 289(23): 3145–51.

Gilroy, P. (1987) *There Ain't No Black in the Union Jack*. London: Hutchinson.

Gittins, D. (1998) *Madness in Its Place*. London: Routledge.

Godfrey, M. and Wistow, G. (1997) The user perspective on managing for health outcomes: the case of mental health. *Health and Social Care in the Community*, 5(5): 325–32.

Goffman, E. (1955) On face work. *Psychiatry*, 18: 213–31.

Goffman, E. (1961) *Asylums*. New York: Anchor.

Goffman, E. (1963) *Stigma: Notes on the Management of Spoiled Identity*. Harmondsworth: Penguin.

Goffman, E. (1971) *Relations in Public*. Harmondsworth: Penguin.

Goldberg, D. and Huxley, P. (1980) *Mental Illness in the Community*. London: Tavistock.

Goldberg, D. and Morrison, S.L. (1963) Schizophrenia and social class. *British Journal of Psychiatry*, 109: 785–802.

Goldberg, D., Gater, R., Sartorius, N. *et al.* (1997) The validity of two versions of the GHQ in the WHO study of mental health in general health care. *Psychological Medicine*, 27: 191–7.

Goldie, N. (1977) The division of labour among mental health professionals: a negotiated or an imposed order?, in M. Stacey and M. Reid (eds) *Health and the Division of Labour*. London: Croom Helm.

Goldie, N., Pilgrim, D. and Rogers, A. (1989) *Community Mental Health Centres: Policy and Practice*. London: Good Practices in Mental Health.

Goldney, R.D., Fisher, L.J. and Wilson, D.H. (2001) Mental health literacy: an impediment to the optimum treatment of major depression in the community. *Journal of Affective Disorders*, 64(2–3): 277–84.

Goldstein, B. and Rosselli, F. (2003) Etiological paradigms of depression: the relationship between perceived causes, empowerment, treatment preferences and stigma. *Journal of Mental Health*, 12(4): 551–64.

Goode, W. (1957) Community within a community: the professions. *American Sociological Review*, 20(1): 194–200.

Gorbien, M.J., Bishop, J. and Beers, M.H. (1992) Iatrogenic illness in hospitalized elderly people. *Journal of American Geriatrics Society*, 40: 1031–47.

Gory, M.L., Ritchey, F.J., Ritchey, J. and Mullis, J. (1990) Depression among homeless people. *Journal of Health and Social Behavior*, 31: 87–101.

Gottesman, I.I. and Shields, J. (1972) *Schizophrenia and Genetics*. London: Academic Press.

Gough, I. (1979) *Political Economy of the Welfare State*. London: Macmillan.

Gould, A. (1981) The salaried middle class in the corporatist welfare state. *Policy and Politics*, 9(4): 401–8.

Gouldner, A.W. (1979) *The Future of Intellectuals and the Rise of the New Class*. London: Macmillan.

Gove, W.R. (1975) The labeling theory of mental illness: a reply to Scheff. *American Sociological Review*, 40: 242–8.

Gove, W.R. (1982) The current status of the labeling theory of mental illness, in W.R. Gove (ed.) *Deviance and Mental Illness*. Beverley Hills, CA: Sage.

Gove, W.R. (1984) Gender differences in mental and physical illness: the effects of fixed roles and nurturant roles. *Social Science and Medicine*, 19(2): 77–91.

Gove, W.R. and Geerken, M. (1977) Response bias in surveys of mental health: an empirical investigation. *American Journal of Sociology*, 82: 1289–317.

Gove, W.R. and Tudor, J.F. (1972) Adult sex roles and mental illness. *American Journal of Sociology*, 78: 812–35.

Graham, H. (2004) Social determinants and their unequal distribution: clarifying policy understandings. *Millbank Quarterly*, 82(1): 101–24.

Granovetter, M. (1973) The strength of weak ties. *American Journal of Sociology*, 78: 1360–80.

Gray, N.S., Snowden, R.J., MacCulloch, S. *et al.* (2004) Relative efficiency of criminological, clinical, and personality measures of future risk of offending in mentally disordered offenders. *Journal of Consulting and Clinical Psychology*, 72: 523–30.

Greenberg, P.E. Kessler, R.C., Birnbaum, H.G. *et al.* (2003) The economic burden of depression in the United States: how did it change between 1990 and 2000? *Journal of Clinical Psychiatry*, 64: 1465–75.

Greenwood, J.D. (1994) *Realism, Identity and Emotion: Reclaiming Social Psychology*. London: Sage.

Grisso, T., Davis, J., Vesselinov, R. Appelbaum, P.S. and Monahan, J. (2000) Violent thoughts and violent behaviour following hospitalization for mental disorder. *Journal of Consulting and Clinical Psychology*, 68(3): 388–98.

Grob, G. (1973) *Mental Institutions in America: Social Policy to 1875*. New York: Free Press.

Grob, G. (1991) Origins of DSM-I: a study in appearance and reality. *American Journal of Psychiatry*, 148: 421–31.

Guidano, G.F. (1987) *Complexity of the Self*. New York: Guilford Press.

Gunnell, D., Middleton, N., Whitley, E., Dorling, D. and Frankel, S. (2003) Why are suicide rates rising in young men but falling in the elderly? A time-series analysis of trends in England and Wales 1950–1998. *Social Science and Medicine*, 57(4): 595–611.

Gunnell, D., Wheeler, B., Chang, S.-S., Thomas, B., Sterne, J.A.C. and Dorling, D. (2012) Changes in the geography of suicide in young men: England and Wales 1981–2005. *Journal of Epidemiology & Community Health*, 66: 536–43.

Guze, S.B. (1989) Biological psychiatry: is there any other kind? *Psychological Medicine*, 19: 315–23.

Ha, J.H., Hong, J., Seltzer, M.M. *et al.* (2008) Age and gender differences in the well-being of midlife and aging parents with children with mental health or developmental problems: report of a national study. *Journal of Health and Social Behavior*, 49(3): 301–16.

Haafkens, J., Nijhof, G. and van der Poel, E. (1986) Mental health care and the opposition movement in the Netherlands. *Social Science and Medicine*, 22: 185–92.

Habermas, J. (1975) *Legitimation Crisis*. Boston: Beacon Press.

Habermas, J. (1981) New social movements. *Telos*, 48: 33–7.

Habermas, J. (1989) The tasks of a critical theory of society, in S.E. Bronner and D.M. Kellner (eds) *Critical Theory and Society: A Reader*. London: Routledge.

Hamid, W. (1991) Homeless People and Community Care: An Assessment of the Needs of Homeless People. Unpublished PhD Thesis. University of London.

Hansen, E.C., Hughes, C., Routley, G. *et al.* (2008) General practitioners' experiences and understandings of diagnosing dementia: factors impacting on early diagnosis. *Social Science and Medicine*, 67(11): 1776–83.

Hardt, R.H. and Feinhandler, S.J. (1959) Social class and mental hospital prognosis. *American Sociological Review*, 24: 815–21.

Hare, R. (1991) *The Hare Psychopathy Checklist: Revised*. Toronto: Multi-Health Systems.

Harkness, E.F., Bower, P., Gask, L. and Sibbald, B. (2005) Improving primary care mental health: survey evaluation of an innovative workforce development in England. *Primary Care Mental Health*, 3(4): 253–60.

Harpham, T. (2008) The measurement of community social capital through surveys, in Kawachi, I., Subramanian, S.V. and Kim, D. (eds) *Social Capital and Health*. New York: Springer.

Harris, E.C. and Barraclough, B. (1998) Excess mortality of mental disorder. *British Journal of Psychiatry*, 173: 11–53.

Harrison, G., Owens, D., Holton, A. *et al.* (1988) A prospective study of severe mental disorder in Afro-Caribbean patients. *Psychological Medicine*, 11: 289–302.

Hassan, L., Weston, J., Senior, J. and Shaw, J. (2012). Prisoners holding their own medications during imprisonment in England and Wales: a survey and qualitative exploration of staff and prisoners' views. *Criminal Behaviour and Mental Health*, 22(1): 29–40.

Hayes, S.C. (1998) Scientific practice guidelines in a political, economic and professional context, in K.S. Dobson and K.D. Craig (eds) *Empirically Supported Therapies: Best Practice in Professional Psychology*. London: Sage.

Hayward, P. and Bright, J.A. (1997) Stigma and mental illness: a review and critique. *Journal of Mental Health*, 6: 345–54.

Healy, D. (1997) *The Anti-Depressant Era*. London: Harvard University Press.

Healy, D. (2004) Psychopathology at the interface between the market and the new biology. In D. Rees and S. Rose. (eds) *The New Brain Sciences: Perils and Prospects*. Cambridge: Cambridge University Press.

Hearing Voices Network (2013) *Press Release: HVN Launches Debate on DSM-5. It's the Bad Things that Happen to you that Drive you Crazy!* London: HVN, www.hearing-voices.org/news/press-release-hvn-launches-debate-on-dsm-5/. (accessed 21 January 2014).

Hearn, J. (1982) Notes on patriarchy, professionalisation and the semi-professions. *Sociology*, 16(2): 184–202.

Heitman, E. (1996) The public's role in the evaluation of health care technology: the conflict over ECT. *International Journal of Technology Assessment in Health*, 12(4): 657–72.

Hemmenki, E. (1977) Polypharmacy among psychiatric patients. *Acta Psychiatrica Scandinavica*, 56: 347–56.

Hemsi, L. (1967) Psychiatric morbidity of West Indian immigrants. *Social Psychiatry*, 2: 95–100.

Henderson, A.S. (1992) Social support and depression, in H.O.F. Veil and U. Baumann (eds) *The Meaning and Measurement of Social Support*. New York: Hemisphere.

Hensing, G., Alexanderson, K., Allebeck, P. and Bjurulf, P. (1996) Sick leave due to psychiatric disorder. *British Journal of Psychiatry*, 169: 740–6.

Herzberg, D. (2009) *Happy Pills in America: From Miltown to Prozac*. Baltimore: Johns Hopkins University Press.

Hiday, V. (1995) The social context of mental illness and violence. *Journal of Health and Social Behavior*, 36: 122–37.

Hirsch, S.R. (1986) Clinical treatment of schizophrenia, in P.B. Bradley and S.R. Hirsch (eds) *The Psychopharmacology and Treatment of Schizophrenia*. Oxford: Oxford University Press.

Hitch, P. (1981) Immigration and mental health: local research and social explanations. *New Community*, 9: 256–62.

Hitch, P. and Clegg, P. (1980) Modes of referral of overseas immigrant and native-born first admissions to psychiatric hospital. *Social Science and Medicine*, 14A: 369–74.

Hochschild, A. (1979) Emotion work, feeling rules and social structure. *American Journal of Sociology*, 85: 551–75.

Hochschild, A. (1983) *The Managed Heart: The Commercialization of Human Feeling*. Berkeley: University of California Press.

Hochstedler-Steury, E. (1991) Specifying 'criminalization' of the mentally disordered misdemeanants.

Journal of Criminal Law and Criminality, 82 (Summer): 334–59.

Hoenig, J. and Hamilton, M. (1969) *The Desegregation of the Mentally Ill*. London: Routledge and Kegan Paul.

Hoggett, B. (1990) *Mental Health Law*. London: Sweet & Maxwell.

Hollander, D. (1991) Homelessness and mental illness in developing countries, in M. Page and R. Powell (eds) *Homelessness and Mental Illness: The Dark Side of Community Care*. London: Concern Publications.

Hollingshead, A. and Redlich, R.C. (1958) *Social Class and Mental Illness*. New York: Wiley.

Hopper, K. (2007) Rethinking social recover in schizophrenia: what a capabilities approach might offer. *Social Science & Medicine*, 65: 868–79.

Horkheimer, M. (1931) Die gegenwärtige Lage der Sozialphilosophie und die Aufgaben eines Instituts für Sozialforschung. *Frankfurter Universitätsreden*, 37: 13–20.

Horne, J. and Wiggins, S. (2009) Doing being 'on the edge': managing the dilemma of being authentically suicidal in an online forum. *Sociology of Health and Illness*, 31(2): 170–84.

Horsfall, J. (1997) Psychiatric nursing: epistemological contradictions. *Advances in Nursing Science*, 20(1): 56–65.

Horwitz, A. (1983) *The Social Control of Mental Illness*. New York: Academic Press.

Horwitz, A. (2002) *Creating Mental Illness*. Chicago: Chicago University Press.

Horwitz, A. and Wakefield, J. (2007). *The Loss of Sadness: How Psychiatry Transformed Normal Sorrow Into Depressive Disorder*. New York: Oxford University Press.

House, J.S., Umberson, D. and Landis, K.R. (1988) Structures and processes of social support. *Annual Review of Sociology*, 14: 293–318.

Howard, M.M. (2003) *The Weakness of Civil Society in Post-Communist Europe*. Cambridge: Cambridge University Press

Howells, J.G. and Guirguis, W.R. (1985) *The Family and Schizophrenia*. New York: International Universities Press.

Huebner, D.M., Rebchook, G.M. and Kegeles, S.M. (2004) Experiences of harassment, discrimination and physical violence among young gay and bi-sexual men. *American Journal of Public Health*, 94(7): 1200–3.

Hughes, E. (1971) *The Sociological Eye: Selected Papers*. Chicago: Aldine Atherton.

Humphrey, M. and Haward, L. (1981) Sex differences in recruitment to clinical psychology. *Bulletin of the British Psychological Society*, 34: 413–14.

Hunt, I.M., Kapur, N., Webb, R. *et al.* (2009) Suicide in recently discharged psychiatric patients: a case-control study. *Psychological Medicine*, 39(3): 443–9.

Hunt, S. (1990) Emotional distress and bad housing. *Health and Hygiene*, 11: 72–9.

Huxley, P. (1990) *Effective Community Mental Health Services*. Aldershot: Avebury.

Hydle, I. (1993) Abuse and neglect of the elderly: a Nordic perspective. *Scandinavian Journal of Social Medicine*, 2(2): 126–8.

Hyndman, S.J. (1990) Housing, dampness and health among British Bengalis in East London. *Social Science and Medicine*, 30: 131–41.

Illich, I. (1974) *Medical Nemesis*. London: Calder & Boyars.

Illich, I. (1977a) *Limits to Medicine*. Harmondsworth: Penguin.

Illich, I. (1977b) Disabling professions, in I. Illich, I.K. Zola, J. McKnight *et al.* (eds) *Disabling Professions*. London: Marion Boyars.

Illsley, R. (1986) Social class, selection and class differences in relation to stillbirths and infant deaths. *British Medical Journal*, 229: 1520–4.

Ineichen, B. (1987) The mental health of Asians in Britain: a research note. *New Community*, 4: 1–2.

Ingleby, D. (1983) Mental health and social order, in S. Cohen and A. Scull (eds) *Social Control and the State*. Oxford: Blackwell.

Inglehart, R.F., Foa, R., Peterson, C. and Welzel, C. (2008) Development, freedom, and rising happiness: a global perspective (1981–2007). *Perspectives on Psychological Science*, 3(4): 264–85.

Ioannidis, J.P.A. (2008) Effectiveness of anti-depressants: an evidence myth constructed from a thousand randomized trials? *Philosophy, Ethics and Humanities in Medicine*, 3:14.

Irwin, E., Mitchell, L., Durkin, L. and Douieb, B. (1972) *The Need for a Mental Patients' Union: Some Proposals*. Available at http://studymore.org.uk/mpu.htm#FishPamphlet (accessed 21 January 2014).

Jackson, P.B. (2004) Role sequencing: does order matter for mental health? *Journal of Health and Social Behaviour*, 45(2): 132–54.

Jahoda, M. (1958) *Current Concepts of Positive Mental Health*. New York: Basic Books.

James, A. and Prout, A. (1990) *The Social Construction of Childhood*. London: Routledge.

James, N. (1989) Emotional labour: skill and work in the social regulation of feelings. *Sociological Review*, 37: 15–42.

James, O. (2008) *Affluenza*. London: Vermillion.

Jamison, K.R. (1998) Stigma of manic depression: a psychologist's experience. *The Lancet*, 352: 1060.

Jefferys, M. (ed.) (1989) *Growing Old in the Twentieth Century*. London: Routledge.

Jehu, D. (ed.) (1995) *Patients As Victims*. London: Wiley.

Jenkins, J.H. and Karno, M. (1992) The meaning of expressed emotion: theoretical issues raised by cross-national research. *American Journal of Psychiatry*, 149: 9–21.

Jenkins, R., Griffiths, S., Wylie, I. *et al.* (eds) (1994) *The Prevention of Suicide*. London: HMSO.

Jenkins, R., Klein, J. and Parker, C. (2005) Mental health in post-communist countries. *British Medical Journal*, 331: 173.

Jodelet, D. (1991) *Madness and Social Representations*. London: Harvester Wheatsheaf.

Johns, L.C., Nazroo, J., Bebbington, P. and Kuipers, E. (2002) Occurrence of hallucinatory experiences in a community sample and ethnic variations. *British Journal of Psychiatry*, 180: 174–8.

Johnson, T. (1977) The professions in the class structure, in R. Scase (ed.) *Industrial Society: Class, Cleavage and Control*. London: Allen and Unwin.

Johnstone, L. (1993) Family management in 'schizophrenia': its assumptions and contradictions. *Journal of Mental Health*, 2: 255–69.

Jones, E.E., Farina, A., Hastorf, A.H., Markus, H., Miller, D.T. and Scott, R.A. (1984) *Social Stigma: The Psychology of Marked Relationships*. New York: Freeman.

Jones, I.R., Ahmed, N., Catty, J. *et al.* (2009) Illness careers and continuity of care in mental health services: a qualitative study of service users and carers. *Social Sciences and Medicine*, 69(4): 632–9.

Jones, K. (1960) *Mental Health and Social Policy 1845–1959*. London: Routledge and Kegan Paul.

Jones, K. (1962) Review. *Sociological Review*, 8: 343–4.

Jones, L. and Cochrane, R. (1981) Stereotypes of mental illness: a test of the labelling hypothesis. *International Journal of Social Psychiatry*, 27: 99–107.

Jones, R. (1991) *Mental Health Act Manual*. London: Sweet & Maxwell.

Junginger, J. (1995) Command hallucinations and the predictions of dangerousness. *Psychiatric Services*, 46: 911–14.

Kaltiala-Heino, R., Marttunen, M., Rantanen, P. and Rimpela, M. (2003) Early puberty is associated with mental health problems in middle adolescence. *Social Science and Medicine*, 57(6): 1055–64.

Karlsen, S. and Nazroo, J. (2002) Agency and structure: the impact of ethnic identity and racism on the health of ethnic minority people. *Sociology of Health and Illness*, 24(1): 1–20.

Karlsen, S. and Nazroo, J. (2004) Fear of racism and health. *Journal of Epidemiology and Community Health*, 58: 1017–18.

Karlsen, S., Nazroo, J.Y., McKenzie, K., Bhui, K. and Weich, S. (2005) Racism, psychosis and common mental disorder among ethnic minority groups in England *Psychological Medicine*, 35: 1795–803.

Karon, B.P. and VandenBos, G.R. (1981) *Psychotherapy of Schizophrenia: The Treatment of Choice*. New York: Jason Aronson.

Kasl, S.V., Rodriguez, E. and Lasch, K.E. (1998) The impact of unemployment on health and well-being, in B.P. Dohrenwend (ed.) *Adversity, Stress and Psychopathology*. Oxford: Oxford University Press.

Kawachi, I. and Berkman, L.F. (2001) Social ties and mental health. *Journal of Urban Health*, 78: 458–67.

Kay, D., Beamish, P. and Roth, M. (1964) Old age mental disorders in Newcastle upon Tyne, part 1, a study of prevalence. *British Journal of Psychiatry*, 110: 146–8.

Kazdin, A.E., Stolar, M.J. and Marciano, P.L. (1995) Risk factors for dropping out of treatment among white and black families. *Journal of Family Psychology*, 9(4): 402–17.

Kellam, A.M.P. (1987) The neuroleptic syndrome, so called: a survey of the world literature. *British Journal of Psychiatry*, 150: 752–9.

Keyes, C.L.M. (2004) The nexus of cardiovascular disease and depression revisited: the complete mental health perspective and moderating role of age and gender. *Aging and Mental Health*, 8(3): 266–74.

Keyes, C.L.M. (2007) Anything Less than Mental Health as Flourishing in Adults. Paper presented to Public Mental Health Leadership Event. Manchester, 15 October.

Khan, N., Bower, P. and Rogers, A. (2007) Guided self-help in primary care mental health: meta-synthesis of qualitative studies of patient experience. *British Journal of Psychiatry*, 191: 206–11.

Kiernan, K.E. and Huerta, M.C. (2008) Economic deprivation, maternal depression, parenting and children's cognitive and emotional development in early childhood. *British Journal of Sociology*, 59(2): 783–806.

Kilian, R., Lindenbach, I., Lobig, U., Uhle, M., Petscheleit, A. and Angermeyer, M.C. (2003) Indicators of empowerment and disempowerment in the subjective evaluation of the psychiatric treatment process by persons with severe and persistent mental illness: a qualitative and quantitative analysis. *Social Science and Medicine*, 57(6): 1127–42.

Killaspy, H., Johnson, S., Pierce, B *et al.* (2009) Successful engagement: a mixed methods study of the approaches of assertive community treatment and community mental health teams in the REACT trial. *Social Psychiatry and Psychiatric Epidemiology*, 44(7): 532–40.

King, M., McKeown, E., Warner, J. *et al.* (2003) Mental health and quality of life of gay men and lesbians in England and Wales: controlled, crosssectional study. *British Journal of Psychiatry*, 183: 552–8.

King, M., Nazroo, J., Weich, S. *et al.* (2005) Psychotic symptoms in the general population of England: a comparison of ethnic groups (the EMPIRIC study). *Social Psychiatry and Psychiatric Epidemiology*, 40(5): 375–81.

Kirk, S.A. (1974) The impact of labeling on rejection of the mentally ill: an experimental study. *Journal of Health and Social Behaviour*, 15: 108–17.

Kirmayer, L.J. and Young, A. (1998) Culture and somatization: clinical, epidemiological, and ethnographic perspectives. *Psychosomatic Medicine*, 60(4): 420–30.

Kirsch, I., Deacon, B.J., Huedo-Medina, T.B., Scoboria, A., Moore, T.J. and Johnson, B.T. (2008) Initial severity and antidepressant benefits: a meta-analysis of data submitted to the Food and Drug Administration. *PLoS Medicine*, 5(2): e45.

Kitwood, T. (1988) The contribution of psychology to the understanding of senile dementia, in B. Gearing, M. Johnson and T. Heller (eds) *Mental Health Problems in Old Age*. London: Wiley.

Kitwood, T. and Bredin, K. (1992) Towards a theory of dementia care: personhood and well-being. *Ageing and Society*, 10: 177–96.

Klassen, D. and O'Connor, W. (1987) Predicting Violence in Mental Patients: Crossvalidation of an Actuarial Scale. Paper presented at the annual meeting of the American Public Health Association.

Kleinman, A. (1986) Some uses and misuses of the social sciences in medicine, in D.W. Fiske and R.A. Shweder (eds) *Metatheory and Social Science*. Chicago: Chicago University Press.

Knapp, M., McDaid, D, and Parsonage, M. (eds). (2011) *Mental Health Promotion and Mental Illness Prevention: The Economic Case*. London: Department of Health 2011.

Kobak, J. (1997) A computer-administered telephone interview to identify mental disorders. *Journal of the American Medical Association*, 278(11): 905–10.

Koenig, H.G., Larson, D.B. and Weaver, A. (1998) Research on religion and serious mental illness. *New Dimensions for Mental Health Services*, 80: 81–95.

Koffman, J., Fulop, N.J., Pashley, D. and Coleman, K. (1997) Ethnicity and the use of psychiatric beds: a one day survey in North and South Thames regions. *British Journal of Psychiatry*, 171: 238–41.

Kokanovic, R. (2011) The diagnosis of depression in an international context, in D. Pilgrim, A. Rogers and B. Pescosolido (eds) *The SAGE Handbook of Mental Health and Illness*. London: SAGE.

Kokanovic, R., Dowrick, C., Butler, E. *et al.* (2008) Lay accounts of depression amongst Anglo-Australian residents and East African refugees. *Social Science and Medicine*, 66(2): 454–66.

Kokanovic, R., Bendelow, G. and Phillips, B. (2013) Depression: the ambivalence of diagnosis. *Sociology of Health and Illness*, 35(3): 377–90.

Koopmans, G.T. and Lamers. L.M. (2007) Gender and health care utilization: the role of mental distress and help-seeking propensity. *Social Science and Medicine*, 64(6): 1216–30.

Krabbendam L. and van Os J (2005) Schizophrenia and urbanicity: a major environmental influence: conditional on genetic risk. *Schizophrenia Bulletin*, 31(4): 795–9.

Kraepelin, E. (1883) *Compendium der Psychiatrie*. Leipzig: Abel.

Kramer, P. (1993) *Listenting to Prozac: The Landmark Book about Antidepressants and the Remaking of the Self*, revised edition. New York: Viking.

Krause, I.B. (1989) Sinking heart: a Punjabi communication of distress. *Social Science and Medicine*, 29(4): 563–7.

Kross, E., Verduyn, P., Demiralp, E., *et al.* (2013) Facebook use predicts declines in subjective well-being in young adults. *PLoS ONE*, 8(8): e69841.

Kubie, S. (1954) The fundamental nature of the distinction between normality and neurosis. *Psychoanalytical Quarterly*, 23: 167–204.

Kvalevaag, A.L., Ramchandani, P.G., Hove, O., Assmus, J., Eberhard-Gran, M. AND Biringer, E. (2013) Paternal mental health and socioemotional and behavioral development in their children. *Pediatrics*, 131(2): E463–E469.

Lacey, R. (1991) *The Complete Guide to Psychiatric Drugs*. London: Ebury Press.

Laing, R.D. (1959) *The Divided Self*. London: Tavistock.

Laing, R.D. (1967) *The Politics of Experience and the Bird of Paradise*. Harmondsworth: Penguin.

Laing, R.D. and Esterson, A. (1964) *Sanity, Madness and the Family*. Harmondsworth: Penguin.

Lamb, J., Bower, P., Rogers, A., Dowrick, C. and Gask, L. (2012) Access to mental health in primary care: a qualitative meta-synthesis of evidence from the experience of people from 'hard to reach' groups. *Health*, 16(1): 76–104.

Lambert, M.J. and Bergin, A.E. (1983) Therapist characteristics and their contribution to psychotherapy outcome, in C.E. Walker (ed.) *The Handbook of Clinical Psychology* (Vol I). Homewood: Dow Jones-Irwin.

Landstedt, E., Asplund, K. and Gadin, K.G. (2009) Understanding adolescent mental health: the influence of social processes, doing gender and gendered power relations. *Sociology of Health and Illness*, 31(7): 962–78.

Lane, C. (2008) *Shyness: How Normal Behavior Became a Sickness*. New Haven: Yale University Press.

Langer, T.S. and Michael, S.T. (1963) *Life Stress and Mental Health*. Glencoe: Free Press.

Lapouse, R., Monk, M. and Terris, W. (1956) The drift hypothesis and socio-economic differentials in schizophrenia. *American Journal of Public Health*, 46: 968–86.

Latour, B. (1987) *Science in Action: How to Follow Scientists and Engineers Through Society*. Cambridge, MA: Harvard University Press.

Law, J. (1992) Notes on the theory of the actor-network: ordering, strategy and heterogeneity. *Systems Practice*, 5: 379–93.

Layard, R. (2005) *Happiness*. London: Penguin

Layard R., Bell S., Clark D.M., Knapp M., Meacher M. and Priebe, S. (2006) The depression report: a new deal for depression and anxiety disorders. London: London School of Economics, http://cep.lse.ac.uk (accessed 21 January 2014).

Lebow, J. (1982) Consumer satisfaction with mental health treatment. *Psychological Bulletin*, 91(2): 244–59.

Lees, S. (1997) How lay is lay? Chinese students' perceptions of anorexia nervosa in Hong Kong. *Social Science and Medicine*, 44(4): 491–502.

Lefley, H.P. (ed.) (1996) *Family Caregiving in Mental Illness*. London: Sage.

Leifer, M., Kilbane, T., Jacobsen, T. and Grossman, G. (2004) A three-generational study of transmission of risk for sexual abuse. *Journal of Clinical Child and Adolescent Psychology*, 33(4): 662–72.

Leighton, A.H. (1959) *My Name is Legion*. New York: Basic Books.

Lelliott, P. and Quirk, A. (2004) What is life like on acute psychiatric wards? *Current Opinion in Psychiatry*, 17(4): 297–310.

Lelliott, P., Audini B. and Duffett, R. (2001) Survey of patients from an inner-London health authority in medium secure psychiatric care. *British Journal of Psychiatry*, 178: 62–6.

Lemert, E. (1974) Beyond reach: the social reaction to deviance. *Social Problems*, 21: 457–67.

Lewis, L. (2009) Politics of recognition: what can a human rights perspective contribute to understanding users' experiences of involvement in mental health services? *Social Policy & Society*, 8(2): 257–74.

Lewis, S. and Leiberman, J. (2008) CATIE and Cutlass: can we handle the truth? *British Journal of Psychiatry*, 192: 161–3.

Levin J. (1988) Intervention in dentention: psychological, ethical and professional aspects. *South African Medical Journal*, 74(5): 460–7.

Liberman, J.A., Scott-Stroup, T., McEvoy, J.P. *et al.* (2005) Effectiveness of antipsychotic drugs in patients with chronic schizophrenia. *New England Journal of Medicine*, 353: 1209–23.

Lidz, C., Meisel, A., Zerubavel, E. *et al.* (1984) *Informed Consent: A Study of Decision Making in Psychiatry*. London: Guilford.

Liegghio, M., Nelso, G. and Evans, S.D. (2010) Partnering with children diagnosed with mental health issues: contributions of a sociology of childhood perspective to participatory action research. *Americal Journal of Community Psychology*, 46(1–2): 84–99.

Lindow, V. (1994) *Self-help Alternatives to Mental Health Services*. London: MIND Publications.

Link, B.G. and Cullen, F.T. (1983) Reconsidering the social rejection of ex-mental patients: levels of attitudinal response. *American Journal of Community Psychology*, 11(3): 261–73.

Link, B. and Phelan, J. (1995) Social conditions as fundamental causes of disease. *Journal of Health and Social Behaviour*, Special No: 80–94.

Link, B.G., Andrews, H.A. and Cullen, F.T. (1992) The violent and illegal behavior of mental health patients reconsidered. *American Sociological Review*, 57: 275–92.

Link, B., Castille, D.M. and Stuber, J. (2008) Stigma and coercion in the context of outpatient treatment for people with mental illnesses. *Social Science and Medicine*, 67(3): 409–20.

Lipsky, M. (1980), *Street-Level Bureaucracy; Dilemmas of the Individual in Public Services*. New York: SAGE.

Littlewood, R. and Cross, S. (1980) Ethnic minorities and psychiatric services. *Sociology of Health and Illness*, 2: 194–201.

Littlewood, R. and Lipsedge, M. (1982) *Aliens and Alienists*. Harmondsworth: Penguin.

Lochner, K., Kawachi, I. and Kennedy, B.P. (1999) Social capital: a guide to its measurement. *Health and Place*, 5: 259–70.

Longo, R. (1982) Sexual learning and experiences among adolescent sexual offenders. *International Journal of Offender Therapy and Comparative Criminology*, 26: 235–41.

Lorant, V., Deliege, D., Eaton, W., Robert, A. and Ansseau, M. (2003) Socio-economic inequalities in depression: a meta-analysis. *American Journal of Epidemiology*, 157: 98–112.

Lowenthal, M. (1965) Antecedents of isolation and mental illness in old age. *Archives of General Psychiatry*, 12: 245–54.

Lundqvist, G., Hansson, K. and Svedin, C.G. (2004) The influence of childhood sexual abuse factors on women's health. *Nordic Journal of Psychiatry*, 58(5): 395–401.

Lupton, D. (1998) *The Emotional Self*. London: Sage.

Lynch, D., Tamburrino, M. and Nagel, R. (1997) Telephone counselling for patients with minor depression: preliminary findings in a family practice setting. *Journal of Family Practice*, 44(3): 293–8.

Lyons, M. (1996) C. Wright Mills meets Prozac: the relevance of 'social emotion' to the sociology of health and illness, in V. James and J. Gabe (eds) *Health and the Sociology of Health and Illness Monograph*. Oxford: Wiley.

Macintyre, S., MacIver, S. and Sooman, A. (1993) Area, class and health: should we be focusing on places or people? *Journal of Social Policy*, 22: 213–34.

Main, T. (1946) The hospital as a therapeutic institution. *Bulletin of the Menninger Clinic*, 10: 64–71.

Maloy, K. (1992) *Critiquing the Empirical Evidence: Does Involuntary Outpatient Commitment Work?* Washington, DC: Mental Health Policy Center.

Mann, A.H., Graham, N. and Ashby, D. (1984) Psychiatric illness in residential homes for the elderly: a survey in one London borough. *Age and Ageing*, 113: 257–65.

Manning, N. (1989) *The Therapeutic Community Movement: Charisma and Routinization*. London: Routledge.

Manning, N. (2002) Actor networks, policy networks and personality disorder. *Sociology of Health and Illness*, 24(5): 644–66.

Marcuse, H. (1964) *One Dimensional Man*. London: Routledge and Kegan Paul.

Markham, D. (2003) Attitudes towards patients with a diagnosis of 'borderline personality disorder': social rejection and dangerousness. *Journal of Mental Health*, 12(6): 595–612.

Marks, I.M. (1987) *Fears, Phobias and Rituals*. Oxford: Oxford University Press.

Marshall, R. (1990) The genetics of schizophrenia: axiom or hypothesis?, in R.P. Bentall (ed.) *Reconstructing Schizophrenia*. London: Routledge.

Marshall, W.L. (1997) Pedophilia: psychopathology and theory, in D.R. Laws and W. O'Donohue (eds) *Sexual Deviance: Theory, Assessment, and Treatment*. New York: Guilford Press.

Martin, J.P. (1985) *Hospitals in Trouble*. Oxford: Blackwell.

Marzano, L., Hawton, K., Rivlin, A. and Fazel, S. (2011) Psychosocial influences on prisoner suicide: a case-control study of near lethal self-harm in women prisoners. *Social Science and Medicine*, 72(6): 874–83.

Marzillier, J. and Hall, J. (1987) *What Is Clinical Psychology?* Oxford: Oxford Medical Publications.

Masson, J. (1985) *The Assault on Truth: Freud's Suppression of the Seduction Theory*. Harmondsworth: Penguin.

Masson, J. (1988a) *A Dark Science: Women, Sexuality and Psychiatry in the Nineteenth Century*. New York: Noonday Press.

Masson, J. (1988b) *Against Therapy*. London: HarperCollins.

Matthews, F., Arthur, A., Barnes, L. *et al.* (2013) A two-decade comparison of prevalence of dementia in individuals aged 65 years and older from three geographical areas of England: results of the Cognitive Function and Ageing Study 1 and II (2013). *The Lancet*, 9902: 1405–12.

Maule, M., Milne, J. and Williamson, J. (1984) Mental illness and physical health in older people. *Age and Ageing*, 13: 349–56.

Maximova, K. and Quesniel-Vallee, A. (2009) Mental health consequences of unintended childlessness and unplanned births: gender differences and life course dynamics. *Social Science and Medicine*, 68(5): 850–7.

May, C., Allison, G., Chapple, A. *et al.* (2004) Framing the doctor–patient relationship in chronic illness: a comparative study of general practitioners' accounts. *Sociology of Health and Illness*, 26(2): 135–58.

Mayall, B. (1998) Towards a sociology of child health. *Sociology of Health and Illness*, 20(3): 269–88.

Mayer-Gross, W., Slater, E. and Roth, M. (1954) *Clinical Psychiatry*. London: Cassell.

McAndrew, S. and Warne, T. (2004) Ignoring the evidence dictating practice: sexual orientation, suicidality and the dichotomy of the mental health nurse. *Journal of Mental Health Nursing*, 11(4): 428–34.

McGovern, D. and Cope, R. (1987) The compulsory detention of males of different ethnic groups with special reference to offender patients. *British Journal of Psychiatry*, 150: 505–12.

McGuire, J. (2008) What's the point of sentencing? Psychological aspects of crime and punishment, in G. Davies, C.R. Hollin and R. Bull (eds) *Forensic Psychology*. Chichester: Wiley.

McLean, C., Campbell, C. and Cornish, F. (2004) Social capital, participation and the perpetuation of health inequalities: obstacles to African-Caribbean participation in 'partnerships' to improve mental health. *Ethnic Health*, 9(4): 313–35.

McLeod, J.D., Pescosolido, B.A., Takeuchi, D.T. and Falkenberg White, T. (2004) Public attitudes toward the use of psychiatric medications for children. *Journal of Health and Social Behavior*, 45(1): 53–67.

McLoone, P. (1996) Suicide and deprivation in Scotland. *British Medical Journal*, 312: 543–4.

McQueen, C. and Henwood, K. (2002) Young men in 'crisis': attending to the language of teenage boys' distress. *Social Science and Medicine*, 55(9): 1493–509.

Medawar, C. (1992) *Power and Dependence*. London: Social Audit.

Meehan, J., Flynn, S., Hunt, I.M. *et al.* (2006) Perpetrators of homicide with schizophrenia: a national clinical survey in England and Wales. *Psychiatric Services*, 57(11): 1648–51.

Melville-Wiseman, J. (2011) Professional sexual abuse in mental health services Capturing practitioner views of a contemporary corruption of care *Social Work and Social Sciences Review*, 15(3): 26–34.

Meltzer, H., Gill, B. and Pettigrew, M. (1994) *The Prevalence of Psychiatric Morbidity Among Adults Aged 16–64 Living in Private Households: OPCS Surveys of Psychiatric Morbidity in Great Britain*. London: HMSO.

Meng, H., Li, J., Loerbroks, A., Wu, J. and Chen, H. (2013) Rural/urban background, depression and suicidal ideation in Chinese college students: a cross-sectional study. *PLoS ONE*, 8(8): e71313.

Mental Health Act Commission (2008) *Risks, Rights and Recovery*, 12th Biennial Report. London: Stationery Office.

Mental Health Foundation (2006) *Cheers? Understanding the Relationship between Alcohol and Mental Health*. London: Mental Health Foundation.

Metzl, J.M. and Angell, J. (2004) Assessing the impact of SSRI antidepressants on popular notions of women's depressive illness. *Social Science and Medicine*, 58(3): 577–84.

Meyer, J.E. (1988) The fate of the mentally ill in Germany during the Third Reich. *Psychological Medicine*, 18: 575–81.

Mheen, H., Stronks, K. and Mackenbach, J. (1998) A life course perspective on socioeconomic inequalities in health. *Sociology of Health and Illness*, 20(5): 754–77.

Miles, R. (1996) Racism and nationalism in the United Kingdom: a view from the periphery. In R. Barot (ed.) *The Racism Problematic: Contemporary Sociological Debates on Race and Ethnicity*. Lewiston: Edwin Mellen Press.

Miller, P. (1986) Critiques of psychiatry and critical sociologies of madness, in P. Miller and N. Rose (eds) *The Power of Psychiatry*. Cambridge: Polity Press.

Miller, P. and Rose, N. (1988) The Tavistock programme: the government of subjectivity and social life. *Sociology*, 22(2): 171–92.

Milligan, C., Gatrell, A. and Bingley, A. (2004) 'Cultivating health': therapeutic landscapes and older people in northern England. *Social Science and Medicine*, 58: 1781–93.

Milliren, J.W. (1977) Some contingencies affecting the utilisation of tranquillisers in the long term care of the elderly. *Journal of Health and Social Behaviour*, 18: 206–11.

Mills, E. (1962) *Living with Mental Illness*. London: Institute of Community Studies/Routledge and Kegan Paul.

Milne, D., McAnaney, A., Pollinger, B., Bateman, K. and Fewster, E. (2004) Analysis of the forms, functions and facilitation of social support in one English county: a way for professionals to improve the quality of health care. *International Journal of Health Care Quality Assurance*, 17(6): 294–301.

MIND (2004) *Ward Watch Report*. London: MIND.

Mitchell, J. (1974) *Psychoanalysis and Feminism*. Harmondsworth: Penguin.

Mitchell, P.B., Slade, T. and Andrews, G. (2004) Twelve-month prevalence and disability of DSM-IV bipolar disorder in an Australian general population survey. *Psychological Medicine*, 34(5): 777–85.

Monahan, J. (1973) The psychiatrization of criminal behaviour: a reply. *Hospital and Community Psychiatry*, 24(2): 105–7.

Moncrieff, J. and Crawford, M.J. (2001) British psychiatry in the 20th century: observations from a psychiatric journal. *Social Science and Medicine*, 53(3): 349–56.

Morgan, C., Mallett, R., Hutchinson, G. and Leff, J. (2004) Negative pathways to psychiatric care and ethnicity: the bridge between social science and psychiatry. *Social Science and Medicine*, 58(4): 739–52.

Morgan, C., Fisher, H., Hutchinson, G. *et al.* (2009) Ethnicity, social disadvantage and psychotic-like experiences in a healthy population based sample. *Acta Psychiatrica Scandinavica*, 119(3): 226–35.

Morgan, H.G. (1994) *Suicide Prevention: The Assessment and Management of Suicide Risk*. Cambridge: Anglia University.

Morris, R.G., Morris, L.W. and Britton, P.G. (1988) Factors affecting the emotional wellbeing of the care-givers of dementia sufferers. *British Journal of Psychiatry*, 152: 147–56.

Morrison, A., Hutton, P., Shiers, D. and Tuckington, D. (2012) Antipsychotics: is it time to introduce patient choice? *British Journal of Psychiatry* 201: 83–4

Moses, T. (2009) Self-labeling and its effects among adolescents diagnosed with mental disorders. *Social Science and Medicine*, 68(3): 570–8.

Mulvany, J. (2000) Disability, impairment or illness? The relevance of the social model of disability to the study of mental disorder. *Sociology of Health and Illness*, 22(5): 582–601.

Muntaner, C., Lynch, J. and Smith, G.D. (2001) Social capital, disorganized communities and the third way: understanding the retreat from structural inequalities in epidemiology and public health. *International Journal of Health Services*, 31(2): 213–37.

Murphy, E. (1982) Social origins of depression in old age. *British Journal of Psychiatry*, 141: 135–42.

Murphy, E. (1988) Prevention of depression and suicide, in B. Gearing, M. Johnson and T. Heller (eds) *Mental Health Problems in Old Age*. London: Wiley.

Myers, D.G. (2000) The faith, friends and funds of happy people. *American Psychologist*, 55: 56–67.

Myers, J. (1975) Life events, social integration and psychiatric symptomatology. *Journal of Health and Social Behavior*, 16: 121–7.

Nairn, R., Coverdale, J. and Claasen, D. (2001) From source material to news story in New Zealand print media: a prospective study of stigmatizing processes in depicting mental illness. *Australian and New Zealand Journal of Psychiatry*, 35(5): 654–9.

Navarro, V. (1979) *Medicine Under Capitalism*. New York: Prodist.

Nazroo, J. (1995) Uncovering gender differences in the use of marital violence: the effect of methodology. *Sociology*, 29(3): 475–9.

Nazroo, J. (1997) *Ethnicity and Mental Health*. London: Policy Studies Institute.

Nazroo, J. (1998) Genetic, cultural or socio-economic vulnerability? Explaining ethnic inequalities in health. *Sociology of Health and Illness*, 20(5): 710–30.

Nazroo, J.Y. (2003) The structuring of ethnic inequalities in health: economic position, racial discrimination, and racism. *American Journal of Public Health*, 93(2): 277–84.

Nazroo, J. and Iley, K. (2011) Ethinicity, race and mental disorder in the UK, in D. Pilgrim, A. Rogers and B. Pescosolido (eds) *The SAGE Handbook of Mental Health and Illness* London: Sage

Nazroo, J.Y. and Karlsen, S. (2003) More about ethnic identity from the British National Survey of Ethnic Minorities, patterns of identity among ethnic minority people: diversity and commonality. *Ethnic and Racial Studies*, 26(5): 902–30.

Nazroo, J.Y., Edwards, A.C. and Brown, G.W. (1998) Gender differences in the prevalence of depression: artifact, alternative disorders, biology or roles? *Sociology of Health and Illness*, 20(3): 3112–330.

Nettleton, S. and Burrows, R. (1998) Mortgage debt, insecure home ownership and health: an exploratory study. *Sociology of Health and Illness*, 20(5): 731–53.

Newton, J. (1988) *Preventing Mental Illness*. London: Routledge.

NHS Hospital Advisory Service (1988) *Report on Broadmoor Hospital*. Sutton: NHS HAS.

Noble, L.M., Douglas, B.C. and Newman, S.P. (2001) What do patients expect of psychiatric services? A systematic and critical review of empirical studies. *Social Science and Medicine*, 52(7): 985–98.

Noble, P. and Rodger, S. (1989) Violence by psychiatric in-patients. *British Journal of Psychiatry*, 155: 384–90.

Nordqvist, P. (2012) Origins and originators: lesbian couples negotiating parental identities and sperm donor conception. *Culture Health & Sexuality*, 14(3): 297–311.

Norris, M. (1984) *Integration of Special Hospital Patients into the Community*. Aldershot: Gower.

North, C.S., Thompson, S.J., Polio, D.E., Ricci, D.A. and Smith, E.M. (1997) A diagnostic comparison of homeless and non-homeless patients in an urban mental health clinic. *Social Psychiatry and Psychiatric Epidemiology*, 32(4): 236–40.

Norton, K. (2004) Re-thinking acute psychiatric inpatient care. *International Journal of Social Psychiatry*, 50(3): 274–84.

Nurse, J., Woodcock, P. and Ormsby, J. (2003). Influence of environmental factors on mental health within prisons: focus group study. *British Medical Journal*, 327(7413): 480.

O'Reilly, M., Taylor, H. and Vostanis, P. (2009) 'Nuts schiz pshyco': an exploration of young homeless people's perceptions and dilemmas of defining mental health. *Social Science and Medicine*, 68: 1737–44.

Obeyesekere, G. (1985) Depression, Buddhism and the work of culture in Sri Lanka, in A. Kleinman and B. Good (eds) *Culture and Depression*. Berkeley: University of California Press.

Odell, S.M. and Commander, M.J. (2000) Risk factors for homelessness among people with psychotic disorders. *Social Psychiatry and Psychiatric Epidemiology*, 35: 9–11.

Offe, C. (1984) *Contradictions of the Welfare State*. London: Hutchinson.

Offe, C. (1993) *Structural Contradictions of the Welfare State*. Cambridge, MA: MIT Press.

Olkkola, K.T. and Ahonen, J. (2008). Midazolam and other benzodiazepines. *Handbook of Experimental Pharmacology*, 182: 335–60.

Olson, M. and Pincus, H. (1994a) Use of benzodiazepines in the community. *Archives of Internal Medicine*, 154(11): 1235–40.

Olson, M. and Pincus, H. (1994b) Outpatient psychotherapy in the US patterns of utilization. *American Journal of Psychiatry*, 51(9): 1289–94.

Olstead, R. (2002) Contesting the text: Canadian media depictions of the conflation of mental illness and criminality. *Sociology of Health and Illness*, 24(5): 621–43.

Oppenheimer, M. (1975) *The Proletarianisation of the Professional*. Sociological Review Monograph 20. Oxford: Wiley-Blackwell.

Orbell, S., Hopkins, N. and Gillies, B. (1993) Measuring the impact of informal care. *Journal of Community and Applied Social Psychology*, 3: 149–63.

Ostamo, A. and Lonnqvist, J. (1992) Parasuicide Rates by Gender in Helsinki, 1988–91. Poster paper at Joint Conference of the British Sociological Association Medical Sociology Group and the European Society of Medical Sociology, Edinburgh.

Ostir, G.V., Markides, K.E., Peek, N.K. and Goodwing, J.S. (2001) The association between emotional wellbeing and the incidence of stroke in older adults. *Psychosomatic Medicine*, 63: 210–15.

Owen, G.S., David, A.S., Richardson, G. *et al.* (2009) Mental capacity, diagnosis and insight in psychiatric in-patients: a cross-sectional study. *Psychological Medicine*, 39(8): 1389–98.

Owens, C., Owen, G., Lambert, H. *et al.* (2009) Public involvement in suicide prevention: understanding and strengthening lay responses to distress. *BMC Public Health*, 9: Art. No. 308.

Padgett, D.K., Patrick, C., Burns, B.J. and Schlesinger, H.J. (1994) Women and out-patient mental health services: use by black, Hispanic and white women in a nationally insured population. *Journal of Mental Health Administration*, 21(4): 347–60.

Padgett, D.K., Gulcur, L. and Tsemberis, S.J. (2006) Housing first services for people who are homeless with co-occurring serious mental illness and substance abuse. *Research on Social Work Practice*, 16: 74–83

Page, M. and Powell, R. (eds) (1991) *Homelessness and Mental Illness: The Dark Side of Community Care*. London: Concern Publications.

Palmier-Claus,J.E.,Rogers,A.,Ainsworth,J.*etal.*(2013) Integrating mobile-phone based assessment for psychosis into people's everyday lives and clinical care: a qualitative study. *BMC Psychiatry*, 13: 34.

Park, R.E. (1936) Human ecology. *The American Journal of Sociology*, 42(1): 1–14.

Parker, I., Georgaca, E., Harper, D., McLaughlin, T. and Stowell-Smith, M. (1995) *Deconstructing Psychopathology*. London: Sage.

Parkhouse, J. (1991) *Doctors' Careers: Aims and Experiences of Medical Graduates*. London: Routledge.

Parkman, S., Davies, S., Leese, M., Phelan, M. and Thornicroft, G. (1997) Ethnic differences in satisfaction with mental health services among representative people with psychosis in South London: PRiSM Study 4. *British Journal of Psychiatry*, 171: 260–4.

Parry, N. and Parry, G. (1977) Professionalism and unionism: aspects of class conflicts in the National Health Service. *Sociological Review*, 25(4): 823–40.

Parsons, T. (1939) The professions and the social structure. *Social Forces*, 17: 457–67.

Parsons, T. (1951) *The Social System*. Glencoe, IL: Free Press.

Patel, V. and Prince, M. (2010) Global mental health: a new global health field comes of age. *Journal of the American Medical Association*, 303 (19): 1976–7.

Patton, G., Coffey, C., Carlin, J., Degenhardt, L., Lynskey, M. and Hall, W. (2002) Cannabis use and mental health in young people: cohort study. *British Medical Journal*, 23(325): 1195–8.

Paveza, G.J., Cohen, J.G., Eisdorfer, C. *et al.* (1992) Severe family violence and Alzheimer's Disease: prevalence and risk factors. *Gerontologist*, 32(4): 493–7.

Pearson, V. (1995) Goods on which one loses: women and mental health in China. *Social Science and Medicine*, 41(8): 1159–73.

Peay, J. (1989) *Tribunals on Trial: A Study of Decision-Making Under the Mental Health Act 1983*. Oxford: Oxford University Press.

Perring, C., Twigg, J. and Atkin, J. (1990) *Families Caring for People Diagnosed as Mentally Ill: The Literature Re-Examined*. London: Social Policy Research Unit.

Perrow, C. (1965) Hospitals: technology, structure and goals, in J.G. March (ed.) *Handbook of Organisations*. Chicago: Rand McNally.

Pescosolido, B.A. (2013) The public stigma of mental illness: what do we think; what do we know;

what can we prove? *Journal of Health and Social Behavior* online first, 16 January.

Pescosolido, B.A. and Wright, E.R. (2004) The view from two worlds: the convergence of social network reports between mental health clients and their ties. *Social Science and Medicine*, 58(9): 1795–806.

Pescosolido, B.A., Perry, B.L., Martin, J.K. *et al.* (2007) Stigmatizing attitudes and beliefs about treatment and psychiatric medications for children with mental illness. *Psychiatric Services*, 58(5): 613–18.

Pescosolido, B.A., Martina, J.K., Lang, A. *et al.* (2008) Rethinking theoretical approaches to stigma: a framework integrating normative influences on Stigma (FINIS). *Social Science and Medicine*, 67(3): 431–40.

Pescosolido, B.A., Medina, T.R., Martin, J.K. and Long, J.S. (2013) The 'backbone' of stigma: identifying the global core of public prejudice associated with mental illness. *American Journal of Public Health*, 103(5): 853–60.

Peters, S., Rogers, A., Salmon, P. *et al.* (2009) What do patients choose to tell their doctors? Qualitative analysis of potential barriers to reattributing medically unexplained symptoms. *Journal of General Internal Medicine*, 24(4): 443–9.

Phillips, D. (1968) Social class and psychological disturbance: the influence of positive and negative experiences. *Social Psychiatry*, 3: 41–6.

Philo, G., Secker, J., Platt, S. *et al.* (1996) Media images of mental distress, in T. Heller *et al.* (eds) *Mental Health Matters: A Reader*. Basingstoke: Macmillan.

Pilger, J. (1989) *A Secret Country*. London: Vantage.

Pilgrim, D. (1988) Psychotherapy in special hospitals: a case of failure to thrive. *Free Associations*, 7: 11–26.

Pilgrim, D. (1992) Psychotherapy and political evasions, in W. Dryden and C. Feltham (eds) *Psychotherapy and Its Discontents*. Milton Keynes: Open University Press.

Pilgrim, D. (1997a) *Psychotherapy and Society*. London: Sage.

Pilgrim, D. (1997b) Some reflections on 'quality' and 'mental health'. *Journal of Mental Health*, 6(6): 567–76.

Pilgrim, D. (1998) Medical sociology and psychoanalysis: a rejoinder to Lupton. *Sociology of Health and Illness*, 20(4): 537–44.

Pilgrim, D. (2000) The real problem for post-modernism. *Journal of Family Therapy*, 22(1): 6–23.

Pilgrim, D. (2001) Disordered personalities and disordered concepts. *Journal of Mental Health*, 10(3): 253–66.

Pilgrim, D. (2002a) The biopsychosocial model in Anglo-American psychiatry: past present and future? *Journal of Mental Health*, 11(6): 585–94.

Pilgrim, D. (2002b) The emergence of clinical psychology as a profession, in J. Allsop and M. Saks (eds) *Regulating the Health Professions*. London: SAGE.

Pilgrim, D. (2005a) Defining mental disorder: tautology in the service of sanity in British mental health legislation. *Journal of Mental Health*, 14(5): 435–43.

Pilgrim, D. (2005b) Protest and cooption: the voice of mental health service users, in A. Bell and P. Lindley (eds) *Beyond the Water Towers: The Unfinished Revolution in Mental Health Services 1985–2005*. London: Sainsbury Centre for Mental Health.

Pilgrim, D. (2007a) The survival of psychiatric diagnosis. *Social Science and Medicine*, 65(3): 536–44.

Pilgrim, D. (2007b) New 'mental health' legislation for England and Wales: some aspects of consensus and conflict. *Journal of Social Policy*, 36(1): 1–17.

Pilgrim, D. (2008a) The eugenic legacy in psychology and psychiatry. *International Journal of Social Psychiatry*, 54(3): 272–84.

Pilgrim, D. (2008b) 'Recovery' and current mental health policy. *Chronic Illness*, 4: 295–304.

Pilgrim, D. (2008c) What is the *British Journal of Clinical Psychology* for? *Clinical Psychology Forum*, 189: 15–18.

Pilgrim, D. (2009) *Key Concepts in Mental Health*. London: Sage.

Pilgrim, D. (2012) The British welfare state and mental health problems: the continuing relevance of the work of Claus Offe. *Sociology of Health and Illness*, 34(7): 1070–84.

Pilgrim, D. (2013) The failure of diagnostic psychiatry and the prospects of scientific progress offered by critical realism. *Journal of Critical Realism*, 12(3): 336–58.

Pilgrim, D. and Bentall, R.P. (1999) The medicalisation of misery: a critical realist analysis of the concept of depression. *Journal of Mental Health*, 8(3): 261–74.

Pilgrim, D. and Carey, T. (2010) Contested professional rationales for the assessment of mental health problems: can social theories help? *Social Theory and Health*, 8: 309–25.

Pilgrim, D. and Guinan, P. (1999) From mitigation to culpability: rethinking the evidence about therapist sexual abuse. *European Journal of Counselling, Psychotherapy and Health*, 2(2): 153–68.

Pilgrim, D. and McCranie, A. (2013) *Recovery and Mental Health: A Critical Sociological Account*. Basingstoke: Palgrave Macmillan.

Pilgrim, D. and Ramon, S. (2009) English mental health policy under New Labour. *Policy and Politics*, 37(2): 273–88.

Pilgrim, D. and Rogers, A. (1994) Something old, something new . . . sociology and the organisation of psychiatry. *Sociology*, 28(2): 521–38.

Pilgrim, D. and Rogers, A. (1997) A confined agenda? Guest editorial. *Journal of Mental Health*, 6(6): 539–42.

Pilgrim, D. and Rogers, A. (2003) Mental disorder and violence: an empirical picture in context. *Journal of Mental Health*, 12(1): 7–18.

Pilgrim, D. and Rogers, A. (2005) Psychiatrists as social engineers: a study of an anti-stigma campaign. *Social Science and Medicine*, 61(12): 2546–56.

Pilgrim, D. and Rogers, A. (2009) Survival and its discontents: the case of British psychiatry. *Sociology of Health and Illness*, 31, 947–61.

Pilgrim, D. and Treacher, A. (1992) *Clinical Psychology Observed*. London: Routledge.

Pilgrim, D. and Waldron, L. (1998) User involvement in mental health service development: how far can it go? *Journal of Mental Health*, 7(1): 95–104.

Pilgrim, D., Rogers, A., Clarke, S. and Clark, W. (1997) Entering psychological treatment: decision-making factors for GPs and service users. *Journal of Interprofessional Care*, 11(3): 313–23.

Pilgrim, D., Kinderman, P. and Tai, S. (2008) Taking stock of the biopsychosocial model in 'mental health care'. *Journal of Social and Psychological Sciences*, 1(2): 1–39.

Pilgrim, D., Rogers, A. and Bentall, R. (2009) The centrality of personal relationships in the creation and amelioration of mental health problems: the current interdisciplinary case. *Health*, 13(2): 235–54.

Pilgrim, D., Tomasini, F. and Vassilev, I. (2011) *Examining Trust in Health Care: A Multidisciplinary Perspective*. Baskingstoke: Palgrave Macmillan.

Pitt, B. (1988) Characteristics of depression in the elderly, in B. Gearing, M. Johnson and T. Heller (eds) *Mental Health Problems in Old Age*. London: Wiley.

Platt, S. (1984) Unemployment and suicidal behaviour: a review of the literature. *Social Science and Medicine*, 39: 93–115.

Pollack, D.A. (2004) *Moving from Coercion to Collaboration in Mental Health Services*. Rockville, MD: Centre for Mental Health Services Research, Substance Abuse and Mental Health Services Administration.

Pollack, S. and Kendall, K. (2005) Taming the shrew: regulating prisoners through women-centered mental health programming. *Critical Criminology*, 13(1): 71–87.

Pols, J. (2001) Enforcing patients' rights or improving care: the interference of two modes of doing good in mental health care. *Sociology of Health and Illness*, 25(4): 325–47.

Portes, A. (1998) Social capital: its origins and application in modern sociology. *Annual Review of Sociology*, 24: 1–24.

Post, F. (1969) The Relationship to Physical Health of the Affective Illnesses in the Elderly. Eighth International Congress of Gerontology Proceedings, Washington, DC.

Potier, M. (1992) *Evidence Recorded by the Report of the Committee of Inquiry About Complaints at Ashworth Hospital*. London: HMSO.

Power, C., Matthews, S. and Manor, O. (1996) Inequalities in self-related health in the 1958 birth cohort: lifetime social circumstances or social mobility? *British Medical Journal*, 313: 449–53.

Power, C., Stansfeld, S.A., Mathews, S., Manor, O. and Hope, S. (2002) Childhood and adulthood risk factors for socio-economic differentials in psychological distress: evidence from the 1958 British birth cohort. *Social Science and Medicine*, 55(11): 1989–2004.

Price, D. (2002) Legal aspects of the regulation of the health professions, in J. Allsop and M. Saks (eds) *Regulating the Health Professions*. London: SAGE.

Priebe, S., Burns, T. and Craig, T. (2013) The future of academic psychiatry may be social. *British Journal of Psychiatry*, 202: 319–20.

Prior, L. (1991) Mind, body and behaviour: theorisations of madness and the organisation of therapy. *Sociology*, 25(3): 403–22.

Pritchard, C. and Hansen, L. (2005) Child, adolescent and youth suicide and undetermined deaths in England and Wales compared with Australia, Canada, France, German, Italy, Japan, and the USA for the 1974–1999 period. *International Journal of Adolescent Medicine and Health*, 17: 239–53.

Prospero, M. and Kim, M. (2009) Ethnic difference in the effects of coercion on mental health and the use of therapy. *Journal of Social Work Practice*, 23(1): 77–91.

Protheroe, J., Rogers, A., Kennedy, A.P., Macdonald, W. and Lee, V. (2009) Promoting patient engagement with self-management support information: a qualitative meta-synthesis of processes influencing uptake. *BMC Implementation Science*; 3: 44.

Protheroe, J., Brooks, H., Chew Graham, C. *et al.* (2012) 'Permission to participate?' A qualitative study of participation in patients from differing socio-economic backgrounds. *Journal of Health Psychology*, 18(8): 1046–55.

Quirk, A. and Lelliott, P. (2001) What do we know about life on acute psychiatric wards in the UK? A review of the research evidence. *Social Science and Medicine*, 53(12): 1565–74.

Rabkin, J. (1979) Criminal behavior of discharged psychiatric patients: a critical review of the research. *Psychological Bulletin*, 86: 1–27.

Rachman, S. (1971) *The Effects of Psychotherapy*. Oxford: Pergamon Press.

Rai, D., Zitko, P., Jones, K., Lynch, J. and Araya, R. (2013) Country- and individual-level socioeconomic determinants of depression: multilevel cross-national comparison. *The British Journal of Psychiatry*, 202(3): 195–203.

Ramon, S. (1985) *Psychiatry in Britain: Meaning and Policy*. London: Gower.

Ramon, S. (1986) The category of psychopathy: its professional and social context in Britain, in P. Miller and N. Rose (eds) *The Power of Psychiatry*. Cambridge: Polity Press.

Ramon, S. (1988) Introduction, in S. Ramon and M.G. Giannichedda (eds) *Psychiatry in Transition: The British and Italian*. Cambridge: Polity Press.

Ramon, S. (2006) British mental health social work and the psychosocial approach in context, in D.B. Double (ed.) *Critical Psychiatry: The Limits of Madness*. Basingstoke: Palgrave.

Ranger, C. (1989) Race, culture and 'cannabis psychosis': the role of social factors in the construction of a disease category. *New Community*, 15(3): 357–69.

Rapaport, J. (2006) New roles in mental health: the creation of the approved mental health practitioner. *Journal of Integrated Care*, 14(5): 37–46.

Read, J. and Bentall, R. (2012) Negative childhood experiences and mental health: theoretical, clinical and primary prevention implications? *British Journal of Psychiatry*, 200: 89–91.

Read, J., Agar, K, Argyle, N. and Aderhold, V. (2003) Sexual and physical abuse during childhood as predictors of hallucinations, delusions and thought disorder. *Psychology and Psychotherapy* 76(1): 1–22.

Reading, R. and Reynolds, S. (2001) Debt, social disadvantage and maternal depression. *Social Science and Medicine*, 53(4): 441–53.

Reed, J. and Lyne, M. (2000) The quality of health care in prison: results of a year's programme of semi-structured inspections. *British Medical Journal*, 320: 1031–4.

Regier, D., Boyd, J., Burke, J. *et al.* (1988) Prevalence of mental disorders in the United States. *Archives of General Psychiatry*, 45: 977–85.

Reich, W. (1933) *The Mass Psychology of Fascism*. London: Pelican, 1975.

Reiner, R. (1986) *The Politics of the Police*. London: Harvester Wheatsheaf.

Rhodes, A. and Goering, P. (1994) Gender differences in the use of outpatient mental health services. *Journal of Mental Health Administration*, 21(4): 338–46.

Rice, M.E., Quinsey, V.L. and Harris, G.T. (1991) Sexual recidivism among child molesters released from a maximum security psychiatric institution. *Journal of Consulting and Clinical Psychology*, 59(3): 381–6.

Rickwood, D.J. and Braithwaite, V.A. (1994) Social psychological factors affecting help seeking for emotional problems. *Social Science and Medicine*, 39(4): 563–72.

Ritzer, G. (1995) *The McDonaldization of Society*. London: Sage.

Ritzer, G. (1997) *The McDonaldization Thesis*. London: Sage.

Roberts, R., O'Connor, T., Dunn, J. and Golding J. (2004) The effects of child sexual abuse in later family life mental health, parenting and adjustment of offspring. *Child Abuse and Neglect*, 28(5): 535–45.

Rogers, A. (1990) Policing mental disorder: controversies, myths and realities. *Social Policy and Administration*, 24(3): 226–37.

Rogers, A. (1993) Coercion and voluntary admissions: an examination of psychiatric patients' views. *Behavioural Sciences and the Law*, 11: 259–67.

Rogers, A.E. and Allison, T. (2004) What if my back breaks? Making sense of musculoskeletal pain among South Asian and African-Caribbean people in the North West of England. *Journal of Psychosomatic Research*, 57(1): 79–87.

Rogers, A. and Pilgrim, D. (1989) Citizenship and mental health. *Critical Social Policy*, 26: 25–32.

Rogers, A. and Pilgrim, D. (1991) 'Pulling down churches': accounting for the British mental health users' movement. *Sociology of Health and Illness*, 13(2): 129–48.

Rogers, A. and Pilgrim, D. (1996) *Mental Health Policy in Britain*. London: Macmillan.

Rogers, A. and Pilgrim, D. (1997) The contribution of lay knowledge to the understanding and promotion of mental health. *Journal of Mental Health*, 6(1): 23–35.

Rogers, A. and Pilgrim, D. (2003) *Mental Health and Inequality*. Basingstoke: Palgrave Macmillan.

Rogers, C.M. and Terry, T. (1984) Clinical interventions with boy victims of sexual abuse, in I. Stuart and J. Greer (eds) *Victims of Sexual Aggression*. New York: Van Nostrand Reinhold.

Rogers, A., Pilgrim, D. and Lacey, R. (1993) *Experiencing Psychiatry: Users' Views of Services*. London: Macmillan.

Rogers, A., Day, J., Williams, B. *et al.* (1998) The meaning and management of medication: perspectives of patients with a diagnosis of schizophrenia. *Social Science and Medicine*, 47(9): 1313–23.

Rogers, A., Hassell, K. and Nicolaas, G. (1999) *Demanding Patients?* Buckingham: Open University Press.

Rogers, A., Pilgrim, D., Brennan, S., Sulaiman, I, Watson, G. and Chew-Graham, C. (2007) Prescribing benzodiazepines in general practice: a new view of an old problem. *Health*, 11: 181–98.

Rogers, A., Bury, M. and Kennedy, A. (2009) Rationality, rhetoric, and religiosity in health care: the case of England's expert patient's programme. *International Journal of Health Services*, 39(4): 725–47.

Romito, P. and Grassi, M. (2007) Does violence affect one gender more than the other? The mental health impact of violence among male and female university students. *Social Science and Medicine*, 65(6): 1222–34.

Romme, M.A., Honig, A., Noorthoorn, E.O. and Escher, S. (1992). Coping with hearing voices: an emancipatory approach. *British Journal of Psychiatry*, 162: 99–103.

Rooke-Matthews, S. and Lindow, V. (1997) *A Survivors' Guide to Working in Mental Health Services*. London: MIND/Joseph Rowntree.

Rose, D. (1998) Television madness and community care. *Journal of Applied Community Social Psychology*, 8: 213–28.

Rose, D. and Barr, M. (2008) The great ambivalence: factors likely to affect service user and public acceptability of the pharmacogenomics of antidepressant medication. *Sociology of Health and Illness*, 30(6): 944–58.

Rose, D., Wykes, T., Leese, M., Bindman, J. and Fleischmann, P. (2003) Patients' perspectives on electroconvulsive therapy: systematic review. *British Medical Journal*, 326: 1363–5.

Rose, D., Fleischman, P. and Wykes, T. (2008) What are mental health service users' priorities for research in the UK? *Journal of Mental Health*, 17(5): 520–30.

Rose, N. (1986) Law, rights and psychiatry, in P. Miller and N. Rose (eds) *The Power of Psychiatry*. Cambridge: Polity Press.

Rose, N. (1990) *Governing the Soul*. London: Routledge.

Rosen, G. (1968) *Madness in Society*. New York: Harper.

Rosen, G. (1979) The evolution of scientific medicine, in H. Freeman, S. Levine and L. Reeder (eds) *Handbook of Medical Sociology*. Englewood Cliffs, NJ: Prentice-Hall.

Rosenfield, S. (2012) Triple jeopardy? Mental health at the intersection of gender, race, and class, *Social Science and Medicine*, 74(1): 1791–6.

Ross, C.E. and Mirowsky, J. (1995) Does employment affect health? *Journal of Health and Social Behavior*, 36: 230–43.

Roth, M. (1973) Psychiatry and its critics. *British Journal of Psychiatry*, 122: 174–6.

Rothman, D. (1971) *The Discovery of the Asylum: Social Order and Disorder in the New Republic*. Boston: Little Brown.

Rothman, D. (1983) Social control: the uses and abuses of the concept in the history of incarceration, in S. Cohen and A. Scull (eds) *Social Control and the State*. Oxford: Basil Blackwell.

Rowe, R., Tilbury, F., Rapley, M. and O'Ferrall, I. (2003) 'About a year before the breakdown I was having symptoms': sadness, pathology and the Australian newspaper media. *Sociology of Health and Illness*, 25(6): 680–96.

Royal College of Psychiatrists (1995) *The ECT Handbook (Council Report 39)*. London: Royal College of Psychiatrists.

Royal College of Psychiatrists (Scottish Division) (1973) *The Future of Psychiatric Services in Scotland*. London: Royal College of Psychiatrists.

Rusch, N., Corrigan, P.W. and Wassel, A. *et al.* (2009) Ingroup perception and responses to stigma among persons with mental illness. *Acta Psychiatrica Scandinavica*, 120(4): 320–8.

Ruskin, P.E., Silves-Aylaiiau, M., Kling, M.A. *et al.* (2004) Treatment outcomes in depression: comparison of remote treatment through telepsychiatry in inpatient treatment. *American Journal of Psychiatry*, 161(8): 1471–6.

Russell, D. (1983) The incidence and prevalence of intrafamilial sexual abuse of female children. *Child Abuse and Neglect*, 7: 133–45.

Rutter, D., Manley, C., Weaver, T., *et al.* (2004) Patients or partners? Case studies of user involvement in the planning and delivery of adult mental health services in London. *Social Science and Medicine*, 58(10): 1973–84.

Rwegellera, G.G.C. (1977) Psychiatric morbidity among West Africans and West Indians living in London. *Psychological Medicine*, 7: 317–29.

Ryan, R.M. and Deci, E.L (2001) On happiness and human potentials: a review on hedonic and eudaimonic wellbeing. *Applied Review of Psychology*, 52: 141–66.

Ryle, A. (1990) *Cognitive-Analytical Therapy: Active Participation in Change*. Chichester: Wiley.

Sainsbury (1998) *Acute Problems: A Survey of the Quality of Care in Acute Psychiatric Wards*. London: Sainsbury Centre for Mental Health.

Sainsbury (2003) *Money for Mental Health*. London: Sainsbury Centre for Mental Health.

Saks, M. (1983) Removing the blinkers? A critique of recent contributions to the sociology of the professions. *Sociological Review*, 33: 1–21.

Saks, M. (ed.) (1992) *Alternative Medicine in Britain*. Oxford: Clarendon Press.

Samson, C. (1992) Confusing Symbolic Events with Realities: The Case of Community Mental Health in the USA. Paper presented at the BSA Medical Sociology Group and European Society of Medical Sociology, Edinburgh.

Sang, B. (1989) The independent voice of advocacy, in A. Brackx and C. Grimshaw (eds) *Mental Health Care in Crisis*. London: Pluto Press.

Sartorius, N. and Henderson, A.S. (1992) The neglect of prevention in psychiatry. *Australian and New Zealand Journal of Psychiatry*, 26(4): 550–3.

Sartre, J.-P. (1963) *Search for a Method*. New York: Knopf.

Sashidharan, S.P. (1986) Ideology and politics in transcultural psychiatry, in J.L. Cox (ed.) *Transcultural Psychiatry*. London: Croom Helm.

Sashidharan, S.P. (1993) Afro-Caribbeans and schizophrenia: the ethnic vulnerability hypothesis re-examined. *International Review of Psychiatry*, 5: 129–44.

Savage, M. *et al.* (2013). A new model of social class: findings from the BBC's great british class survey experiment. *Sociology*, online first, 2 April.

Sayce, L. (1989) Community Mental Health Centres: rhetoric or reality?, in A. Brackx and C. Grimshaw (eds) *Mental Health Care in Crisis*. London: Pluto.

Sayce, L. (2000) *From Psychiatric Patient to Citizen: Overcoming Discrimination and Social Exclusion*. Basingstoke: Macmillan.

Scambler, A. (1998) Gender, health and the feminist debate on post-modernism, in G. Scambler and P. Higgs (eds) *Modernity, Medicine and Health*. London: Routledge.

Scambler, A., Scambler, G. and Craig, D. (1981) Kinship and friendship networks and women's demand for primary care. *Journal of the Royal College of General Practitioners*, 26: 746–50.

Scambler, G. (2009) Health related Stigma. *Sociology of Health and Illness*, 31(3): 441–55.

Scheff, T. (1966) *Being Mentally Ill: A Sociological Theory*. Chicago: Aldine.

Schilling, E.A., Aseltine, R.H. and Gore, S. (2008) The impact of cumulative childhood adversity on young adult mental health: measures, models, and interpretations. *Social Science and Medicine*, 6(5): 1140–51.

Schnitzer, P.K. (1996) 'They don't come in': stories told, lessons taught about poor families and therapy. *American Journal of Orthopsychiatry*, 66(4): 572–82.

Schoener, G.R. and Lupker, E.L. (1996) Boundaries in group settings: ethical and practical issues, in B. DeChant (ed.) *Women and Group Psychotherapy*. New York: Guilford Press.

Schulze, B. (2007) Stigma and mental health professionals: a review of the evidence on an intricate relationship. *International Review of Psychiatry*, 19(2): 137–55.

Schutt, R.K. and Rogers, E.S. (2009) Empowerment and peer support: structure and process of self help in a consumer-run centre for individuals with mental illness. *Journal of Community Psychology*, 37(6): 697–710.

SCMH (2000) *Finding and Keeping: Review of Recruitment and Retention of the Mental Health Workforce*. London: SCMH.

Scott, A. (1990) *Ideology and the New Social Movements*. London: Unwin Hyman.

Scott, M.B. and Lyman, S.M. (1968) Accounts. *American Journal of Sociology*, 33: 12–18.

Scott, R.D. (1973) The treatment barrier, part 1. *British Journal of Medical Psychology*, 46: 45–53.

Scourfield, J. (2005) Suicidal masculinities. *Sociological Research Online*, 10(2).

Scourfield, J., Dicks, B., Holland, S. *et al.* (2006) The significance of place in middle childhood: qualitative research from Wales. *British Journal of Sociology*, 57(4): 577–95.

Screech, M.A. (1985) Good madness in Christendom, in W.F. Bynum, R. Porter and M. Shepherd (eds) *The Anatomy of Madness* (Vol. 1). London: Tavistock.

Scull, A. (1977) *Decarceration: Community Treatment and the Deviant – A Radical View*. Englewood Cliffs, NJ: Prentice-Hall.

Scull, A. (1979) *Museums of Madness*. Harmondsworth: Penguin.

Secker, J. and Harding, C. (2002) Users' perceptions of an African and Caribbean mental health resource centre. *Health and Social Care in the Community*, 10(4): 270–6.

Sedgwick, P. (1982) *Psychopolitics*. London: Pluto Press.

Seedat, S., Scott, K.M., Angermeyer, M.C. *et al.* (2009) Cross-national associations between gender and mental disorders in the World Health Organization World Mental Health Surveys. *Archives of General Psychiatry*, 66(7): 785–95.

Seligman, M.E.P. (1975) *Helplessness: On Depression, Development and Death*. San Francisco: Freeman.

Shah, A. (2009) Eight years of controversy: has it made any difference? Will the amendments contained in the Mental Health Act 2007 (UK) result in more patients being subject to compulsion? *Psychiatry, Psychology and Law*, 16(1): 60–8.

Shaikh, A. (1985) Cross-cultural comparison: psychiatric admission of Asian and indigenous patients in Leicestershire. *International Journal of Social Psychiatry*, 31(1): 3–11.

Shaw, J., Hunt, I.M., Flynn, S. *et al.* (2006) Rates of mental disorder in people convicted of homicide. National clinical survey. *British Journal of Psychiatry*, 188: 143–7.

Shaw, M., Dorling, D. and Brimblecombe, D. (1998) Changing the map: health in Britain 1951–1991. *Sociology of Health and Illness*, 20(5): 694–709.

Sheppard, G., Boardman, G. and Slade, M. (2007) *Making Recovery a Reality*. London: Sainsbury Centre for Mental Health.

Sheppard, M. (1990) Social work and psychiatric nursing, in P. Abbott and C. Wallace (eds) *The*

Sociology of the Caring Professions. London: Falmer Press.

Sheppard, M. (1991) General practice, social work and mental health sections: the social control of women. *British Journal of Social Work*, 21: 663–83.

Shiner, M., Scourfield, J., Fincham, B *et al.* (2009) *Social Science and Medicine*, 69(5): 738–46.

SHSA (1990) *Inquiry into the Death of Joseph Watts*. London: Special Hospital Service Authority.

SHSA (1993) *Big Black and Dangerous? Report of the Inquiry into the Death in Broadmoor Hospital and a review of two other African-Caribbean patients* London: Special Hospital Service Authority.

Sibicky, M. and Dovidio, J.F. (1986) Stigma of psychological therapy: stereotypes, interpersonal reactions, and the self fulfilling prophecy. *Journal of Counseling Psychology*, 33: 148–54.

Sieff, E.M. (2003) Media frames of mental illnesses: the potential impact of negative frames. *Journal of Mental Health*, 12(3): 259–69.

Silove, D., Austin P. and Steel, Z. (2007) No refuge from terror: the impact of detention on the mental health of trauma affected refugees seeking asylum in Australia. *Transcultural Psychiatry* 44(3): 359–94.

Silver, E., Mulvey, E. and Monahan, J. (1999) Assessing violence risk among discharged psychiatric patients: an ecological approach. *Law and Human Behavior*, 23(2): 237–47.

Sjostrom, S. (1997) *Party or Patient? Discursive Practices Relating to Coercion in Psychiatric and Legal Settings*. Borea: Spinettstraket.

Skeem, J.L., Monahan, J. and Mulvey, E.P. (2002) Psychopathy, treatment involvement and subsequent violence amongst civil psychiatric patients. *Law and Human Behaviour*, 26(3): 577–603.

Skinner, L.J., Berry, K.K., Griffith, S.E. and Byers, B. (1995) Generalizability and specificity associated with the mental illness label: a reconsideration twenty-five years later. *Journal of Community Psychology*, 23: 3–17.

Skultans, V. (2003) From damaged nerves to masked depression, inevitability and hope in Latvian psychiatric narratives. *Social Science and Medicine*, 56(12): 2421–31.

Slater, P. (1977) *Origin and Significance of the Frankfurt School*. London: Routledge.

Sleath, B. and Shih, Y.C.T. (2003) Sociological influences on antidepressant prescribing. *Social Science and Medicine*, 56(6): 1335–44.

Smail, D. (1996) *Getting By Without Psychotherapy*. London: HarperCollins.

Smaje, C. (1996) The ethnic patterning of health: direction of theory and research. *Sociology of Health and Illness*, 18: 139–66.

Smelser, N. (1962) *A Theory of Collective Action*. New York: Free Press.

Smith, M. (2013) Anti-stigma campaigns: time to change *British Journal of Psychiatry* (202): s49–s50.

Smith, R. (2002) In search of 'non-disease'. *British Medical Journal*, 324: 883–5.

Snow, D., Baker, S., Anderson, L. and Martin, M. (1986) The myth of pervasive mental illness amongst the homeless. *Social Problems*, 33: 407–23.

Snowden, J. and Donnelly, M. (1986) A study of depression in nursing homes. *Journal of Psychiatric Research*, 20: 327–33.

Society of Humanistic Psychologists (2011) Open letter to DSM–5, www.ipetitions.com/petition/dsm5 (accessed 21 January 2014).

Soskis, D.A. (1978) Schizophrenia and medical inpatients as informed drug consumers. *Archives of General Psychiatry*, 35: 645–7.

Soyka, M. (2000) Substance misuse, psychiatric disorder and violent and disturbed behaviour. *British Journal of Psychiatry*, 176: 345–50.

Spagnoli, A., Foresti, G., MacDonald, A. and Williams, P. (1986) Dementia and depression in Italian geriatric institutions. *International Journal of Geriatric Psychiatry*, 1: 15–23.

Spandler, H. and Calton, T. (2009) Psychosis and human rights: conflicts in mental health policy and practice. *Social Policy and Society* 8(2): 245–56.

Spector, M. and Kitsuse, J. (1977) *Constructing Social Problems*. Menlo Park, CA: Cummings.

Speed, E. (2006) Patients, consumers and survivors: a case study of mental health service user discourse. *Social Science and Medicine*, 62(1): 28–38.

Spielmans, G. (2009) The promotion of Olanzapine in primary care: an examination of internal industry documents. *Social Science and Medicine*, 69: 14–20.

Spitzer, R.L. (2003) Can some gay men and lesbians change their sexual orientation? 200 participants reporting a change from homosexual to heterosexual orientation. *Archives of Sexual Behaviour*, 32(5): 403–17.

Sproston, K. and Nazroo, J. (2002) *Ethnic Minority Psychiatric Illness Rates in the Community*. London: HMSO.

Srole, L., Langer, T.S., Michael, S.T. *et al.* (1962) *Mental Health in the Metropolis: The Midtown Manhattan Study*. New York: McGraw-Hill.

Stafford, D.M., De Silva, M., Stansfeld, S. and Marmot, M. (2008) Testing the effects of gender, motor skills and play area on the free play activities of 8–11 year old school children. *Health and Place*, 14(4): 386–92.

Stansfeld, S., Head, J., Bartley, M. *et al.* (2008) Social position, early deprivation and the development of attachment. *Social Psychiatry and Psychiatric Epidemiology*, 43(7): 516–26.

Stansfeld, S.A., Head, J., Fuhrer, R., Wardle, J. and Cattell, V. (2003) Social inequalities in depressive symptoms and physical functioning in the Whitehall II study: exploring a common cause explanation. *Journal of Epidemiology and Community Health*, 57: 361–7.

Starr, P. (2009) Professionalization and public health: historical legacies, continuing dilemmas. *Journal of Public Health Management and Practice*, 15(6): 26–30.

Steadman, H.J., Mulvey, E.P., Monahan, J. *et al.* (1998) Violence by people discharged from acute psychiatric inpatient facilities and by others in the same neighbourhoods. *Archives of General Psychiatry*, 55: 393–401.

Stein, J., Golding, J., Seigel, J. *et al.* (1988) Long term psychological sequelae of child sexual abuse: the Los Angeles epidemiologic catchment area study, in G.E. Wyatt and G.J. Powell (eds) *Lasting Effects of Child Sexual Abuse*. Thousand Oaks: SAGE.

Stein, L. (1957) 'Social class' gradient in schizophrenia. *British Journal of Preventative and Social Medicine*, 11: 181–95.

Steptoe, A., Gibson, E.L., Hamer, M. and Wardle, J. (2007) Neuroendocrine and cardiovascular correlates of positive affect measure by ecological momentary assessment and by questionnaire. *Psychoneuroendocrininology*, 32(1): 56–64.

Stevenson, P. (1992) *Evidence Cited in Report of the Committee of Inquiry into Complaints about Ashworth Hospital*. London: HMSO.

Stoller, N. (2003) Space, place and movement as aspects of health care in three women's prisons, *Social Science & Medicine*, 56(11): 2263–75.

Stone, L. and Finlay, W.M.L. (2008) A comparison of African-Caribbean and white European young adults' conceptions of schizophrenia symptoms and the diagnostic label. *International Journal of Social Psychiatry*, 54(3): 242–61.

Stone, M. (1985) Shellshock and the psychologists, in W.F. Bynum, R. Porter and M. Shepherd (eds) *The Anatomy of Madness* (Vol. 2). London: Tavistock.

Strand, M. (2011) Where do classifications come from? The DSM-III, the transformation of American psychiatry, and the problem of origins in the sociology of knowledge. *Theory and Society*, 40(3): 273–313.

Summerfield, D. (2008) How scientifically valid is the knowledge base of global mental health? *British Medical Journal*, 336: 992–4.

Swami, V. (2012) Mental health literacy of depression: gender differences and attitudinal antededents in a representative British sample. *PLoS ONE*, 7(11): e49779.

Swanson, J.W., Holzer, C.E., Granju, I.K. and Jono, R.T. (1990) Violence and psychiatric disorder in the community: evidence from the epidemiological catchment area surveys. *Hospital and Community Psychiatry*, 41: 761–70.

Swartz, M.S., Swanson, J.W., Hiday, V.A. and Borum, R. (1998) Taking the wrong drugs: the role of substance use and medication non-compliance in violence among severely mentally ill individuals. *Social Psychiatry and Psychiatric Epidemiology*, 33: 75–80.

Sweeting, H. and Gilhooly, M. (1997) Dementia and the phenomenon of social death. *Sociology of Health and Illness*, 19(1): 93–117.

Szasz, T.S. (1961) The uses of naming and the origin of the myth of mental illness. *American Psychologist*, 16: 59–65.

Szasz, T.S. (1963) *Law, Liberty and Psychiatry*. New York: Macmillan.

Szasz, T.S. (1971) *The Manufacture of Madness*. London: Routledge and Kegan Paul.

Szasz, T.S. (1992) Crazy talk: thought disorder or psychiatric arrogance? *British Journal of Medical Psychology*, 65: 38–44.

Taylor, P.J. (1985) Motives for offending among violent psychotic men. *British Journal of Psychiatry*, 147: 491–8.

Teasdale, K. (1987) Stigma and psychiatric day care. *Journal of Advanced Nursing*, 12: 339–46.

Tedeschi, J.T. and Reiss, M. (1981) Verbal strategies in impression management, in C. Antaki (ed.) *The Psychology of Ordinary Explanations of Social Behaviour*. London: Academic Press.

Teeson, M., Hodder, T. and Buhrich, N. (2000) Substance use disorders among homeless people in inner Syndey. *Social Psychiatry and Psychiatric Epidemiology*, 35(10): 451–6.

Teghtsoonian, K. (2009) Depression and mental health in neoliberal times: a critical analysis of policy and discourse. *Social Science and Medicine*, 69: 28–35.

Teplin, L.A. (1984) Managing disorder: police handling of the mentally ill, in L.A. Teplin (ed.) *Mental Health and Criminal Justice*. Beverly Hills: SAGE.

Teplin, L.A., Abram, K.M. and McLelland, G.M. (1994) Does psychiatric disorder predict violent crime among released jail detainees: a 6-year longitutdinal study. *American Psychologist*, 49(4): 335–42.

Thoits, P.A. (1985) Self-labeling processes in mental illness: the role of emotional deviance. *American Journal of Sociology*, 91: 221–49.

Thomas, P. and Longden, E. (2013) Madness, childhood adversity and narrative psychiatry: caring and the moral imagination. *Journal of Medical Humanities*, 39(2): 119–25.

Thomas, S., McCrone, P. and Fahy, T. (2009) How do psychiatric patients in prison healthcare centres differ from inpatients in secure psychiatric inpatient units? *Psychology Crime and Law*, 15(8): 729–42.

Thompson, A., Shaw, M., Harrison, G., Davidson, H., Gunnell, D. and Veue, J. (2004) Patterns of hospital admission for adult psychiatric illness in England: analysis of hospital episode statistics data. *British Journal of Psychiatry*, 185: 334–41.

Tietze, C., Lemkau, P. and Cooper, M. (1941) Schizophrenia, manic depressive psychosis and socio-economic status. *American Journal of Sociology*, 47: 167–75.

Timimi, S. (2002) *Pathological Child Psychiatry and the Medicalization of Childhood*. Hove: Brunner-Routledge.

Toch, H. (1965) *The Social Psychology of Social Movements*. New York: Bobbs Merrill.

Tolmac, J. and Hodes, M. (2004) Ethnic variation among adolescent in-patients with psychotic disorders. *British Journal of Psychiatry*, 184: 428–31.

Tones, K. and Tilford, S. (1994) *Health Education: Effectiveness, Efficiency and Equity*. London: Chapman Hall.

Toro, P.A. (1998) Homelessness, in A.S. Bellack and M. Hersen (eds) *Comprehensive Clinical Psychology* (Vol. 9). New York: Pergamon.

Torrey, E.F. and Zdannowicz, M. (2001) Outpatient commitment: what, why and for whom? *Psychiatric Services*, 52(3): 337–41.

Townsend, P. (1981) The structured dependency of the elderly: a creation of social policy in the twentieth century. *Ageing and Society*, 1: 1–28.

Tribe, R. and Patel, N. (2007) Editorial Special Issue on Refugees and Asylum Seekers, *The Psychologist*, 20(3): 149–51.

Truman, C. and Raine, P. (2002) Experience and meaning of user involvement: some explorations from a community mental health project. *Health and Social Care in the Community*, 10(3): 136–43.

Tseng, W.-S. (2003) *Clinician's Guide to Cultural Psychiatry*. New York: Academic Press.

Tudor, K. (1996) *Mental Health Promotion: Paradigms and Practice*. London: Routledge.

Turner, B.S. (1986) *Equality*. London: Tavistock.

Turner, B.S. (1987) *Medical Power and Social Knowledge*. London: SAGE.

Turner, B.S. (1990) The inter-disciplinary curriculum: from social medicine to post modernism. *Sociology of Health and Illness*, 12(1): 1–23.

Turner, J.R. and Marino, F. (1994) Social support and social structure: a descriptive epidemiology. *Journal of Health and Social Behavior*, 35: 193–212.

Tyrer, P. (1987) Benefits and risks of benzodiazepines. *Proceedings of the Royal Society of Medicine*, 114: 7–11.

Tyrer, P. (2000) *Personality Disorders: Diagnosis, Management and Course*. Oxford: Butterworth-Heinemann.

Tyrer, P. (2008) Editorial. *British Journal of Psychiatry*, 192: 242.

Unger, R. (1984) *Passion: An Essay on Personality*. New York: Free Press.

Ussher, J. (1994) Women and madness: a voice in the dark of women's despair. *Feminism and Psychology*, 4(2): 288–92.

Van den Berg, W. and van Marle, H. (1997) Offenders who can and who cannot be treated in the Netherlands, In H. van Marle (ed.) *Challenges in Forensic Psychotherapy*. London: Jessica Kingsley.

Van Hoecken, D., Lucas, A.R. and Hoek, H.W. (1998) Epidemiology, in H.W. Hoek, J.L. Treasure and M.A. Kazman (eds) *Neurobiology in the Treatment of Eating Disorders*. Chichester: Wiley.

Varese, F., Smeets, F., Drukker, M. *et al.* (2012) Childhood adversities increase the risk of psychosis: a meta-analysis of patient-control, prospective- and cross-sectional cohort studies. *Schizophrenia Bulletin*, 38(4): 661–71.

Veling, W., Selten, J.P., Veen, N., Laan, W., Blom, J.D. and Hoek H.W. (2006) Incidence of schizophrenia among ethnic minorities in the Netherlands:

a four-year first-contact study. *Schizophrenia Research*, 86: 189–93.

Verbrugge, L. and Wingard, D. (1987) Sex differentials in health and mortality. *Women and Health*, 12: 103–45.

Verhaeghe, M. and Bracke, P. (2012) Associative stigma among mental health professionals: implications for professional and service user well-being *Journal of Health and Social Behavior*, 53: 17.

Victor, C.R., Scambler, S.J., Marston, L., Bond, J. and Bowling, A. (2006). Older people's experiences of loneliness in the UK: does gender matter? *Social Policy and Society*, 5: 27–38.

Wahl, O.F. (1995) *Medic Madness: Public Images of Mental Illness*. New Brunswick, NJ: Rutgers University Press.

Wahl, O.F. (2000) Obsessive-compulsive disorder in popular magazines. *Community Mental Health Journal*, 36(3): 307–12.

Waldron, I. (1977) Increased prescribing of Valium, Librium and other drugs: an example of economic and social factors in the practice of medicine. *International Journal of Health Services*, 7: 41–7.

Walker, A. (1980) The social creation of poverty and dependency in old age. *Journal of Social Policy*, 9: 49–75.

Wallcraft, J. (1996) Some models of asylum and help in times of crisis, in D. Tomlinson and J. Carrier (eds) *Asylum in the Community*. London: Routledge.

Wallcraft, J. with Read, J. and Sweeney, A. (2003) *On Our Own Terms*. London: Sainsbury Centre for Mental Health.

Wallcraft, J., Amering, M., Freidin, J. *et al.* (2011) Partnerships for better mental health worldwide: WPA recommendations on best practices in working ith service users and family carers. *World Psychiary*, 10(3): 229–36 www.wpanet.org/detail.php?section_id=7&content_id=1056 (accessed 21 January 2014).

Walters, V. (1993) Stress, anxiety and depression: women's accounts of their health problems. *Social Science and Medicine*, 36(4): 393–402.

Warner, R. (1985) *Recovery from Schizophrenia: Psychiatry and Political Economy*. London: Routledge.

Warner, R. (2003) How much of the burden of schizophrenia is alleviated by treatment? *British Journal of Psychiatry*, 183: 375–6.

Warren, F. and Dolan, B. (2001) *Perspectives on Henderson Hospital*. Sutton: Henderson Hospital.

Watkins, T.R. and Callicutt, J.W. (1997) Self-help and advocacy groups in mental health, in T.R.

Watkins and J.W. Callicutt (eds) *Mental Health Policy and Practice*. London: SAGE.

Watters, C. (1996) Representations of Asians' mental health in psychiatry, in C. Samson and N. South (eds) *The Social Construction of Social Policy*. London: Macmillan.

Watters, E. (2010) *Crazy Like Us: The Globalization of the American Psyche*. New York: Free Press.

Weich, S., Nazareth, I., Morgan, L. *et al.* (2007) Treatment of depression in primary care: socioeconomic status, clinical need and receipt of treatment. *British Journal of Psychiatry*, 191: 164–9.

Weinberg, S.K. (1960) Social psychological aspects of schizophrenia, in J. Appleby (ed.) *Chronic Schizophrenia*. Glencoe, IL: Free Press.

Weller, P. (2013) The social model of disability in the CRPD: from theory to practice. Presentation given at the 2013 International Conference on Mental Health Law: The United Nations Convention on the Rights of Persons with Disabilities (CRPD): What Does It Mean for Mental Health Law and Practice?

Wenger, G.C. (1989) Support networks in old age: constructing a typology, in M. Jeffries (ed.) *Growing Old in the Twentieth Century*. London: Routledge.

West, P. and Sweeting, H. (2004) Evidence on equalization in health in youth from the West of Scotland. *Social Science and Medicine*, 59(1): 13–27.

Westermeyer, J. and Kroll, J. (1978) Violence and mental illness in a peasant society: characteristics of violent behaviours and 'folk' use of restraints. *British Journal of Psychiatry*, 133: 529–41.

Whittington, C., Kendall, T., Fonagy, P., Cottrell, D., Cotgrove, A. and Boddington, E. (2004) Selective serotonin reuptake inhibitors in childhood depression: systematic review of published versus unpublished data. *The Lancet*, 24: 1341–5.

Whitton, A., Warner, R. and Appleby, L. (1996) The pathway to care in post-natal depression: women's attitudes to post-natal depression and its treatment. *British Journal of General Practice*, 46(408): 427–8.

Whooley, O. (2010) Diagnostic ambivalence: psychiatric workarounds and the Diagnostic and Statistical Manual of Mental Disorders. *Sociology of Health and Illness*, 32(3): 552–469.

Wiggins, R.D., Schoeld, P., Sacker, A., Head, J. and Bartley, M. (2004) Social position and minor psychiatric morbidity over time in the British Household Panel Survey 1991–1998. *Journal of Epidemiology and Community Health*, 58: 779–87.

Wilkinson, R.G. (1996) *Unhealthy Societies: The Afflictions of Inequality*. London: Routledge.

Wilkinson, R.G. (2005) *The Impact of Inequality: How to Make Sick Societies Healthier*. London: Routledge.

Williams, P., Tarnopolosky, A., Hand, D. and Sheperd, M. (1986) Minor psychiatric morbidity and general practice consultations: the West London Survey. *Psychological Medicine Monograph*, Supplement: 9–14.

Williams, S.J. (1995) Theorising class, health and lifestyles: can Bourdieu help us? *Sociology of Health and Illness*, 17(5): 577–604.

Williams, S.J. (1998) Capitalising on emotions? Rethinking the inequalities in health debate. *Sociology*, 32(1): 121–40.

Williams, S. (1999) Is anybody there? Critical realism, chronic illness and the disability debate. *Sociology of Health & Illness*, 21: 797–819.

Wilson, C., Nairn, R., Coverdale, J. and Panapa, A. (1999) Constructing mental illness as dangerous: a pilot study. *Australian and New Zealand Journal of Psychiatry*, 33(2): 240–7.

Wilson, M. (1993) DSM-III and the transformation of American psychiatry: a history *American Journal of Psychiatry*, 150(3): 399–410.

Wilson, W.P. (1998) Religion and psychosis, in H. Koenig (ed.) *Handbook of Religion and Mental Health*. San Diego: Academic Press.

Wing, J.K. (1962) Institutionalism in mental hospitals. *British Journal of Social and Clinical Psychology*, 1: 38–51.

Wing, J.K. (1978) *Reasoning about Madness*. Oxford: Oxford University Press.

Wing, J.K. and Freudenberg, R.K. (1961) The response of severely ill chronic schizophrenic patients to social stimulation. *American Journal of Psychiatry*, 118: 311–13.

Winnicott, D.W. (1958) The doctor, his patient and the illness. *International Journal of Psychoanalysis*, 39: 425–7.

Woolfe, J. and Tumin, S. (1990) *Prison Disturbances 1990* (The Tumin Report), Cmnd 1456. London: HMSO.

Woolgar, S. and Pawluch, D. (1985) Ontological gerrymandering: the anatomy of social problems' explanations. *Social Problems*, 32: 214–27.

Workforce Action Team (2001) *Adult Mental Health National Service Framework (and the NHS Plan) Underpinning Programme: Workforce Education and Training*. London: Department of Health.

World Health Organization (1979) *Schizophrenia: An International Follow-Up Study*. Chichester: Wiley.

World Health Organization (1986) *Health Promotion: Concepts and Principles in Action*. Copenhagen: WHO.

World Health Organization (1991) *Implications for the Field of Mental Health of the European Targets for Attaining Health for All*. Copenhagen: WHO.

World Health Organization (1992) *The ICD-10 Classification of Mental and Behavioural Disorders*. Geneva: WHO.

World Health Organization (2001) *Mental Health a Call for Action*. Geneva: WHO.

Wright, E.R., Gronfein, W.P. and Owens, T.J. (2000) Deinstitutionalization, social rejection, and the self-esteem of former mental patients. *Journal of Health and Social Behaviour*, 41(1): 68–90.

Wright Mills, C. (1959) *The Sociological Imagination*. Oxford: Oxford University Press.

Wrong, D.H. (1961) The over-socialised conception of man in modern sociology. *American Sociological Review*, 26(2): 183–93.

Wyatt, G.E. and Powell, G.J. (eds) (1988) *Lasting Effects of Child Sexual Abuse*. Thousand Oaks: SAGE.

Wykes, T. and Callard, F. (2010) Diagnosis, diagnosis, diagnosis: towards DSM-5. *Journal of Mental Health*, 19(4): 301–4.

Yates, A. (1970) *Behaviour Therapy*. New York: Wiley.

Yoon. J. (2011) Effect of increased private share of inpatient psychiatric resources on jail population growth: evidence from the United States. *Social Science & Medicine*, 72(4): 447–55.

Ziersch, A.M., Baum, F.E., MacDougall, C. and Putland, C. (2005) Neighbourhood life and social capital: the implications for health. *Social Science & Medicine*, 60(1): 71–86.

Zimmerman, F.J., Christakis, D.A. and Vander Stoep, A. (2004) Tinker, tailor, soldier, patient: work attributes and depression disparities among young adults. *Social Science & Medicine*, 58(10): 1889–901.

Index